D1619058

高等教育出版社　中國·北京
Higher Education Press, Beijing, China

英漢實用中醫藥大全

趙樸初題

14

ORTHOPEDICS
AND TRAUMATOLOGY

骨傷科學

THE ENGLISH–CHINESE ENCYCLOPEDIA OF PRACTICAL TRADITIONAL CHINESE MEDICINE

Chief Editor	Xu Xiangcai	
Assistants	You Ke	Kang Kai
	Bao Xuequan	Lu Yubin

英汉实用中医药大全

主　编	徐象才	
主编助理	尤　可	康　凯
	鲍学全	路玉滨

Higher Education Press
高等教育出版社

14

骨 伤 科 学

	中文	英文
主　编	曹贻训	雷希濂
副主编	张志刚	
	陈广祯	
编　者		顾建安　林雅
		汪洁

ORTHOPEDICS AND TRAUMATOLOGY

	English	Chinese
Chief Editor	Lei Xilian	Cao Yixun
Deputy Chief Editors		Zhang Zhigang
		Chen Guangzhen
Editors	Gu Jianan	
	Lin Ya	
	Wang Jie	

The Leading Commission of Compilation and Translation
编译领导委员会

Honorary Director 名誉主任委员	Hu Ximing 胡熙明		
Honorary Deputy Directors 名誉副主任委员	Zhang Qiwen 张奇文	Wang Lei 王镭	
Director 主任委员	Zou Jilong 邹积隆		
Deputy Director 副主任委员	Wei Jiwu 隗继武		
Members 委员 (以姓氏笔划为序)	Wan Deguang 万德光	Wang Yongyan 王永炎	Wang Maoze 王懋泽
	Wei Guikang 韦贵康	Cong Chunyu 丛春雨	Liu Zhongben 刘中本
	Sun Guojie 孙国杰	Yan Shiyun 严世芸	Qiu Dewen 邱德文
	Shang Chichang 尚炽昌	Xiang Ping 项平	Zhao Yisen 赵以森
	Gao Jinliang 高金亮	Cheng Yichun 程益春	Ge Linyi 葛琳仪
	Cai Jianqian 蔡剑前	Zhai Weimin 翟维敏	
Advisers 顾问	Dong Jianhua 董建华	Huang Xiaokai 黄孝楷	Geng Jianting 耿鉴庭
	Zhou Fengwu 周凤梧	Zhou Ciqing 周次清	Chen Keji 陈可冀

The Commission of Compilation and Translation
编译委员会

Director 主任委员	Xu Xiangcai 徐象才

Deputy Directors 副主任委员	Zhang Zhigang 张志刚	Zhang Wengao 张文高	Jiang Zhaojun 姜兆俊
	Qi Xiuheng 亓秀恒	Xuan Jiasheng 宣家声	Sun Xiangxie 孙祥燮
Members 委员 （以姓氏笔划为序）	Yu Wenping 于文平	Wang Zhengzhong 王正忠	Wang Chenying 王陈应
	Wang Guocai 王国才	Fang Tingyu 方廷钰	Fang Xuwu 方续武
	Tian Jingzhen 田景振	Bi Yongsheng 毕永升	Liu Yutan 刘玉檀
	Liu Chengcai 刘承才	Liu Jiaqi 刘家起	Liu Xiaojuan 刘晓娟
	Zhu Zhongbao 朱忠宝	Zhu Zhenduo 朱振铎	Xun Jianying 寻建英
	Li Lei 李 磊	Li Zhulan 李竹兰	Xin Shoupu 辛守璞
	Shao Nianfang 邵念方	Chen Shaomin 陈绍民	Zou Jilong 邹积隆
	Lu Shengnian 陆胜年	Zhou Xing 周 行	Zhou Ciqing 周次清
	Zhang Sufang 张素芳	Yang Chongfeng 杨崇峰	Zhao Chunxiu 赵纯修
	Yu Changzheng 俞昌正	Hu Zunda 胡遵达	Xu Heying 须鹤瑛
	Yuan Jiurong 袁久荣	Huang Naijian 黄乃健	Huang Kuiming 黄奎铭
	Huang Jialing 黄嘉陵	Cao Yixun 曹贻训	Lei Xilian 雷希濂
	Cai Huasong 蔡华松	Cai Jianqian 蔡剑前	

Preface

I am delighted to learn that THE ENGLISH–CHINESE ENCYCLOPEDIA OF PRACTICAL TRADITIONAL CHINESE MEDICINE will soon come into the world.

TCM has experienced many vicissitudes of times but has remained evergreen. It has made great contributions not only to the power and prosperity of our Chinese nation but to the enrichment and improvement of world medicine. Unfortunately, differences in nations, states and languages have slowed down its spreading and flowing outside China. At present, however, an upsurge in learning, researching and applying Traditional Chinese Medicine (TCM) is unfolding. In order to maximize the effect of this upsurge and to lead TCM, one of the brilliant cultural heritages of the Chinese nation, to the world for it to expand and bring benefit to the people of all nations, Mr. Xu Xiangcai called intellectuals of noble aspirations and high intelligence together from Shandong and many other provinces in China and took charge of the work of both compilation and translation of THE ENGLISH–CHINESE ENCYCLOPEDIA OF PRACTICAL TRADITIONAL CHINESE MEDICINE. With great pleasure, the medical staff both at home and abroad will hail the appearance of this encyclopedia.

I believe that the day when the world's medicine is fully

developed will be the day when TCM has spread throughout the world.

I am pleased to give it my preface.

Prof. Dr. Hu Ximing

Deputy Ministerof the Ministry of Public Health of the People's Republic of China,

Director General of the State Administrative Bureau of Traditional Chinese Medicine and Pharmacology,

President of the World Federation of Acupuncture —Moxibustion Societies,

Member of China Association of Science & Technology,

Deputy President of All—China Association of Traditional Chinese Medicine,

President of China Acupuncture & Moxibustion Society.

December, 1989

Preface

The Chinese nation has been through a long, arduous course of struggling against diseases and has developed its own traditional medicine—Traditional Chinese Medicine and Pharmacology (TCMP). TCMP has a unique, comprehensive, scientific system including both theories and clinical practice. Some thousand years since its—beginnings, not only has it been well preserved but also continuously developed. It has special advantages, such as remarkable curative effects and few side effects. Hence it is an effective means by which people prevent and treat diseases and keep themselves strong and healthy.

All achievements attained by any nation in the development of medicine are the public wealth of all mankind. They should not be confined within a single country. What is more, the need to set them free to flow throughout the world as quickly and precisely as possible is greater than that of any other kind of science. During my more than thirty years of being engaged in Traditional Chinese Medicine(TCM), I have been looking forward to the day when TCMP will have spread all over the world and made its contributions to the elimination of diseases of all mankind. However it is to be deeply regretted that the pace of TCMP in extending outside China has been unsatisfactory due to the major difficulties in expressing its concepts in foreign languages.

Mr. Xu Xiangcai, a teacher of Shandong College of TCM, has sponsored and taken charge of the work of compilation and translation of The English—Chinese Encyclopedia of Practical Traditional Chinese Medicine—an extensive series. This work is a great project, a large—scale scientific research, a courageous effort and a novel creation. I deeply esteem Mr. Xu Xiangcai and his compilers and translators, who have been working day and night for such a long time, for their hard labor and for their firm and indomitable will displayed in overcoming one difficulty after another, and for their great success achieved in this way. As a leader in the circles of TCM, I am duty—bound to do my best to support them.

I believe this encyclopedia will be certain to find its position both in the history of Chinese medicine and in the history of world science and technology.

Mr. Zhang Qiwen

Member of the Standing Committee of
All—China Association of TCM,
Deputy Head of the Health Department
of Shandong Province.

March, 1990

Publisher's Preface

Traditional Chinese Medicine(TCM) is one of China's great cultural heritages. Since the founding of the People's Republic of China in 1949, guided by the farsighted TCM policy of the Chinese Communist Party and the Chinese government, the treasure house of the theories of TCM has been continuously explored and the plentiful literature researched and compiled. As a result, great success has been achieved. Today there has appeared a world—wide upsurge in the studying and researching of TCM. To promote even more vigorous development of this trend in order that TCM may better serve all mankind, efforts are required to further it throughout the world. To bring this about, the language barriers must be overcome as soon as possible in order that TCM can be accurately expressed in foreign languages.

Thus the compilation and translation of a series of English—Chinese books of basic knowledge of TCM has become of great urgency to serve the needs of medical and educational circles both inside and outside China.

In recent years, at the request of the health departments, satisfactory achievements have been made in researching the expression of TCM in English. Based on the investigation into the history and current state of the research work mentioned above, the English—Chinese Encyclopedia of Practical TCM has been published to meet the needs of extending the knowledge of TCM around the world.

The encyclopedia consists of twenty—one volumes, each dealing with a particular branch of TCM. In the process of compilation, the distinguishing features of TCM have been given close attention and great efforts have been made to ensure that the content is scientific, practical, comprehensive and concise. The chief writers of the Chinese manuscripts include professors or associate professors with at least twenty years of practical clinical and / or teaching experience in TCM. The Chinese manuscript of each volume has been checked and approved by a specialist of the relevant branch of TCM. The team of the translators and revisers of the English versions consists of TCM specialists with a good command of English professional medical translators, and teachers of English from TCM colleges or universities. At a symposium to standardize the English versions, scholars from twenty—two colleges or universities, research institutes of TCM or other health institutes probed the question of how to express TCM in English more comprehensively, systematically and accurately, and discussed and deliberated in detail the English versions of some volumes in order to upgrade the English versions of the whole series. The English version of each volume has been re—examined and then given a final checking.

Obviously this encyclopedia will provide extensive reading material of TCM English for senior students in colleges of TCM in China and will also greatly benefit foreigners studying TCM.

The assiduous efforts of compiling and translating this encyclopedia have been supported by the responsible leaders of the State Education Commission of the People's Republic of China, the State Administrative Bureau of TCM and Pharmacy, and the Education Commission and Health Department of Shandong

Province. Under the direction of the Higher Education Department of the State Education Commission, the leading board of compilation and translation of this encyclopedia was set up. The leaders of many colleges of TCM and pharmaceutical factories of TCM have also given assistance.

We hope that this encyclopedia will bring about a good effect on enhancing the teaching of TCM English at the colleges of TCM in China, on cultivating skills in medical circles in exchanging ideas of TCM with patients in English, and on giving an impetus to the study of TCM outside China.

Higher Education Press
March, 1990

Foreword

The English—Chinese Encyclopedia of Practical Traditional Chinese Medicine is an extensive series of twenty—one volumes. Based on the fundamental theories of traditional Chinese medicine(TCM) and with emphasis on the clinical practice of TCM, it is a semi—advanced English—Chinese academic works which is quite comprehensive, systematic, concise, practical and easy to read. It caters mainly to the following readers: senior students of colleges of TCM, young and middle—aged teachers of colleges of TCM, young and middle—aged physicians of hospitals of TCM, personnel of scientific research institutions of TCM, teachers giving correspondence courses in TCM to foreigners, TCM personnel going abroad in the capacity of lecturers or physicians, those trained in Western medicine but wishing to study TCM, and foreigners coming to China to learn TCM or to take refresher courses in TCM.

Because Traditional Chinese Medicine and Pharmacology is unique to our Chinese nation, putting TCM into English has been the crux of the compilation and translation of this encyclopedia. Owing to the fact that no one can be proficient both in the theories of Traditional Chinese Medicine and Pharmacology and the clinical practice of every branch of TCM, as well as in English, to ensure that the English versions express accurately the inherent meanings of TCM, collective translation measures have been taken. That is, teachers of English familiar with TCM, professional medical translators, teachers or physicians of TCM and even teachers of palaeography with a strong command of English were all invited together to co-translate the Chinese manuscripts and, then, to co-deliberate and discuss the English versions. Finally English-speaking foreigners studying TCM or teaching English in China were asked to polish the English versions. In this way, the skills of the above translators and foreigners were merged to ensure the quality of the English versions. However, even using this method, the uncertainty that the English versions will be wholly accepted still remains. As for the Chinese manuscripts, they do reflect the essence, and give a general picture, of traditional Chinese medicine and pharmacology. It is not asserted, though, that they are perfect, I whole-heartedly look forward to any criticisms or opinions from readers in order to make improvements to future editions.

More than 200 people have taken part in the activities of compiling, translating and revising this encyclopedia. They come from twenty-eight institutions in all parts of China. Among these institutions, there are fifteen colleges of TCM:Shandong, Beijing, Shanghai, Tianjin, Nanjing, Zhejiang, Anhui, Henan, Hubei, Guangxi, Guiyang, Gansu, Chengdu, Shanxi and Changchun, and scientific research centers of TCM such as China Academy of TCM and Shandong Scientific Research Institute of TCM.

The Education Commission of Shandong province has included the compilation and translation of this encyclopedia in its scientific research projects and allocated funds accordingly. The Health Department of Shandong Province has also given financial aid together with a number of pharmaceutical factories of TCM. The subsidization from Jinan Pharmaceutical Factory of

TCM provided the impetus for the work of compilation and translation to get under way.

The success of compiling and translating this encyclopedia is not only the fruit of the collective labor of all the compilers, translators and revisers but also the result of the support of the responsible leaders of the relevant leading institutions. As the encyclopedia is going to be published, I express my heartfelt thanks to all the compilers. translators and revisers for their sincere cooperation, and to the specialists, professors, leaders at all levels and pharmaceutical factories of TCM for their warm support.

It is my most profound wish that the publication of this encyclopedia will take its role in cultivating talented persons of TCM having a very good command of TCM English and in extending, rapidly, comprehensive knowledge of TCM to all corners of the globe.

Chief Editor   Xu Xiangcai

Shandong College of TCM

March, 1990

Contents

Notes

Orthopedics and Traumatology is the 14th volume of the English—Chinese Encyclopedia of Practical Traditional Chinese Medicine.

TCM orthopedics and traumatology has unique methods in diagnosis and treatment. Fractures, if treated with these methods, will be rapidly healed and the limb and / or body functions will be satisfactorily restored. For this reason, it is more and more highly appreciated both in and outside China.

This volume consists of the following five chapters: General Introduction, Fractures, Dislocations, Injuries of Soft Tissues and Osteoarticular Infections. In addition, it includes 129 related illustrations and 83 recipes for the convinience of the readers. In this volume, the merits of TCM orthopedics and traumatology are stressed and the clinical diagnosis and treatment is the main consideration. Great efforts have been made to render its text simple, clear, practical and easy to understand.

The Chinese manuscript was checked and approved by Prof. Liu Bailing from Changchun College of Traditional Chinese Medicine, and the English version was once revised by Mr. Li Lei from Zhejiang College of Traditional Chinese Medicine during Taian Symposium for Standardizing the English Versions of the Encyclopedia.

The Editors

1 General Introduction

1.1 Manipulation of Bone—setting

Manipulation of bone—setting is of great importance in TCM orthopedics and traumatology. If fractures occur and the ends happen to have some relative displacement from each other or to form angular deformity, there is always a need of restoration of anatomical or functional position through manipulative maneuvers so as to lay a beneficial basis for healing and functional restoration. The more accurately the ends are reset, the more stable the fixation will be; the patient will also be enabled to perform functional rehabilitation exercises as early as possible and earlier healing can be expected.

Time for Reduction

As long as the general condition of the patient permits, earlier reduction is recommended because during the initial stage of fracture there is but slight local swelling and mild pain, and spasms of the muscles have not yet taken place. This provides the best possibility for successful reduction by merely one attempt. Moreover, within 4—6 hours after the fracture, the local blood stasis will remain un—coagulated and unhardened, and it is easier to reduce the fracture ends at this stage. Delayed operation will meet greater difficulties in reduction. As a rule, successful reduction by manipulative maneuvers can be achieved within 7—10 days after the fracture.

However, if the patient suffers from shock, coma or injuries to internal organs, the operation must be deferred until the patient's condition becomes stable, though, in order to relieve the patient from pain and to prevent secondary injuries, wellmanaged fixation at the fracture site is quite necessary. When there is notable swelling or any blister, the exudation must be extracted with sterilized apparatuses under disinfected condition, and the affected extremity lifted higher than the body, with temporary splint fixation. Reduction can only be performed after extinction of the swelling. Open fractures ought to be well reduced once for all with precise apposition after debridement and suturing.

Pre—operative Preparations

1. Choice of Anesthesia.

This is determined by the general condition of the patient. Local injection of 0.5—2% procaine at the hematoma site will be effective in relieving the pain for patients who have been suffering from the wound for not more than 6—8 hours. For those cases with displaced ends which have been delayed for reduction for a considerable period of time, the setting will meet with greater difficulty and will cause severe pains. Generally, block anesthesia at brachial plexus is selected in the case of fractures of upper extremities, block anesthesia at nervus femoralis or nervus ischiadicus or lumbar anesthesia in the case of fractures of lower extremities.

2. The Surgeon and the Assistant (s)

The surgeon and the assistants must learn very well about the patient's general condition, the mechanism of the wound, the pattern of the fracture and the degree of displacement, etc. On the basis of the state of the fracture in X—ray films and the true condition of the patient and through careful analysis, decision can be made as to what manipulative maneuvers for reduction are to be prescribed and how the assistants should cooperate with the surgeon. In the operation, they must see that the patient, especially the injured bone, is kept at an appropriate position. It is important to have the patient's close cooperation by convincing him / her of the necessity of doing so for successful reduction.

3. Materials

Materials needed for the operation are dependent upon the part where the fracture occurs, the type of fracture and the size of the wounded part. These include such things as cardboard, splints, cotton pads, laces, bandage, adhesive plaster and small compresses. Essential necessaries for first aid must be ready at hand in case unpredictable emergency occurs during reduction.

TCM Manipulative Maneuvers for Reduction and their Indications

In traditional Chinese medicine, manipulative reduction is one of the most effective methods in treatment of fractures. To reduce the ends that are displaced, certain maneuvers must be employed, and how the manipulation is performed will decide whether the treatment is successful or not . There are various maneuvers for reduction of fractures in TCM orthopedics and traumatology. To sum up, the most commonly used are as follows:

1. Palpating and Feeling

This is the first chosen maneuver in clinical practice. The doctor feels the surface of the wounded part and the areas around it with the thumb, or thumb plus the forefinger and middle finger of a hand and presses slightly so as to make sure how the displacement between the ends is like. With reference to what is manifested in X−ray films , the doctor can then analyze all aspects of the fracture and gain a perspective view of the condition, thus assuring a better basis for the next step of treatment.

2. Pulling and Stretching

This means that, in order to restore the normal length of the injured extremity, the overriding ends should be brought to the right position by pulling carefully(to overcome the contraction force of the muscles), as is expressed in a conclusion in TCM classics: "Reunion follows remedial separation and remedial separation makes reunion". This maneuver can also be used as an auxiliary means in reduction of angular or rotatory displacement. Performance of this maneuver generally requires collaboration of both the surgeon and his assistants. The surgeon holds firmly in both hands the corresponding parts to the fracture ends and the assistants respectively fix the distal end and proximal end of the extremity; by gradual simultaneous exertion of force, they can perform stretching traction. The extremity should initially be kept in its existing position and the tracting force is exercised along the vertical axis of the injured bone to bring about countertraction so that the ends inserting the soft tissues can be slowly pulled out. Then, according to the steps of reduction, the extremity can be placed to the desired direction and be extended through exertion of a much greater force. How great the force for extension should be exercised depends upon the strength of muscles of the patient. For children, females and the aged, the force must be properly controlled whereas for young males at their prime of life, powerful extension is necessary as their well-developed muscles are much stronger. While pulling traction is performed, the direction and position of the extremity must be adjusted accordingly to achieve high rate of successful reduction and avoid deformity.

The assistants responsible for traction should be very careful in keeping constant and steady pulling. No sudden exertion of force is allowed (Fig. 1).

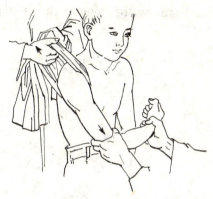

Fig. 1   Reduction of a fracture of the surgical neck of the humerus

(Adduction Type) by pulling—stretching maneuver

3. Pushing and Pressing

This maneuver requires the operator to press forcefully the protruding end with thumbs or palmbases " to flatten the jutting". The surgeon then has to hold tightly the displaced end with the thumb, forefinger and middle finger of a hand and push it back to its original position, and make sure that it will not move away (Fig. 2).

This maneuver is generally used in coordination with elevating and up—supporting maneuver in practice.

4. Elevating and Up—supporting

The direction of the force to be exerted in this method is just the opposite to that of Pushing and Pressing maneuver. In operation, the doctor either directly raises the sinking end with the fingers (except the thumb) of a hand and endevours to bring it up in combination with Pushing and Pressing maneuver by the other hand or uses something else(for example, a proper piece of cloth) as an auxiliary means and lifts the end up with it. Elevating and Up-supporting maneuver is primarily used to reduce lateral displacement of fracture ends by "bringing up the sinking"(Fig. 3).

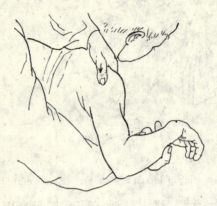

Fig. 2   Reduction of a fracture of the great tuberosity of the

humerus by pushing-pressing maneuver

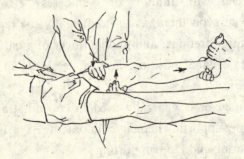

Fig. 3   Reduction of a fracture of the humeral shaft by

elevating-up-supporting and pushing-pressing

5. Pinching

This maneuver is usually employed to reduce fracture ends of minor bones such as those of the fingers or toes. In performance, the surgeon has to take the fracture ends in a hand with the thumb on one side and the forefinger and middle finger on the opposite, and squeezes the ends until the displaced fragment returns to its right position. (Fig. 4). Occasionally, the operator may find it necessary to use his palmbases to press the two sides of the fractured bone forcibly by clasping the fingers to correct the displacement. This maneuver has proved safe and effective in reduction of such ends as those in a calcaneum fracture.

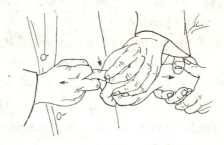

Fig. 4   Reduction of a phalangeal fracture by finger–pinching maneuver

6. Separating Parallel Bones

When a fracture occurs in a part where there are parallel bones, for example, the ulna and the radius, the tibia and the fibula, the metacarpal bones, and the metatarsal bones, the parallel ends may get very close to each other due to contraction of the musculi interossei or membrane interossei. In reduction, the doctor should put his fingers on the medial side of the ends and thumbs on the dorsal aspect in between the bones and press energetically so as to separate the ends that have drawn near each other. This will restore their normal distance and the fracture ends thus regain stable and natural apposition. (Fig. 5)

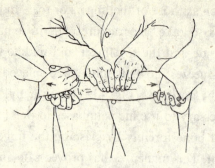

Fig. 5　Reduction of fractures of the shafts of the radio–ulnar

bones by bonesseparating maneuver

7.　Contra–angular Flexing

This method can be applied to two conditions: (1) The fracture ends remain in good apposition, but there is certain angular deformity. In this case, the maneuver begins with Pullling and Stretching. Then the operator has to hold firmly the angular protrusion with one hand and seize the distal terminal of the extremity with the other. By exercising a contra–angular flexing force, he can correct the deformity and restore the normal anatomical alignment. (2) The fracture occurs at a part where the muscles are powerful, and greater displacement exists that usual pulling and stretching force cannot set the overriding ends right as in the case of fractures of the fermoral shaft and fractures of both bones of the forearm. Manipulative reduction of this type of fractures requires more efforts and greater force. The operator and the assistants have to begin the reduction with increasing degrees of the angular deformity and endevour to stretch the fractured part by pulling energetically while pressing the distal end to make it move towards the distal direction so as to cause the ends to meet on cortex. Then, by a sudden exertion of contra–flexing force on the distal terminal of the extremity, they can restore the normal axial alignment of the bone and complete the reduction. The performance requires great reliability, precise swiftness and harmonious coordination between the operator and the assistants. Care must be taken to prevent the ends from injuring the vessels, nerves or skin (Fig. 6).

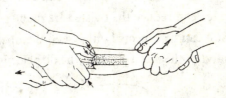

6-1   Increasing the degrees of the angular deformity

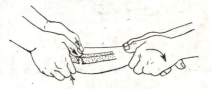

6-2   Pushing the ends back to the normal position

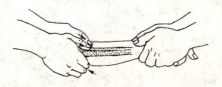

6-3   Restoring good apposition

Fig. 6   Reduction of a double fracture of the radio-ulnar bones by contra-angular

8. Contra-rotating

When a spiral fracture occurs, or when the fracture fragments are displaced in a back-to-back way by external force, the reduction needs contra-rotating to retrack the rotated fragment so as to give good apposition. In certain parts, the fracture fragments may be twisted by contraction of the muscles. Correction of this condition demands complicated operation based on Pulling and Stretching plus Pushing and Pressing, Elevating and Up-supporting. By proper application of the maneuvers, with the assistants contra-rotating the distal end around the vertical axis, the operator can reduce the twisted fragments (Fig.7). However, good result can be expected only when the operator has had a good command of the mechanism of the displacement.

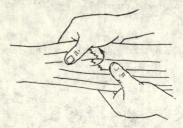

7-1　Contra-rotating for back-to-back displacement of the ends

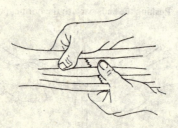

7-2　Completion of the reduction

Fig. 7　Reduction of an obloque fracture of the radius with back-to-back displacement of the ends by contra-rotating maneuver

9. Flexing and / or Extending

This maneuver is usually used in reduction of articular frac-

tures such as those of the elbow, wrist and ankle joints. It generally follows the initial Pulling and Stretching maneuver. To correct
the displacement of the fragments, the operator has to decide, according to the type of fracture, whether to flex or extend (or both,
each after the other, for several times) the joint while performing
Pushing and Pressing as a coordinative maneuver (Fig. 8).

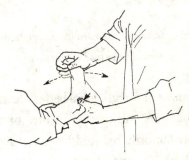

Fig. 8   Reduction of an ankle fracture by flexing—extending maneuver

10. Rocking

Nearly all types of common fractures can be reduced by one
or some or all of the maneuvers described above. However, a
transverse fracture or serrated fracture may have a small gap between the ends. In order to make the ends in close contact with
each other, the operator has to hold firmly the fracture part and
have the assistants keep tracting and gently rocking the distal
terminal of the affected limb. When the crepitus becomes less and
less audible or completely disaapears, successful reduction is
achieved and will remain stable. If it happens to be an
intraarticular fracture, Rocking maneuver may as well be employed as it has a function of remoulding the articular surface,
which will restore the original articular shape and smoothness
and thus prevent traumatic arthritis (Fig. 9).

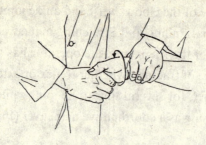

Fig. 9 . Reduction of a comminuted fracture of the distal part
of the radius by rocking maneuver

11. Clapping

In order to make the ends gain better steady impaction in certain type of fractures, such as a fracture of the metaphysis, that have been satisfactorily reduced by manipulative maneuvers and fixed with splints, the operator can further employ Clapping maneuver. He himself firmly fixes the fracture part with both hands and has the assistant gently clap the distal terminal of the distal end. This maneuver helps healing considerably.

12. Pneumatic Supporting

This is particularly effective in reducing fractures of the ribs. When diagnosis shows that there is anteroposterior displacement of the ends in a rib fracture, this maneuver proves necessary. The operator presses the torus with a thumb while the assistant depresses the upper abdomen with his palms. The patient is told to do deep breathing and then coughing. At the instant of the coughing, both the operator and the assistant exert force energetically, and this usually results in good reduction. (Fig.10).

13. Stroking

This is frequently the last step of reduction. The operator mildly presses the affected part with a thumb, sometimes plus the forefinger, and strokes it to and fro along the direction of the muscles or of the bone vertical axis. The maneuver has the effect of relaxing the ligaments, smoothing the bone, eliminating stasis and relieving pains. It can also be used as a means of examining how the result of the previous manipulative reduction is. Bandage splint fixation and bandaging should be applied after satisfactory reduction.

Requirements for Good Reduction

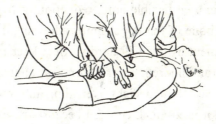

Fig. 10 Reduction of a rib fracture by pneumatic supporting maneuver

1. Anatomical Apposition

This means complete correction of deformity and displacement, complete restoration of the original anatomical shape and position. Anatomical apposition makes the fracture ends stable, ascertains early healing and good functional restoration. In any case, every necessary means should be tried to bring about good anatomical apposition.

2. Functional Apposition

This means non-existance of overriding displacement, complete correction of rotatory / angular deformity, and good restoration of normal functional alignment (including the length) after the reduction. Moreover, when the fracture heals, the physical functions of the limb or other part of the body must be restored so well that the patient's daily life and work will not be affected.

The standard for functional apposition is relative. Requirements vary with different parts, different aging groups and different professional need. The elders often feel much less affected in their daily life even without satisfactory apposition; on the other hand, dancers and athletes find it extremely important to have good apposition after fracture, for poor apposition may cause malfunction, which will ruin their career thereafter. Intraarticular fractures demand precise apposition, but , since the treatment aims at maintaining a flexible limb, reduction of fractures at the shaft of a long bone of the upper limbs allow slight angular and lateral displacement as this will hardly affect later restoration of functions. As for children, no rotatory or angular deformity should be neglected though slight overriding and mild lateral displacement do not need much concern because these can be naturally corrected in the course of their growth.

Principles for Operators and Their Assistants in Reduction

1. Serve the patients wholeheartedly, be full of warmth, pay special attention to the patient's desires and worries, and work confidently so as to gain the patient's close cooperation.

2. Never make any sudden exertion of force during performance of maneuvers. In performing stretching countertraction, apply a most proper force slowly (that is, neither too powerful nor too weak). Make sure that the point or area for maneuvers is precisely located and that the force applied and the direction of the force are absolutely appropriate for the patient's condition. Never rub the wounded part with fingers in case the soft tissues get injured.

3. Highly concentrate on what you are performing; try to perceive whatever you feel by the contact of you hand with the

target part of the patient and pay attention to any external changes of the injured site; carefully watch the patients reflection so as to judge the result of the operation; be always on guard against any accident.

4. Try every means to achieve successful reduction in only one attempt, for repeated operation will cause more injuries to the soft tissues and lead to severer swelling, which may give rise to more difficulties for another reduction or even to delayed healing or stiff articulation.

5. Be extremely careful in treating petients of weak constitution, or with complicated fractures in several parts, or with other severe complications, or in treating pregnant female patients. In all these cases, the reduction should be postponed until the condition is made favourable after proper medical measures have improved the health state of the patient;always keep in mind the general condition of the patient when treating local problems.

1.2 Bandage—splint Fixation

To maintain good apposition after reduction and assure normal healing, proper immobilization must be made, which has proved a significant measure in treatment of fractures. Beneficial fixation must be able

(1) to keep the injured limb at a suitable position so that the fracture site may rest at relaxation and in a relatively stable state, making a better basis for healing.

(2) to retain the effect of reduction, protect the fracture site from any harmful force, and prevent re—displacement of the ends.

(3) to provide favourable conditions for rehabilitation.

(4) to correct gradually remaining deformity and / or dis-

placement after reduction.

(5) to protect the wound, relieve pains and prevent new injuries.

Types of Local External Immobilization

1. Local External Splint Fixation

This is mainly applied to fractures such as those of the humeri, the radii and ulnae, the tibiae and fibulae.

2. Super–articular Splint Fixation

This is applied to intra–articular fractures with complete articular surface or metaphysial fractures adjacent to joints, such as a surgical neck fracture, a supercondylar fracture of the humeri and an ankle fracture.

3. External Local Splint Fixation / Super–articular Splint Fixation in Combination with Skeletal Traction

Local splint fixation combined with skeletal traction is applied to fractures of the fermoral diaphysis where there are abundant soft tissues and the muscles are powerful, and to unstable fractures of the tibiae or fibulae. Super–artucilar splint fixation combined with skeletal traction is applied to intraarticular fractures with damage to the articular surface, such as an intra–condylar fracture of the humeri.

4. Small Bamboo–curtain / Cardboard / Bone–dieresis Pad Fixation

This is applied to fractures of the metacarpal bones or metatarsal bones.

5. Small Bamboo–splint / Cardboard Slice Fixation

This applied to fractures of the finger bones or metatarsal bones.

6. Bandage and Adhesive Plaster Fixation

This is applied to fractures of the ribs or clavicles.

Function of Splint Fixation

1. External Effect of Binding Laces, Splints and Compresses

Binding with laces can provide a force which will pass on to the fracture segment or the ends through the splints, compresses and the soft tissues as a means of resistance to re–displacement of the fracture fragments. Fixation with 3 compresses will produce a compressing function and a lever force which can prevent angular re–displacement, and fixation with 2 compresses will provide a compressing function and a wrenching force which can prevent lateral re–displacement. In a word, use of binding laces, splints and compresses can effectively avoid lateral and angular re–displacement of the ends whereas continuous traction can prevent new overriding.

2. Internal Force Produced by Muscular Contraction

Splint fixation after reduction only immobilizes local part, usually not beyond the adjacent upper or lower joint, and articular flexion and extension as well as other functional movement are possible. Vertical muscular contraction is free and this contraction along the diaphysis can provide a vertical compressing force on the fracture ends, which will make the ends closely anastomose, thus reinforcing the stability of them. On the other hand, as the muscles become thicker in diameter when they contract, the perimeter of the limb will expand accordingly, a pressure upon the compresses and the splints is therefore produced. Simultaneously, a counter–pressure produced by the splints and compresses will in turn act upon the fracture ends. This will reinforce the stability of the ends, thus resulting in correction of the retained displacement of the ends. When the muscles relax, the limb perimeter will return to its normal state and the splints to their usual tightness. Based on this phenomenon, the disadvantageous action of muscular contraction can be changed into a favourable factor for fracture healing if compresses and splints are applied to proper position and kept in suitable tightness according to the type of fracture and condition of the displacement. Intentional contractive activitiy of the muscles as a rehabilitating exercise can only be practised under close supervision of the doctors and nurses. Unrestricted exercise is in no case advisable, re—displacement may occur otherwise. If the doctor thinks it necessary to prescribe rehabilitating exercises for the patient, he must be well aware of the fact that it depends upon what type the fracture is, where the fracture occurs, what stage the case is at and how old the patient is. The pattern of exercises greatly varies with different cases.

3. Necessity of an Opposite Position

The injured limb must be put at an opposite position to the direction of the displacement. Displacement after the fracture may be caused by the direction of the injury force, the traction of the muscles and the gravity of the distal terminal of the limb. So the tendency of re—displacement due to limb gravity posterior to reduction must be avoided and that is why the injured limb must be seated at a position opposite to the direction of the displacement. If this is done and followed by necessary mobilization, it will be very beneficial in maintaining good apposition and alignment and in correcting remaining angular displacement. For example, in the case of extension type of supracondylar fractures of the humerus, the fixation must be done with the elbow joint at a flexion position.

Requirements for Quality of the Materials of Splints

Plasticity The materials must be plastic as the splints may have to be in various flexing forms according to the specific shape of the injured part.

Tenacity The materials must be tenacious as the splints have to be strong enough to maintain their given shape without breaking or cracking.

Elasticity The materials must be elastic as the splints have to accommodate to the change of the internal pressure of the limb during muscular contraction and relax—ation so that they may keep their supporting and fixing action when the limb flexes.

The splints must also be absorbent and ventilative so as to allow the limb to discharge heat from its surface under the splints and to avoid dermatitis of the skin.

The splints must be of possibly less weight. If the splints are too heavy, the injured limb will have to bear too much weight and to meet increased shearing force, which will hinder rehabilitation exercises.

The splints must be penetrable to X—rays for easy radiative examination.

Besides, the materials must be of abundant resources and low prices.

Clinically, the commonly—used materials include willow sheet, bamboo sheet, cypress cortex, cardboard, veneer, aluminum sheet, plastic sheet, etc.

Manufacture of Splints

The splints must be of proper size and thickness and they must be carefully made and shaped according to the outline of the injured part where they are to be applied. If the material ready for use happens to be a bamboo sheet, it must first be planed smooth, generally about 1.5—2.5 mm thick. The length and width vary with different needs. For forearm fixation, it is normally about 12—18 cm long by 3—5 cm wide on the palm and dorsal aspects and about 2 cm wide on the medial and lateral sides.

The manufacturing steps are as follows:

(1) Get all the edges and corners smoothly rounded.

(2) Soak the sheet in warm water for a few hours before taking out for moulding.

(3) Heat it on an alcohol burner until it becomes soft.

(4) Shape it according to clinical need on a specially designed shaper (Fig. 11).

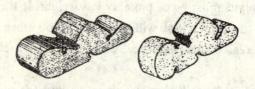

Fig. 11 Wood—made splint shapers

In non—superarticular immobilization for a fracture of the diaphysis, the length of the splints is just the same or approximately the same as that of the fractured limb as long as movement of the upper or lower joint is not hindered. For superarticular immobilization, the splints are required to be 2—3 cm beyond the articulation in length so as to fix the binding, the total width of the splints being approximately four fifths or five sixths of the perimeter of the limb that is to be fixed. There must be certain space between each two splints, and between the splints and the skin is needed a smooth—surfaced pad or stockinet which is soft, water—absorbent, heat—diffusive, non—irritating to the skin, and 0.2 cm thick.

Clinically, three sizes (large, middle and small) of splints applicable to different parts of the body or limbs should be available (Fig. 12).

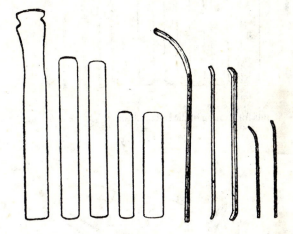

12—1 Splints for fixation of the fractured surgical neck of the humerus

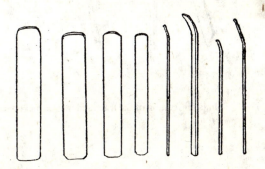

12—2 Splints for fixation of the fractured distal segment of the radius

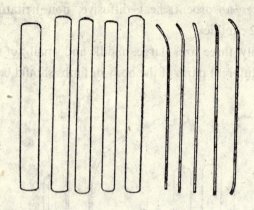

12–3　Splints for fixation of the fractured shaft(s) of the tibia and / or fibula

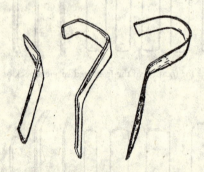

12–4　Splints for fixation of the fractured metacarpal bone

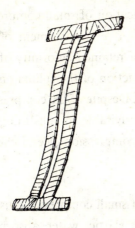

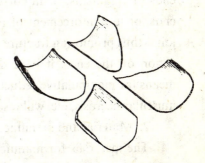

12–5 A splint for fixation of the
fractured lumbar vertebra
(an I–shape bamboo splint with
bandage–cotton covering)

12–6 Arch–shape cardboard
splints for fixation of the
fractured elbow

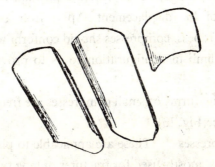

12–7 Arch–shape cardboard splints for fixation of the fractured ankle

Fig. 12 Splints of various sizes and shapes

Application of Compresses

1. Use of Small Compresses

Small compresses in certain forms can reinforce local fixation strength of the splints. Application of small compresses will produce an effect in prevention of re–displacement of the ends or fragments, or in correction of retained deformity of the ends, or in reinforcement of fixation action of the splints on the joint, thus promoting fracture healing. Despite of the compressive action on the ends, it is in no case advisable to substitute this means for manipulative reduction, or compression ulcer, ischemic muscular necrosis, etc. will result.

2. Material and manufacturing

The materials for manufacture of small compresses must be soft, and, to some extent, tenacious, elastic, water–absorbent, heat–diffusive, and non–irritating to the skin. They must also be able to keep certain shape and maintain certain strength. The commonly used materials include tissue paper, cotton, cotton felt, bandage gauze, etc. The specific shape, thickness and size of small compresses all depend upon the fracture position and the type and condition of the displacement. Apart from suitable size, thickness and hardness, compresses should conform with the part of the body or limb in configuration so as to provide an even pressure.

The following forms of small compresses are frequently used in clinical practice(Fig. 13):

Plane Compresses   These are applicable to plane parts of the body or limbs, mostly used for fractures of long tubular bones. of the extremities.

Terrance–shaped Compresses   These are applicable to the concave parts of joints such as the elbow joint and the ankle joint.

Flight–shaped Compresses   These are applicable to slope parts of the body or limbs, such as the dorsal aspect of the elbow and the ankle.

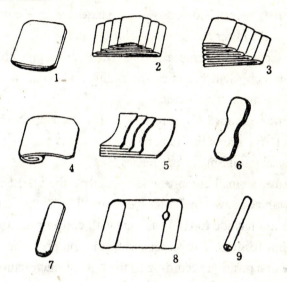

13–1   A plane compress   13–2   A terrace–shape compress
13–3   A flight–shape compress   13–4   A note–shape compress
13–5   A bone–embracing compress 13–6   A gourd–shape compress
13–7   A transverse compress   13–8   A bones–regathering compress
13–9   A bones–separating compress

Fig. 13   Various tissue–paper–made compresses

Note–shape Compresses   These are applicable to fractures of the clavicles or of the radii and / or ulnae with unstable reposition of displacement.

Bone–embracing Compresses   These are applicable to fractures of the olecranon bones or patellae. The compresses are in most instances made of flannel felt.

Gourd–shaped Compresses   These are applicable to radius capitulum fractures.

Transverse Compresses   These are applicable to distal terminal of the radius.

Bone—regathering Compresses   These are applicable to separation of the lower radius—ulna joint.

Bone—separating Compresses   These are applicable to fractures of such small bones as the radius and ulna, the palm bones, and the metatarsal bones.

Mushroom—shaped Compresses   These are applicable to surgical neck fracture of the humeri.

3. Placement of Small Compresses

As a rule, a small compresse is applied to the affected part and fixed with adhesive tapes after reduction. The further steps of immobilization include to bind the part with cotton padding and provide splint fixation. The placement of the compress should be right at the due position according to the type of the fracture and condition of the displacement. There are three ways of compress placement.

(1) 1—compress Fixation is mostly applied to fractures of epicondylus medialis or lateral condyle of the humerus as a means of direct pressure on the fracture site.

(2) 2—compress Fixation is applied to transverse fractures with lateral displacement. After reduction, two compresses are placed on the displaced aspect of the ends on either side of the fracture line, and make sure that neither of them extends across the line in case re—displacement occurs.

(3) 3—compress Fixation is applied to fractures with angular deformity. One of the compresses is placed at the point of the angle whereas the other two, on the opposite side, respectively at a

position as near one of the terminals of the diaphysis as possible. The three compresses then provide a force of lever action that can prevent recurrence of angular displacement (Fig. 14).

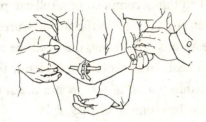

14-1   Fixation with one compress

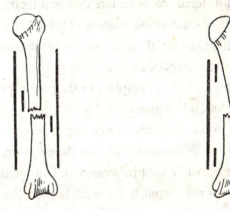

14-2   Fixation with two compresses   14-3   Fixation with three compresses

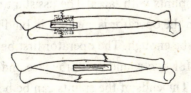

14-4   Application of a bones—separating compress (a roll) for a double fracture

Fig. 14

4. Cautions in Application of Compresses

The size and thickness of compresses and the diameter and length of compress rolls, are all dependent upon what part they are applied to. Too thin a compress or a roll can provide very little fixation effect because of insufficient pressure. On the other hand, if the pressure is too strong, there will be a danger of injuring the skin. Local dark scarlet skin posterior to fixation may probably be a manifestation of too great a pressure by the compresses and it must be promptly corrected.

Methods of Immobilization with Small Splints

Fractures at different parts require different fixations. To illustrate this, we take small splint fixation at long diaphyses as an example. All things essential must be ready at hand before fixation. The procedures related are as follows:

(1) If necessary, apply a compress to the proper position after successful reduction is achieved.

(2) Encircle the injured part with cotton padding.

(3) Arrange the splints evenly outside the cotton padding. A space of 1—1.5cm must be kept between each two splints and the terminals of the splints should not extend beyond the padding. The fracture line should be made rightly across the middle line of the splints.

(4) Bind the splints with laces. The assistant(s) must firmly fix the splints when the operator is engaged in binding. Generally, three bindings will be enough. The operator first binds the middle part of the splints for two rounds with the lace and makes a knot to fix the binding. The ends of the splints can be bound later and a distance of 1.5 cm from the terminals must be left in case the lace slips off. The tightness of the binding should be most appro-

priate(for plump persons, greater tightness may be necessary) as can allow the laces to move in either directions along the splints when they are drawn. If long slabs are needed as a means of support for the limb, they can be bandaged over the splints. In some cases, traction may be essential, and proper traction management should be made. In 3—5 days after the fixation, the binding is inclined to become tighter and tighter due to tumefaction and then gradually gets looser and looser due to subsiding of the swelling. This requires timely adjustment.

Cautions Posterior to Splint Fixation

1. The affected limb of the patient should be elevated to a proper height and maintained there until the tumefaction subsides.

2. Pay full attention to the circulatory condition of the patient's affected limb. If there is any disturbance of blood circulation, the binding must be promptly unfastend or serious consequence will occur.

3. Any apophysical pain must be carefully examined in case compression ulcer occurs.

4. Frequent adjustment of tightness of the binding is essential.

5. Let the patient and his / her family know the effect and problems likely to follow the fixation. Advise the patient to come for medical help whenever any of the problems occurs.

6. Timely exercises under the direction of the doctor is of great importance.

1.3 Administration of Chinese Medicines on the Basis of Overall Analysis and Differentiation of Symptoms and Signs

One of the characteristics of TCM orthopedics and traumatology in treatment of fracture is to prescribe for the patient certain Chinese medicines to help healing. Clinical practice has proved that treatment of fracture by administration of certain Chinese medicines can produce such beneficial results as quicker alleviation of pains and swelling, earlier growth of callus, better healing and more satisfactory restoration of functions.

In traditional Chinese medicine, it is deemed that the human body is an integrated organism. The five solid viscera and six hollow viscera, the limbs and the skeleton, *Qi* and blood, the meridian system, the skin, flesh, tendons and bones are all closely correlated to each other. The bones, for example, grow on essential substances which are provided by the viscera after they have taken them in from the food, drink and air. The whole bone system also gets nourished and moistened in *Qi* and blood and is interconnected by the meridians. If any part of the body is impaired, the other parts are usually involved, and, as a result, there will be dysfunction in the solid and hollow viscera, in the meridian channels and collaterals as well as in *Qi* and blood. Hence, in following holism, treatment of fractures in TCM begins with overall analysis and differentiation of symptoms and signs so as to establish correct diagnosis and proper principles of treatment, and lays emphasis on regulation of physiological functions of the body for elimination of all pathological responses resulting from the fracture. The explanation lies in that the impairment of any part of the body will inevitably injure somewhere in the meridian system, which will in turn lead to stoppage of mechanism of Qi-flow, usher in diviation of $Ying$ Qi and Wei Qi systems from the right channels , and cause stagnancy of stasis in the tendons and flesh. One conclusion in classic TCM theory affirms that " impediment brings about pains while free passage relieves them" . In accordance with this, emphasis in treatment of fractures is laid on regulation of the flow of Qi and blood. The first and foremost consideration is to invigorate circulation of blood to remove the stasis, for if blood circulation is not invigorative enough to remove the stasis, the union of the ends will be impossible. Clinically, The condition of injury can be divided into 3 stages each of which has its own characteristics and particularities that demand proper prescriptions based on differentiation of symptoms and signs.

The Initial Stage (within 1—2 weeks after fracture)

During this stage, the principles for prescription are as follows:

1. Promoting the Flow of Qi and Invigorating Circulation of the Blood so as to Allay Swelling and Eliminate Blood Stasis

This principle is applicable for patients suffering from impediment of Qi and stagnancy of stasis that result in pains and swelling. The commonly prescribed medicines are mostly of blood—flow—invigorating and stasis—removing properties, frequently accompanied with those of Qi—flow—promotive and meridian—passage dredging effect. The usually prescribed recipes are *Fuyuan Huoxue Tang* (1), *Huoxue Zhitong Tang* (2), *Huoxue Quyu Tang* (3), etc.

2. Activating Circulation of the Blood, Subduing Swelling and Clearing Away Heat and Toxic Materials

This principle is applicable for patients with local stasis, pains, swelling, red skin, and systemic fever as a result of rise of body temperature. The commonly prescribed recipes are *Qingxing Yao* (4) and modified *Wuwei Xiaodu Yin* (5).

3. Promoting the Flow of *Qi*, Removing Stagnancy and Eliminating Extravasated Blood by Catharsis

Trauma is often complicated with dysfunction of the internal organs. If the symptoms happen to be stomach distention, anorexia and vomiting, the principle for prescription should be activating circulation of the blood and promoting the flow of *Qi* so as to remove stagnancy, and the recipe to be prescribed will be *Shunqi Huoxue Tang* (6). If the symptoms are distention of and pains in the abdomen, vomiting, constipation, with signs of red tongue and yellow tongue fur, the principle should be eliminating extravasated blood by catharsis and the recipes may be *Dacheng Tang* (7) or *Taoren Chengqi Tang* (8).

4. Activating *Ying* System and Regulating the Flow of *Qi*

Trauma is usually followed by a choke sensation in the chest complicated with coughing (but there is some difficulty or even hemoptysis in coughing) and stabbing pain in the sternocostal part which becomes severer with breathing. These symptoms are mostly due to disorder of the liver—*Qi* and obstruction of lung—*Qi* resulting from rib fracture. The usual prescriptions are *Liqi Zhitong Tang* (9) and *Heying Liqi Tang* (10) .

The Intermediate Stage

Generally, swelling and pain around the fracture site subside within 3—6 weeks after the fracture. The ends may become practically stable and the systemic symptoms will disappear. In addition to maintaining the stability of the ends, the prescription should be able to help formation of callus and reunion of the ends. The commonly prescribed recipe at this stage is *Jiegu Dan*(11).

The Natural Cure Stage

As a rule, porosis will occur in 7 weeks after the fracture. This can be deemed as clinical healing. The primary principles at this stage are as follows:

1. Tonifying *Qi* and Blood

This method is applicable for cases with both traumatic injuries of bones and soft tissues and internal injuries of *Qi* and blood, or for cases with deficiency of *Qi* and blood and flaccidity of muscles and bones due to long—term bed rest. The commonly prescribed recipes are *Sijunzi Tang* (12), *Siwu Tang* (13), *Bazhen Tang* (14) , etc.

2. Tonifying the Spleen and Stomach

This method is applicable for cases with indigestion, limb fatigue, enfeebled physique, muscular atrophy and weak pulse. All these symptoms are ascrible to dysfunction and debility of the spleen and stomach in transformation and transportation caused by injury of considerably long duration that may result in excessive consumption of vital *Qi*, deficiency of both *Qi* and blood and ineffectiveness of the viscera. The principle of treatment is therefore to tonify the spleen and stomach so as to strengthen mourishment of *Qi* and blood, which will in turn speed up restoration of functions of the muscles, tendons and bones. The common prescriptions are *Sheng–ling Baizhu San* (15), *Yangpi Jinshi Tang* (16), *Guipi Tang* (17), etc.

3. Tonifying the Liver and Kidney

This method is also termed as Strengthening Muscles, Tendons and Bones. According to TCM theory, the liver dominates the tendons and the kidney governs the bones as well as the loins and lower limbs. This explains why fractures at the Natural Cure Stage heals slow in elderly patients. Old people are normally less strong with osteoporosis and limb fatique, a manifestation of insufficiency of both the liver and kidney. The treatment should therefore be based on tonification of the liver and kidney. Among the common prescriptions are *Bushen Huoxue Tang*(18), *Zhuangjin Yangxue Tang*(19), *Jianbu Huqian Tang*(20), etc.

4. Warming the Channels to Promote the Flow of *Qi*

This method aims at elimination of pathogenic wind and dampness that are stagnating in the body by administration of medicines of warming property that can expel wind and clear away cold. Drugs that can regulate the flow of *Qi* and blood are also necessary. The combined effect of the above mentioned medicines can restore normal flow of *Qi* and blood and relieve rigidity of the joints. The common prescriptions include *Huoxue Shujin Tang*(21), *Magui Wenjin Tang* (22), etc.

1.4　Medicinal Preparations for External Use

Preparations used by Mounting Method

These preparations are applied directly to the injured site to treat the trauma with the medicinal substances contained in them.

The following are the usual forms:

1. Ointment

This form is prepared in the following processes:Grind the drugs into a fine powder, add to the powder any or some such substances as maltose, honey, sesame oil, water, liquor, vinegar and vaseline to form a pasty preparation which can then be applied to the injured site. Ointments used for close injuries are often made of certain medicinal powder and maltose in a ratio of 1 (powder) to 3 (maltose). The portion of maltose can also be changed into a mixture of maltose and vinegar in a ratio of 8 to 2. For open injuries , the preparations are frequently made of certain medicinal powder and sesame oil or the like to produce an ointment, for it is not only soft but moistening. According to their effects, ointments consist of several types.

(1) Ointments Used to Eliminate Extravasated Blood

This type can be precribed for cases with fractures or injuries to soft tissues who frequently suffer from swelling and pains. The usually used prescriptions are *Xiaozhong Zhitong Yiaogao* (23), *Shuangbai San* (24), etc.

(2) Ointments Used to Promote Reunion of Bones and Repairment of Muscles and Ligaments   In some cases apposition of ends is good enough, but, at the intermediate stage, the fracture heals very slow or there is even non—union of the ends despite that the swelling has subsided. This type is usually prescribed for those cases. The commonly used prescriptions are *Jiegu Shujin Gao* (25) and *Waiyong Jiegu Gao*(26) .

(3) Ointments Used to Clear Away Pathogenic Heat and Toxic Materials   This type can be prescribed for cases with infection posterior to the injury who have the symptoms of local

redness, swelling, fever and pain. The commonly used are *Jinhuang Gao* (27) and *Sihuang Gao* (28).

(4) Ointments Used to Promote Regeneration of Tissues, Draw out Toxic Substances and Enhance Scabbing   This type is usually prscribed for cases whose wounds remain unhealing though the swelling has subsided. The commonly used are *Shengji Xiangpi Gao* (29), *Shengji Yuhong Gao* (30), etc.

2. Plaster

This form is prepared by refining mixture of the powder of needed medicinal sbstances and seasmae oil, yellow lead or beeswax. For patients with pains in the muscles at the intermediate and late stages of fracture, *Shenjin Gao* (31) or *Jiangu Zhuangjin Gao* (32) can be prescribed to alleviate the pain. Those who suffer from adhesive joints resulting in restricted activities of the involved joints can be given *Huajian Gao*(33) for external application. *Goupi Gai* (34) is effective to rheumatism whereas *Taiyi Gao* (35) is helpful to ulcerative wounds.

3. Remedial Powder

This is a fine powder of medicinal substances that can be directly spread over the wound or added to plasters for use. The common types are:

(1) Powder Used to Arrest Bleeding and Promote Wound Healing This type is generally prescribed for cases with bleeding wounds. The frequently used recipes include *Taohua San* (36), *Huarushi San* (37), etc.

(2) Powder Used to Remove Necrotic Tissues and Draw Out Toxins   This type is generally prescribed for cases with layers of necrotic tissues over the wound or with hypersarcosis. The frequently prescribed recipe is *Jiuyi Dan* (38).

(3) Powder Used to Promote Repairment of the Wound   This type is generally prescribed for cases with little pus and delayed formation of scab at the wound. The best choice is *Shengji Yuhong San* (30).

(4) Powder Used to Warm Up the Meridian Channels and Expel Pathogenic Cold   This type is generally prescribed for cases at the late stage of the injury who suffer from local accumulation of cold and dampness that causes stagnated *Qi* and blood and thus pains. The commonly prescribed recipe is *Dinggui San* (39) and *Guishe San* (40).

4. Lotion   This form of liquid preparation is usually prescribed for external application.

Type of Alcoholic or Aqueous liniment   This may be a medicated liguor in TCM, such as *Huoxue Jiu*(41), or a water solution of certain medicinal substances such as *Shujin Zhitong Sui*(42). They are effective in activating circulation of the blood, relieving pains, relaxing muscles and tendons, promoting the flow of *Qi* and blood in the channels and collaterals and expelling pathogenic wind and cold.

Type of Oil Solution   The solution is made by heating mixture of seasame oil and medicinal substances for some time, and , then, removing the residues through filtration. If beeswax is added to the oil solution, an ointment can be produced. This type of preparations has such effects as expelling pathogenic cold from the channels, eliminateing extravasated blood , etc. The commonly prescribed recipes include *Shangyou Gao* (43) and *Dieda Wanhua You* (44).

5. Drugs for Fumigation or Washing Use

Fumigation with drug decoction stream and / or washing

with drug decoction is used in TCM as a therapy which plays an important part in treatment of traumatic injuries at the late stage. This therapy requires to boil the drugs in water and fumigate the affected part in the steam. When the decoction cools to a temperature where the heat will not hurt, the patient should soak the part into the decoction or wash the part with it. It is advised to do fumigation and soaking / washing two times a day, 30—40 minutes a time. This method has such effects as relaxing muscles and tendons, activating circulation of the blood, easing the joints in functional movement, etc. The therapy is applicable for patients suffering from ankylosis, joint spasms, aches or numbness complicated with invasion of pathogenic wind and cold (in most cases the joints involved are those of the limbs). The usually prescribed recipes are *Huoxue Zhitong San* (45), No. 1 Washing Recipe (46), No. 2 Washing Recipe (47), etc.

6. Drugs for Fomentation

The drugs used in this therapy are mostly those of the properties of expelling pathogenic cold from the channels, promoting the flow of *Qi* and activating circulation of the blood. Wrap the drugs with a piece of cloth and heat them for external application to the affected part while the pack is hot.

(1) *Kanli Sha* (48)　　This is a mixture of heated iron pellets and water—vinegar decoction of the drugs for external application. Administration:Pack some of the mixture in a cloth bag, add to it a small amount of vinegar and stir the new mixture thoroughly. A few minutes later, the bag will naturally become very warm and it can then be applied to the affected part. This therapy is generally prescribed for patients with old trauma accompanied by wind—cold syndrome.

(2) Drugs for Pyrogenic Dressing　　Pack the drugs in a cloth bag and steam the bag hot in a steamer. Apply the hot bag to the injured part. This method is effective in treatment of wind-cold-dampness syndrome and painful swelling. The usual prescription is *Zhenggu Tangyao* (49).

(3) Others　　Such substances as raw salt and quarts sand can also be used for fomentation. Heat some salt or sand and put it into a cloth bag. Apply the bag to the injured part while it is hot.

1.5　Exercises for Rehabilitation

Significance of Exercises for Functional Rehabulitation

Exercises signify in treatment of injuries of bone joints and soft tissues. They can help improve the curative effect and reduce sequelae. That is why they are used as an important means of management of fractures. In the course of treatment of fractures or other injuries, rehabilitation of the muscles, tendons, joints and other parts of the body should be exercised for functional restoration on the basis of sequential progress and according to individual condition at each different stage. These exercises can improve the flow of *Qi* and blood throughout the body, build up constitutions and restore normal functions of the joints. Through rehabilitation exercises right relationships between local parts and the body as an integral, and between mobility and immobility, can be re-established. Proper functional exercises will produce the following effects:

1. Improving the Health Condition or Eliminating Local / General Symptoms　　By doing exercises under the doctor's supervision, the patient can realize better that he / she may as well perform certain exercises though he / she is fractured and

immobilized. The patient will also become self-confident, optimistic and free from depression, which helps considerably in improving the general condition. Local activities of the injured limbs and wounded trunk will enhance circulation of the blood and alleviate swelling and pain. On the contrary, if the patient is treated with extensive plaster immobilization without functional exercises, swelling and pain will hesitate in subsiding.

2. Promoting Fracture Healing   Articular exercises of the injured limb and general exercises can promote circulation of the blood, thus providing sufficient nutrients to meet the need of repairment for materials. As a result, the body metabolism will be reinforced and this will enhance fracture healing. Besides, this will lay a basis for synchronous healing and functional recovery and reduce the course of treatment.

3. Preventing Muscular Atrophy and Articular Rigidity   Organs of the body will degenerate if they do not work. So will the muscles, Long-term inactivity of a muscle will lead to its atrophy and ineffectiveness. Rational active exercises can prevent muscular atrophy. Similarly, long-term immobilization of the joints may cause rigidity and regular exercises will help the patient avoid adhesion between the joint capsule and the ligaments. This guranttees constant secretion and circulation of intraarticular synovial fluid, thus preventing the joint cartilages from degenerating; and when the fracture heals and the immobilization is discarded, satisfactory restoration of functions can be expected.

4. Preventing Osteoporosis   Osteoporosis is also a result of durative inactivity. Clinical studies have proved that a patient with immobilization of the trunk and the limbs will lose 1% of

the total amount of bone calcium within 5—6 weeks even if he / she is given the most ideal diet and sufficient vitamines. If the patient's body weight is 70 kg, with a corresponding total amount of 1 200 g of calcium, for example, the loss of calcium will amount to 12—14 g . This is known as disuse atrophy, which is more prominent in cases with local superarticular plaster immobilization. What is discussed here shows that inactivity or lack of functional exercises is one of the important causes leading to osteoporosis.

5. Preventing Other Complications   It has been proved that active exercises play an important role in prevention of such complications as hypostatic pneumonia, lithiasis of the urinary tract, etc.

Cautions in Practising Exercises

1. It is recommended to have active exercises of the muscles and joints instead of having them pulled or tracted passively.

2. No exercise should cause pain or further injury to the wounded part, so shearing, turning or injury—mechanism—repeating movements must never be tried.

3. The exercises must be practised under the doctor's correct instruction. The practical movements are dependent upon the condition of the patient and must be performed step by step. The patient can increase the times gradually, augment the mobile amplitude deliberately and prolong the time of a set of exercises properly. When doing exercises, the doer must get his / her mind completely concentrated on it and do the exercises slowly. In addition, local exercises and systemic exercises should be well combined.

Ways and Procedures in Performing the Exercises

Exercises of the upper limbs are designed for the purpose of restoring the functions of all the joints of the hands, especially the functions of the metacarpophalangeal joints and the interphalangeal joints. Exercises of the lower limbs aim at restoring the function of weight—bearing and walking and maintaining the stability of all relevant joints. In order to keep normal walking manner, strength of all the muscles of the lower limbs, especially the strength of the musculi glutaeus maximus, musculi quadratus femoris and musculi triceps surae, must be reinforced.

1. Exercises at Different Stages

(1) At the initial stage, there is local pain and distention;the fracture ends are not stable and the injury of the soft tissue needs repairing, therefore the purposes of doing exercises at this stage are to promote the subsidence of distention of the soft tissues and to prevent muscular atrophy and articular adhesion. So the main exercise should be a training of muscular contraction. Movements of certain joints can also be performed as long as they are not too energetic to benefit the local immobilization. For instance, exercises of fist—making of the fingers and mild movement of the shoulder joint and the elbow joint can be recommended for patients with stable forearm fracture. However, rotatory movement of the forearm must be excluded strictly. For patients with fractures of the lower limbs, femoral shaft, tibia or fibula, activities of the ankle joint and phalangeal joint should be emphasized and due attention paid to exercises of muscular contraction and relaxation of the quadriceps, but raising or turning movement can never be attempted. General exercises of the body are dependent upon the condition of the patient. As a rule, there is no need of absolute bed rest. Patients with fractures of the up-

per limbs should do all exercises as long as they do not cause any hurt to the injured limb. In cases with fractures of the lower limbs, none of the parts other than the injured limb should be restrained from free movements.

(2) The intermediate stage is characterized by alleviation of pains, extinction of distention, repairment of soft tissue injuries, stabilization of the ends and formation of callus. Therefore, in addition to beneficial exercises for muscular contraction and relaxation, patients with upper—limb fractures are encouraged to practise certain autonomous articular movements simultaneously at several joints in greater amplitude than at the initial stage as long as the muscles are strong enough and the fractured part is not hurt. Patients with lower—limb fractures can gradually start practice of raising the affected limb;and if there is no pain or trembling, they can go on with the exercises, from one—joint movement gradually to coordinative movements of a number of articulations. Cases who have been treated with traction are allowed to do systemic movements that can mobilize the joints of the injured limb whereas those who remain untracted can begin to practise crutch—walking with the help of crutches.

(3) At the natural cure stage, the soft tissues have already recoverd functionally. The muscles are now strong and powerful and fracture healing has realized clinically. However, exercises for rehabilitation are of extreme importance. Attention should be paid mainly to enlarged amplitude of movement of all the joints and to normal ability of weight—bearing of the limb or trunk. Active exercises will still be the primary form and massage can be applied as a means of auxiliary treatment. Patients with injuries at the lower limbs can begin to practise walking with support of

crutches and gradually initiate exercises for restoration of normal functions of the knees and ankles, without any weight—bearing at first, but with small weights later. On the other hand, every means possible should be tried for patients with injuries at the upper limbs to activate all the joints so as to restore their functions as early as possible.

2. Methods in Doing Exercises of different Parts

(1) Exercises of the Neck

When doing the exercises, the patient can take the posture of standing or sitting. In the former posture, the patient should stand with the arms akimbo and the feet apart in a width approximately the same as that between the acromia.

a. Bowing and Raising the Head   Do deep breathing before performing the exercise. Then bow the head down so hard as to make the chin get very close to the upper border of the manubrium of the sternum when exhaling and raise the head, looking up to the utmost, when inhaling, and repeat the process 6—7 times (Fig. 15–1).

b. Flexing the Neck Bilaterally   Do deep breathing before performing the exercise. First flex the head leftward when inhaling and restore it to the normal position when exhaling;and, then, flex the head rightward when inhaling and restore it to the normal position when exhaling. This exercise needs repeating the above process 6—7 times (Fig. 15–2).

c. Extending the Neck   Extend the neck as hard as possible to the left front direction when doing deep inhalation and restore it to the normal position when exhaling;and, then, extend the neck to the right front direction when doing deep inhalation and restore it to the normal position when exhaling. Repeat the processes 6—7 times (Fig. 15—3).

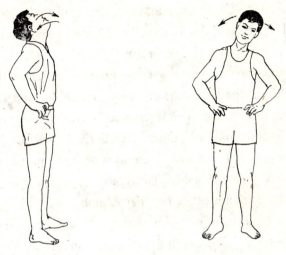

15—1   Bowing and raising the head alternately   15—2   Flexing the neck bilaterally

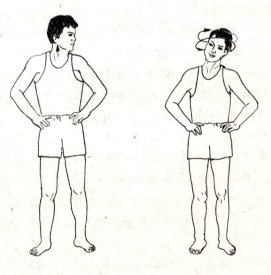

15—3   Extending the neck   15—4   Turning the head

Fig. 15   Exercises of the neck

d. Turning the Head   Turn the head to the left, restore it to the normal position, and, then, turn it to the right and restore it again. Repeat this process 1—2 times. Then, move the head levorotatorily and vice versa (Fig. 15—4).

By practising the above mentioned exercises of the neck,the strength of the neck muscles can be reinforced and the joints of the neck activated. The exercises will also regulate the flow of Qi and blood and an inner equillibrium will be established therefrom. This method is curative to neck sprain and bruise, stiffneck, cervical spondylopathy, etc.

(2) Exercises of the Lumbar Region

a. Bending Forward and Slightly Over—stretching Backward   Stand with the feet apart and hands supporting the hypochondria, bend forward and stretch the backbone backward moderately beyond the normal position (Fig. 16—1). Be sure to relax the muscles as much as possible when doing the exercise. This exercise can activate the lumbosacaral joint and allow the lumbar muscles to contract and relax alternately and spasms of the muscles will then be alleviated, producing an effect of relieving rigidity of the muscles and tendons and allaying pains and swelling.

b. Flexing the Backbone Bilaterally   Stand with the feet apart and hands supporting the hypochondria, and bend the backbone first to the left as hard as possible before restoring it to the normal position, and then to the right. Do these alternately (Fig. 16—2). This method can produce the same effect as the above one.

c. Rotating   Stand with the feet apart in shoulder—to—shoulder width and hands supporting the hypochondria. By exerting force of the lumbar portion and the lower limbs, rotate the lumbar portion clockwise and counterclockwise alternately (Fig. 16—3). Be sure to do the exercise in a soft, harmonious and rhythmic way. This method can make the lumbosacaral joint and sacaral—iliac joint move freely;it can also promote the flow of *Qi* and blood in the meridians.

d. Exercise of the Lumbodorsal Muscles and Gluteal Muscles   Lie in dorsal position with the legs flexing and clinging to each other, and both hands under the head, elbow joints touching the bed. By exerting force through the feet and the elbows, the belly, the loins and buttocks can be raised. Keep them at the possibly highest position for a short while and then let them down slowly (Fig. 16—4). Be sure not to cease breathing when raising these parts. As a rule, a raising and falling process can be completed in three respirations. This exercise has an effect of strengthening the lumbosacaral and gluteal muscles. Besides, it can also be employed for patients with simple compression fractures at the lumbovertebrae, being helpful for replacement of the fragments.

e. Exercise of the Back Muscles   Lie in prone position with the legs stretching straight and hands extending by the sides of the body (Fig. 16—5). By raising the head and legs, the back muscles can be made in a strain state and the back pulled straight to the utmost. This exercise has the same effect as the last one mentioned above.

f. Exercise of the Gluteal Muscles and the Abdominal Muscles   Lie in dorsal position with both the hip joints and the knee joints flexing, and arms embracing the legs. First do extension—flexion exercise of the hip joint. The extension should reach

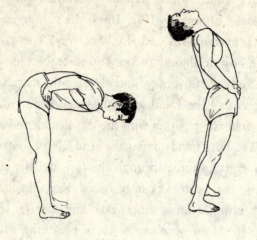

16-1   Bending forward and overstretching backward

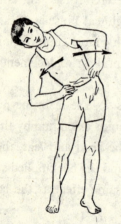

16-2   Bending the backbone sideward bilaterally

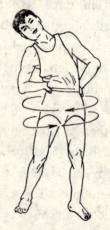

16-3   Rotating the lumbar portion

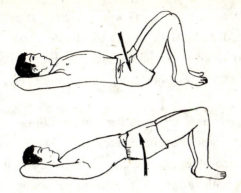

16-4　Raising the lumbar portion in the dorsally lying position

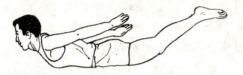

16-5　Exercise of the back muscles

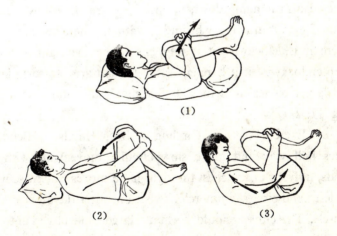

(1)

(2)　　　　　　　　　　　(3)

16-6　Extension-flexion of the hip joint and rocking of the whole body

Fig. 16　Exercises of the lumbar portion

the position where the arms are stretched straight while the flexion should make both thighs touch the chest. This exercise should be followed by a rocking exercise (Fig. 16—6). This method is designed to strengthen the gluteal muscles and the abdominal muscles.

(3)　Exercises of the Shoulder and the Elbow

a.　Extendion—flexoin Exercises　　Stand with the feet apart from each other and the arms hanging down naturally and, then, raise both arms in the front direction to a height approximately to the shoulder level and keep them extending straight. When these preparatory postures are ready, begin withdrawing and re—extending one arm after the other alternately. This exercise is designed to expand the range of movement of the shoulder and the elbow joints (Fig. 17—1).

b.　Whirling Exercise　　Stand with the feet apart from each other and, then, bend forward to form a right angle with the affected arm hanging down naturally. When these postures are ready, begin " drawing whirlings" with the hanging arm from where it is, clockwise if it happens to be the right arm and counterclockwise if it happens to be the left arm, to form larger and larger circles until the possible maximum range is reached (Fig. 17—2).

c.　Exercise of Slow Circling of Both Hands　　Bend the knees half way and make slow circular movements with the hands, in front of the chest;the right hand moves clockwise while the left hand circles counterclockwise, one after the other by half a circle. The circles should be made larger and larger until the possible maximum range is reached and the legs should be kept swaying / extending—flexing synchronously with the movement

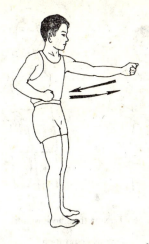

17-1 Extending–withdrawing of
the arms

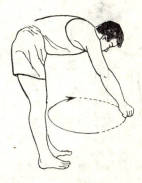

17-2 Whirling of the hanging
arm

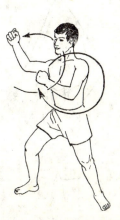

17-3 Slow cycling of the hands
and the whole upper limbs

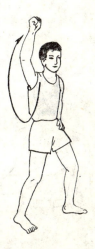

17-4 Swaying the upper limb

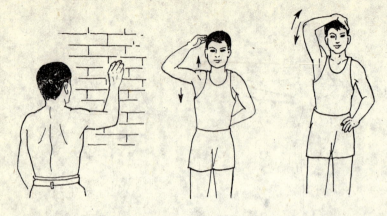

17—5　Finger—creeping

17—6　Flexing the elbow joint in

the raising position

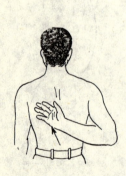

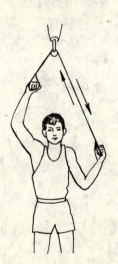

17—7　Backward reaching and

intortion of the right

shoulder joint

17—8　Raising the affected limb

through the pulley device

Fig. 17　Exercises of the shoulder joint and elbow joint

of the hands (Fig.17—3).

     d. Exercise of the Shoulder Joint   Stand with the feet apart from each other. Then swing one hand (which is in fist—making state) around the shoulder joint from the front to the back and vice versa while keeping the other hand supporting the other hypochondrium(Fig. 17—4).

     e. Exercise of Finger "Creeping"   Stand facing a wall and lay the fingers, except the thumb, of the affected hand on the wall and let them " creep" slowly upward until the arm is fully stretched, and then "creep" back (Fig. 17—5).

     f. Exercise of Elbow Flexion   Raise the affected arm with the elbow joint flexing and rub with the palm the homolateral top—side of the head and then the contralateral side (Fig. 17—6).

     g. Exercise of the Shoulder and the Forearm   Pronate the right forearm and press the dorsal aspect of the palm against the back of the body (Fig. 17—7) so as to pracitse backward stretching and intorsion of the shoulder joint.

     h. Exercise of Shoulder—raising through Pulley Device   Stand directly under the pulley and hold the ends of the pulley rope, each in one hand, and raise the affected limb by pulling the other end of the rope with the unaffected hand(Fig. 17—8). Be sure not to pull too forcefully.

    (4) Exercises of the Hand and the Wrist

     The physiological functions of the wrist joint and other joints of the hand is of great importance. Not only the normal functional position but also the capability of free turning and flexibility in wilful movement muts be maintained. These exercises are generally prescribed for cases with fractures of the hand or wrist at the natural cure stage.

a. Exercise of Finger Clenching   Stretch out the fingers energetically and then clench them tight to form a fist.

b. Exercise of Forearm—rotating   Press the forearm against the costal parts and raise them to a level position with a short stick in each hand. Do rotatory movements with the fore-arms forwardly and backwardly around the contacting areas (Fig. 18—1).

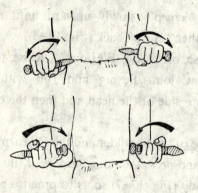

18—1   Turning of the forearms

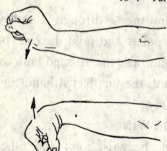

18—2   Dorsal—extension and
palmar—flexion of the
wrist joint

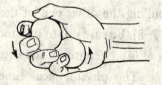

18—3   Rolling steel balls in
the hand

Fig. 18   Exercises of the wrist joint and the hand

c. Exercise of Dorsal Extension and Palmar Flexion of the Wrist　　Do movements of dorsal extension and palmar flexion of the wrist joint with the fingers clenching tight energetically to form a fist (Fig. 18−2).

d. Exercise of the Fingers　　Hold two wulnuts or small steel balls in the hands and roll them unceasingly (Fig. 18−3).

(5) Exercises of the Hips

Hips, knees and ankles are the most important joints of the body in weight−bearing. Satisfactory restoration of the functions of these joints after traumatic injuries is most significant in future as regars weight−bearing, walking manner and labour capability. Sequela at the knee or ankle after injury is quite common and exercises for restoration of functions of these joints should therefore be performed possibly earlier as long as they prove harmless to recovery.

a. Exercise of Muscular contraction　　Atrophy of quadriceps femoris frequently occurs after a fracture of the femoral shaft or after an injury of the knee, so exercise of muscular contraction of the quadriceps femoris should never be neglected whether at the initial stage or at the natural cure stage.

b. Exercises of Raising Extending Legs　　Lie dorsally on a bed with the lower limbs exteding straight, slowly raise them to a certain height and, then, let them down gradually. This will help restore the strength of muscular contraction. Increase the times of performing the exercises to reinforce endurance . If the raising can be done easily, extra weight may be added by attaching it to the foot soles.

c. Exercise of Flexion−extension of the Hip Joints and the Knee Joints　　Lie in dorsal position with the legs stretching straigh. First do flexion−extension movements of the ankle joints and, then, flex both the hip joints and the knee joints energetically for subsequent lateral upward extension as if to pedal something (Fig.19—1).

d. Exercise of Moving the Knees Rotatorily   Stand with the knees flexing half way and the hands on the knees, and move the knees rotatorily. While moving the knees, the knee joints can slowly extend and flex alternately (Fig. 19—2).

e. Exercise of Stepping up and Down a Flight   This exercise is very helpful for restoration of functions of the hip joints, knee joints and ankle joints(Fig. 19—3).

f. Exercise of "cycle—pedaling"   Ride on a medical cycle and pedal it with the healthy foot so as to drive the affected limb to move passively. This exercise will provide an extra chance of functional activities for the major joints of the affected limb (Fig. 19—4).

g. Exercise of Roller—pedaling   Tread on a wood roller and roll it to and for with the feet(Fig 19—5).

h. Exercise of Dorsal Extension and Instep Flexion of the Ankle Joint   Lie in dorsal position or sit on a stool and do exercises of instep flexion and sole flexion as hard as possible.

i. Exercise of Ankle Rotating   Lie in dorsal positon or sit on a stool and do exercise of ankle—rotating, first clockwise and then counterclockwise.

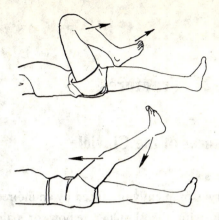

19—1　Flexion—extension of the hip joints and the knee joints

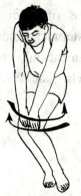

19—2　Moving the knees rotatorily

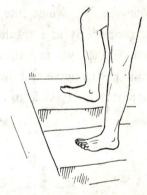

19—3　Stepping up and down a flight

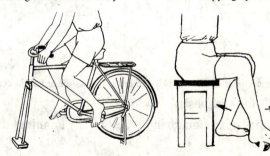

19—4　Pedaling a medical cycle　19—5　Roller—pedalling

Fig. 19　Exercises of the hip, the knee and the ankle

2　Fractures

2.1　Fractures of the Clavicle

Pathogenesis

The injury is frequently produced by an indirect force. When a person falls with the shoulder, elbow or palm against the ground, the injury is likely to occur, mostly at the middle 3rd of the clavicle, in which the proximal end is often displaced posterosuperiorly as a result of traction by sternocleidomastoid muscle (Fig. 20) whereas the distal end or fragments may stab the brachial plexus nerve and the subclavian vessels. Fractures at the distal part of the clavicle are rare.

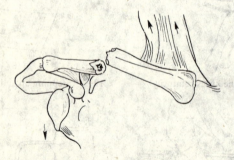

Fig. 20　Displacement of the ends in a fracture of the middle 3rd of the clavicle

Essentials for Diagnosis

1. A history of traumatic injury, especially an injury due to a fall.

2. Swelling and pain at the clavicle part with the affected shoulder in a collapsing position;hindrance to the raising of the

homolateral arm due to hurting.

3. Local tenderness with bony crepitus and displacement of the proximal fragment that can easily be felt.

4. Careful examination of the affected limb for better information about its blood circulation, sense of perception and ability to move helps to make sure whether there is any injury to the brachial plexus nerve or to the vessels.

5. X—ray films of the clavicle in anteroposterior view helps to establish the diagnosis:Greenstick fractures occur more often in children while oblique or comminuted fractures more often in adults.

Treatment

Reduction   The patient sits on a stool, supporting the costal sides with hands. An injection of 1% procaine into the local hemotoma is necessary. An assistant stands behind the patient, a foot on the stool with the knee supporting the patient by the part between the scapulae, fixes both of the patient's forearms with hands, and proceeds to pull the patient's arms posterosuperiorly and laterally by exerting force gradually while the patient throws his / her chest out and inclines his / her head to the affected side as required. The operator stands in front of the patient and lays the thumbs, forefingers and middle fingers on both the distal and proximal fracture ends. By pressing the proximal end while simultaneously raising the distal end, reduction of the ends will be achieved(Fig. 21).

Immobilization

1. "∞—shape" Bandaging Fixation   A cotton pad is applied to the affected armpit and the bandaging begins from the injured part, goes through the armpit to the opposite shoulder, past

under the opposite armpit and back to the upside of the affected shoulder. Repeat the process a few times before the bandage is fastened tight. Then apply a U—shaped compress at the fracture site and a square plain compress at the proximal end and cover them with a proper piece of cardboard that is pad—lined inside. The bandage now goes above the cardboard and is knotted tight through the bandage ring at the chest (Fig. 22).

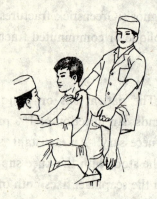

Fig. 21   Manipulative reduction of a fracture of the clavicle

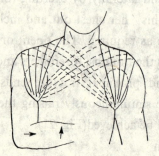

Fig. 22   ∞—shape bandaging fixation for a fracture of the clavicle

2. Bandage—ring Fixation   A cotton pad is applied to each of the armpits. Make two bandage rings and put them

around the shoulders, one for each. Tighten the rings with two bandages respectively on the back side.

3. Adhesive-plaster Fixation   Apply an adhesive tape, 6cm in width, to the affected limb, the elbow precisely at the middle part of the tape, and firmly fix the elbow and the shoulder with the tape from the anterior to the posterior and vice versa (Fig. 23). This method is applicable to fractures of the distal segment of the clavicle.

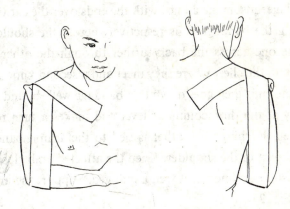

23-1   The anterior view   23-2   The posterior view

Fig. 23   Adhesive plaster fixation for a fracture of the clavicle

4. Cardboard-compress Fixation with an " armpit-roll"
This method is applied immediately after manipulative reduction. The patient sits on a stool and is given local anesthesia. By supporting the patient's affected upper arm with a forearm from under it and pressing the outer part of the affected scapula with the ulnar ridge of the hand, the operator can make the patient's shoulder stretch posteriorly so as to correct overriding displacement. Then the operator begins to press the posteriorly protruding proximal end of the fracture with the thumb and forefin-

ger of the other hand to complete the reduction (Fig. 24). The assistant now applies the "armpit roll" (a cardboard—made tube, 12 cm long and 8 cm in diameter, wrapped with cotton matress and bandage;a long bandage being set through it for binding) to the armpit of the affected limb and a square compress to the proximal end of the fracture. And, then, the operator can proceed to perform the immobilization:Cover the compress with a cotton pad, ride on the pad with a piece of cardboard, fasten the rollbandageends, make a knot with the ends over the cardbopard, and bring the bandage ends respctively across the shoulder and back, the one across the back further through the other armpit and back to the chest where they meet and a second knot is made. One of the ends then goes down to a bandage well—bound around the body at the thoracolumbar level and makes a turn round it before self—hitching. The other is tied to the armpit bandage at the front part of the shoulder. Keep the affected limb close to the sternocostal part and get it well bandaged. Support the arm with a sling (Fig. 25).

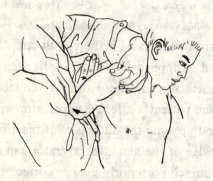

Fig. 24   Reduction of a fracture of the distal segment of the clavicle

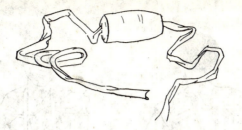

25-1　The armpit roll

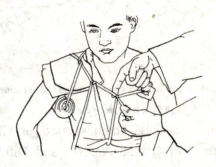

25-2　3, 4, 5, 6 Steps of the fixation

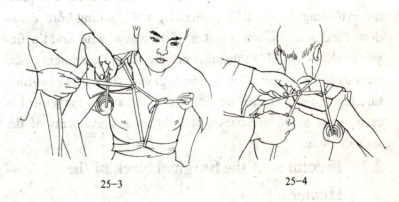

25-3　　　　　　　　　　　　　　25-4

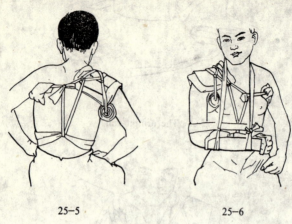

25-5   25-6

Fig. 25   Cardboard-compress fixation with an armpit

roll for a fracture of the clavicle

Medication   See 1.3:Administration of Chinese Medicines on the Basis of Overall Analysis and Differentiation of
Symptoms and Signs

Exercises   At the initial stage, it is recommended to practise extending the shoulder posteriorly and squaring both shoulders. Flexion-extension activities of the elbow, wrist and the fingers are also helpful. At the intermediate stage, the amount of exercises can be increased. At the natural cure stage when the fracture has healed and the immobilization discarded, the patient is
encouraged to do exercises of all-direction movements of the
shoulder joint.

2.2   Fractures of the Surgical Neck of the
   Humerus

Pathogenesis

This fracture is in most instances caused by an indirect force.

The injury mostly befalls adults. When an adult falls on the elbow or palm, the resultant axial or torsional load may be transmitted up to the shoulder and produce the facture.

Essentials for Diagnosis

1. Swelling, pain, tenderness at the shoulder, impact pain at the elbow, and inability to lift the affected limb.

2. Fractures without apparent displacement just presenting vague deformity, indistinct bony crepitus and little pseudo—activities;abducent fractures showing a plump shoulder despite of palpable bone protrusion in the armpit, which differentiates from dislocation (Fig. 26);adducent fractures manifesting a palpable protruding fracture end at the lateral part of the proximal segment of the upper arm;fractures complicated with dislocation of the shoulder joint presenting an angular shoulder with palpable displaced clavicular head at the armpit in spite of a negative result in Dugar's test which differentiates it from simple dislocation of the shoulder joint.

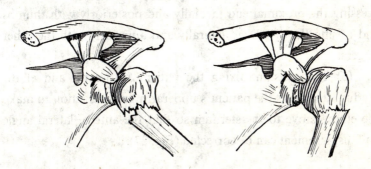

26—1   The abduction type.   26—2   The adduction type.

Fig. 26   A fracture of the surgical neck of the humerus

3. X—ray films in anteroposterior and lateral views is help-

ful in establishment of the diagnosis.

Treatment

Reduction

1. Fractures without Displacement   *Shenjin Gao* (31) can be externally applied to the affected shoulder before shoulder—coaptation splint immobilization is given and the affected forearm should be supported with a sling for 3—4 weeks.

2. Abducent Fractures   The patient sits on a stool or lies in dorsal position, Under local anesthesia, the operation is performed in the following steps:

(1) An assistant fixes the forearm and elbow of the patient's affected limb, making the elbow flex in 90 degrees.

(2) Another assistant gets hold of a cloth—strap loop that has been set with a cotton pad as a support from under the armpit of the patient's affected limb.

(3) The two assistants perform traction along the alignment of the distal end of the fracture for 10 minutes or so.

(4) The operator fixes the fracture ends with both hands, pressing the proximal end medially and posteriorly with thumbs and raising the distal end laterally and anteriorly with the other fingers.

(5) The assistant fixing the patient's forearm and elbow gradually adducts the patient's upperarm under traction to make the elbow move to the sternum so that the antero—lateral angle and displacement can be corrected (Fig. 27).

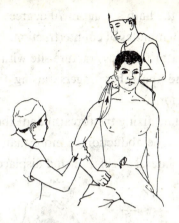

27-1   An abducent fracture of the surgical neck of the humerus managed

with abducent traction

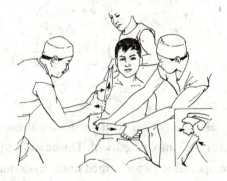

27-2   Reduction of an abducent fracture of the surgical neck of the humerus

Fig. 27

3. Adducent Fractures   The preparations are all the same as in reduction of abducent fractures. The procedures are as follows:

(1) An assistant does the same as in (1) above for reduction of an abducent fracture.

(2) Another assistant fixes the patient's affected forearm and

elbow and makes the limb abduct in 70 degrees and flex forward in 30 degrees for 10 minutes of countertraction.

(3) The operator fixes the fracture site with thumbs pressing the distal end and the other fingers raising the proximal end laterally and anteriorly.

(4) The assistant fixing the forearm and elbow of the patient gradually increases the abduction to more than 90 degrees so as to correct anterio–lateral angulation and displacement (Fig. 28).

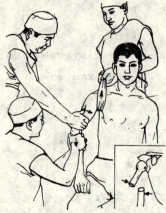

Fig. 28   Reduction of an adducent fracture of the surgical neck of the humerus

4.   Fractures Complicated with Dislocation of the Shoulder Joint   The operation is performed under systemic anesthesia.

(1) The assistant keeps the patient's affected shoulder joint in an abducent position of 90—150 degrees to make the distal end precisely align to the proximal end, as will allow the broken joint sac to open for easy replacement of the head of the humerus.

(2) The operator pushes the anterior lower border of the humeral head upwardly, posteriorly and outwardly with thumbs from the armpit while fixing the shoulder with all the other fingers.

(3) The assistant slightly moves the injured limb in a favourable direction and gradually makes it adduct so as to reposit the humeral head. The steps for reduction of the fracture ends are the same as for adducent fractures.

Immobilization   An abducent fractures is immobilized with a shoulder—coaptation splint and the forearm is supported with a sling. An adducent fracture is immobilized with an abducent supportor. A fracture complicated with shoulder dislocation is immobilized with shoulder—coaptation splint fixation and a sling is applied to support the forearm.

Medication   See 1.3:Administration of Chinese Medicines on the Basis of Overall Analysis and Differentiation of the Symptoms and Signs. If there is severe swelling or distention at the initial stage, the dosage of blood—flow—activating drugs should be increased and heat—clearing and detoxifying drugs should be added. A compound prescription based on modified *Fuyuan Huoxue Tang*(1) and *Wuwei Xiaodu Yin* (5) will prove most effective.

Exercises   As long—term immobilization of the injured shoulder due to contuse tends to cause adhesion of the shoulder joint, functional exercises of this joint should never be neglected. At the initial stage, the patient should be advised to do flexion—extension exercises of the fingers and the wrist. At the intermediate stage when the fracture becomes stable, the patient can begin flexion—extension and turning exercises of the elbow and forearm and all—direction movements of the shoulder joint. When the fracture heals at the natural cure stage, the range of all—direction movements of the shoulder joint should be increased in case adhesion occurs.

2.3　Fractures of the Humeral Shaft

Pathogenesis

Fractures of the humeral shaft occur in people of all ages, but, mostly in adults. The injury frequently results from a direct force in birth trauma, machine impact or crush and so on. Occasionally, an indirect force in a fall or in throwing an object may also cause the fracture. The common forms are transverse or spiral fractures. If the radial nerve is injured, it may be in a fracture of the middle 3rd of the humerus.

Essentials for Diagnosis

1. Swelling and pain in the upper arm, deformity in the lateral process, and inability to raise the affected arm high.

2. Crush pain with pseudo—activities and bony crepitus, and impact pain at the elbow.

3. X—ray films can help reveal the position, type and degree of the displacement in the fracture.

4. Wrist dropping, failure of the hand in stretching straight, anesthesia between the thumb and the forefinger on the dorsal aspect of the hand may suggest injury of the radial nerve.

Treatment

Fractures of the humeral shaft do not require complete reposition. Slight over—riding and / or angular deformity hardly affects the functions of the upper extremity.

Reduction

The operation is performed under brachial plexus anesthesia or local anesthesia. The patient sits on a stool with the elbow flexing at 90 degrees. Two assistants respectively fix the upper segment and the elbow of the patient's injured limb and perform mild traction. The operator lays his hands on the fracture site to grasp it firmly and begins the reduction.

(1) A fracture at the Upper Segment of the Humerus (a position just above the lower border of the deltoid muscle)　　The assistant fixing the the patient's affected elbow lets it drop down and places it at a position close to the chest. The operator presses the distal fragment with thumbs and pushes up the proximal fragment with the other fingers. This combined performance will reduce the ends.

(2) A Fracture at the Middle Part of the Humerus (a position below the lower border of the deltoid muscle)　　The assistant fixing the patient's affected elbow abducts the injured limb by 40—50 degrees and the operator presses the proximal fragment with thumbs and pushes up the distal fragment with the other fingers to complete the reduction (Fig. 29). If there is notable sliding of the ends without crepitus during the reduction, it suggests that there is soft tissue insertion into the crack between the ends. This will require oscilations or circlings to release the inlaying tissue.

(3) A Fracture at the Lower 3rd in the Middle of the Humerus　　The proper maneuvers to be used are Pulling—stretching and Pushing—pressing instead of Angular—flexing and oscillation, or the radial nerve will be injured. When there is no overriding but some separating displacement, the best way to reduce it is to bring together the ends so as to make the ends into contact with each other. Slight injury to the radial nerve will generally heal without any management. However, care must be taken in performing the reduction. Mild and soft manipulation is of great importance in order not to worsen

the injury.

Immobilization

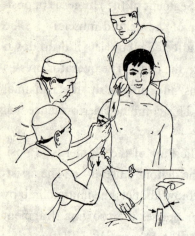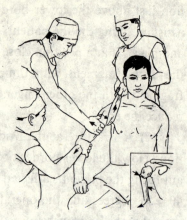

29-1   Reduction of a fracture of the   29-2   Reduction of a fracture of the
upper 3rd of the humeral shaft   middle 3rd of the humeral shaft

Fig. 29

1. Splint Fixation   For fractures of the upper part of the humerus, shoulder-coaptation splint fixation should be applied. The injured arm is placed against the lateral part of the chest and bandage-bound along with the chest. Support the forearm with a sling. For fractures of the middle segment of the humerus, splint fixation is applied to the part, but the shoulder joint and the elbow joint are left free. Between the injured arm and the chest, a cotton compress is necessary to keep the arm in an abducent position of about 30 degrees. For fractures of the middle lower 3rd of the humerus, superarticular splint fixation is utilized with the affected arm suspended with a sling.

2. Splint Fixation Plus Suspending Skin-traction   This is applicable for cases with severe swelling of the upper arm and

overriding displacement. The patient lies in dorsal position, the shoulder of the injured limb forming a forward right angle and the elbow joint flexing in 90 degrees. The forearm is pronated and skin—traction along the alignment is provided in combination with an overhead suspending traction. Four splints are applied and bound with laces.

3. Plaster—and—Splint Fixation   This method is applicable to fractures with separate displacement of the ends. The operator fixes the ends firmly. An assistant pushes the distal end upward while another assistant applies a cotton pad to the affected joint and sticks a plaster tape, 4—6 cm in width, to the arm, extending from the acromionclavicular part, posteriorly up to and across the shoulder, down along the posterior aspect of the upper arm, around the elbow, up along the anterior of the upper arm, toward the posterior direction and to the spine of scapula. After the plaster is well affixed, the splints can be applied to finish the fixation.

Mediciation

See 1.3:Administration of Chinese Medicines on the Basis of Overall Anlysis and Differentiation of Symptoms and Signs.

Exercises

At the initial stage, flexion—extension exercises of the wrist joint and fist—forming of the hand are recommended. All—direction movements of the elbow joint and the shoulder joint can be initiated at the intermediate stage. When the injury enters the natural cure stage, increase the range of movement of the shoulder and elbow. Special attention must be paid to prevention of stiff shoulder. Exercises of mobility of the shoulder joint should be gradually started once the fracture ends become stable.

2.4 Supracondylar Fractures of the Humerus

Pathogenesis

Supracondylar fractures are clinically common. Most of the victims are children at the age of 4—8 years old. With regard to the violence that causes the fracture, these fractures are clinically divided into two types:Extension Type and Flexion Type. In the case of Extension Type, severe displacement frequently causes serious consequences due to ischemia of the forearm resulting from direct pressure on or injury to the brachial arteries and / or veins by the proximal fracture end. Besides, the proximal end may also injure the intermediate nerve and the radial and ulnar nerves. This requires high vigilence in examination.

Essentials for Diagnosis

1. Swelling and pain at the elbow, crush pain at the supracondyle.

2. Presense of remarkable crepitus and complete loss of the functions of the elbow joint despite of normal specific osseous equilateral triangle at the elbow.

3. In cases with vascular injuries, the radial and ulnar arteriopulses will become weak or unpalpable, resulting in poor peripheral circulation and low temperature of the relevant part.

4. In cases with nervous injuries, there will be corresponding signs of injuries of the median , radial and ulnar nerves.

5. X—ray films in the anteroposterior and lateral views will help establish the diagnosis. Be cautious to differentiate a supracondylar fracture from a dislocation of the elbow or from separation of epiphysis of captillum.

Treatment

Reduction

1. There is no need of reduction for undisplaced fractures or mild greenstick fractures. The treatment is just to prescribe external application of *Shenjin Gao* (31) and a triangular sling to support the affected arm for two weeks. Severe greenstick fractures do require restitution, but be sure to get aware of the normal presence of an anteverting angle of 25 degrees at the lower segment of the humerus. For Extension Type of fractures, the operator should

(1) fix with one hand the forearm of the patient's affected limb, making it flex at 90 degrees,

(2) push the elbow apex with the thumb of the other hand and raise the upper part of the cubital fossa with the other fingers so as to form an angle less than 90 degrees at the elbow joint, and.

(3) apply ∞ −shape bandage−fixation or U−shape cardboard bandage fixation for 2—3 weeks.

2. For displaced fractures, the reduction is performed under local anesthesia or brachial plexus anesthesia. The patient sits on a stool or lies in dorsal position. An assistant fixes the upper arm of the patient's affected limb and another assistant holds the wrist and forearm and makes the patient's elbow slightly flex. By performing continual countertraction, the two assistants can correct overriding displacement of the ends. In addition, if there is prone deformity of the distal fracture end, the affected forearm should be made supinated under traction by the assistants, and vice versa. In reducing medial displacement, the operator needs to lay the fingers of both hands on the lateral aspect of the patient's injured forearm, fixing the distal end, and put the thumbs on the medial aspect, and pushes the inwardly displaced end outward. In

the performance, the operator must direct the parts between the thumbs and forefingers toward the distal terminal of the affected limb. Reduction of anteroposterior displacement can be done next.

(1) Extension Type   In management of this type of fractures, the operator should push the patient's affected elbow apex with thumbs (the parts between the thumbs and the forefingers towards the distal end) while pressing the upper part of the cubital fossa with the other fingers and have the patient's elbow flexed slowly by an assistant under traction. But the force exerted for the performance can never be too powerful and the flexion of the elbow must be of sufficient degrees in case the fracture stability is impaired as a result of subsequent forward displacement of the distal end (Fig. 30).

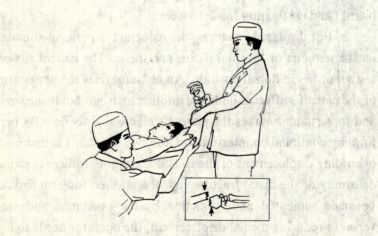

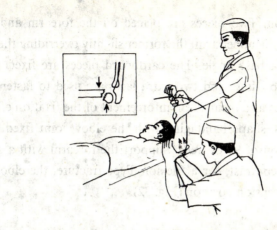

Fig. 30　Reduction of a supracondylar fracture (Extension Type) of the humerus

(2) Flexion Type　　In treatment of fractures of Flexion Type, the operator should press the cubital fossa of the patient's injured limb with thumbs (the parts between the thumbs and the forefingers towards the distal end) and raise the posterior upper part of the affected elbow while an assistant slowly extends the patient's elbow joint straight under traction. If the flexion is toward the ulnar side, slight overcorrection is allowable. After the ends have been reduced, the operator still needs to fix the fracture site with both hands, and the assistant holds the patient's elbow joint, keeping it stretching straight slightly and extending the forearm to the radial side so as to make the bone cortex of the end on the radial side inlay properly. This will prevent occurrence of cubitus varus.

Immobilization

1. Arch−shaped Cardboard Fixation　　After reduction of an abducent fracture, apply a broad cotton pad to the apex of the elbow and the corresponding opposite. Four long trapezoidal pieces of cardboard moulded in arch−shape are needed for

immobilization. Two pieces are placed on the forearm and the other two on the upper arm, the former slightly overriding the latter, each by a base angle. The cardboard pieces are fixed with four—bonds—binding, and two extra laces are used to fasten the inner two ones as a means of reinforcement of the fixation effect. Then apply 8—shape bandaging with the elbow joint fixed in a flexion position of 90 degrees. Support the forearm with a sling (Fig. 31). In contrast, for a Flexion Type fracture, the elbow is fixed in an extension position (Fig. 32).

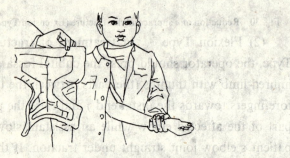

31—1 A thin cotton—compress used in the fixation

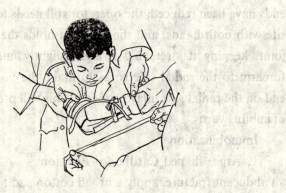

31—2 3, 4, 5 Steps of the fixation

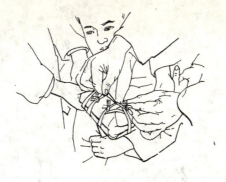

31-3

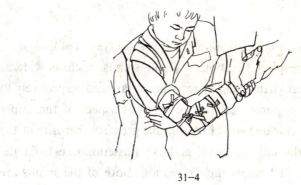

31-4

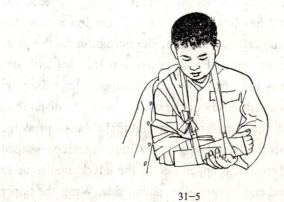

31-5

Fig. 31   Fixation for a supracondylar fracture

(Extension Type) of the humerus

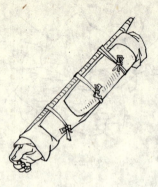

Fig. 32   Fixation for a supracondylar fracture(Flexion Type) of the humerus

2.   Four−splint Fixation   Four splints, each as wide as 1 / 5 the largest girth of the upper arm, are applied respectively to the anterior, posterior, lateral, and medial aspect of the upper arm. The anterior one stretches from the greater tuberosity of the humerus to the cubital fossa, and the posterior one from the armpit to the part below the olecreanon. Both of the splints are heat−processed into an anterior arch−shape at the lower end. The medial splint stretches from the axilla to 3 cm lower than the tuberosity, and the lateral one from the acromion to the same reach as the medial splint. For an extension fracture with displacement towards the ulna, two flight−shaped compresses are needed, one on the tuberosity of the ulna to press the distal fracture end forward, the other on the medial malleolus to press the distal end towards the lateral side. In addition, a terrace−shaped compress is applied to the upper side of the lateral malleolus to press the proximal end towards the medial side. Wrap the upper part of the elbow with a cotton pad and apply the splints rightly above the compresses and get them fastened with three laces.

Support the forearm with a sling (Fig. 33).

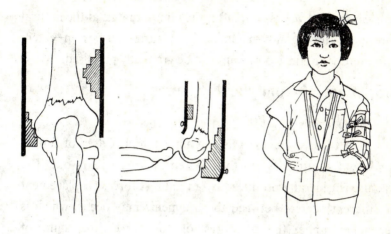

33-1　Placement of the compresses
and position of the forearm

33-2　After the fixation

Fig. 33　Fixation for a supracondylar fracture

(Extension Type) of the humerus

Medication

Huoxue Quyu Pian(54) should be prescribed for oral admini-stration at the initial stage. If there is severe swelling and distention, prescription of *Fuyuan HuoxueTang* (1) plus Rhizoma Ligustici Chuanxiong and Rhizoma Curcumae Longae for oral intake will be the remedy. At the intermediate stage, oral admini-stration of *Jiegu Dan* (11) is helpful. The natural cure stage re-quires No. 2Washing Recipe for fumigation and washing and *Shenjin Pian* (50) for oral intake.

Exercise

Extension-flexion exercises of the wrist and the fingers are of great importance at the initial stage. At the intermediate stage, the patient can begin to do exercises of the shoulder in all directions. When healing of the fracture begins and the immobilization is discarded in 4 weeks or so after the injury, that is, at the natural cure stage, turning movements of the forearm and flexion—extension exercises of the elbow joint can be gradually practised.

2.5 Lateral Condylar Fractures

Pathogenesis

This type of fractures is not uncommon. Cases of lateral condylar fractures are mostly children of 5—10 years old. The fracture is generally produced by an indirect force. Displacement of different degrees between the fragments may occur, which is dependent upon the greatness of the force, the state of introversion or extroversion of the elbow joint and the rotatory direction of the forearm at the time when the injury takes place. Clinically, these fractures can be classified as undisplaced fractures, displaced fractures and rotatorily displaced fractures.

Essentials for Diagnosis

1. A history of trauma, especially a history of trauma due to a fall.

2. Lateral swelling and pain at the elbow joint, loss of functions of this joint which is frequently at a half—flexion position (about 130 degrees).

3. Local tenderness and presence of bony crepitus at times.

4. X—ray films in anteroposterior and lateral views can help determine the state of displacement. However, attention must be paid to the fact that the fragments are mostly of cartilage and that they are actually larger than they appear to be in the films as cartilages are almost transparent to X—rays.

Treatment

Reduction

1. For cases of undisplaced condylar fractures, Shenjin Gao (31) is usually prescribed for external application. The affected elbow is immobilized at a flexion position of 90 degrees with 8—shape bandaging. Support the forearm with a sling for as long as 3 weeks or so.

2. For cases of condylar fractures with simple displacement of the ends, manipulative reduction is routine. The patient lies in a dorsal position.

(1) An assistant fixes the upper arm of the patient's affected limb.

(2) The operator fixes the affected forearm of the patient with one hand, makes a proper supination of it while keeping the elbow at a half—flexion position and the wrist extending dorsally so as to relax the traction by the extensor muscles, holds the elbow of the jnjured limb with the other hand, and presses the fracture fragment with the thumb while raising the medial side of the elbow with the other fingers so as to make the elbow invert and give a larger lateral joint space. Then, by direct pressure on the fragment with the thumb, the operator can reduce the displaced ends.

(3) Subsequent flexion—extension exercises of the elbow at a position of 135 degrees are undertaken to help stabilize the effect of reposition(Fig. 34).

3. For cases of condylar fractures with resupinate displacement of the ends, there are 3 methods of reduction.

(Assuming that the fracture occurs in the right upper limb.)

Method 1   (1) The patient lies in dorsal position and is given brachial plexus anesthesia. (2) Two assistants fix the upper arm and forearm of the patient's affected limb respectively and perform mild pulling. (3) The operator first pushes with his right thumb the fragment towards the lateral–posterior space at the distal terminal of the humerus, and, then, presses the trochlear end of the fragment inwardly and downwardly with the left thumb so as to make the fragment insert into the right position of the fracture surface. By pushing the lateral condylar end of the fragment from the lateral–downward position to lateral–upward direction with the right thumb and the forefinger, the operator can reduce the resupinate displacement. (4) The next steps are the same as in reduction of condylar fractures with simple displacement.

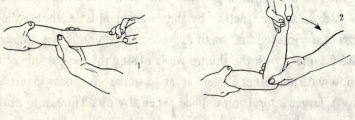

34–1 Pinching at the extension
position

34–2 Pinching at the flexion
position

Fig.34 Reduction of a condylar fracture of the humerus

Method 2   The patient's posture, the preparations for the operation, and the coordinative performances by the assistant are all the same as in Method 1.

The operator (1) presses with his left forefinger the trochlear end of the fragment and fixes with the thumb the external humeral epicondylar end, slightly pushing the fragment to move posteriorly, the trochlear end towards the posterior inward direction and the external humeral epicondular end from lateral downward position to lateral upward direction. and, (2)pushes and presses the fragment medially with the right thumb to bring it up to the level of the upper ridge of the external humeral epicondylar to present a plane surface, which shows good replacement of the fragment (Fig. 35).

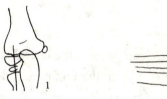

35–1 The anteroposterior view   35–2 The lateral view

Fig. 35 Normal longitudinal axis of the radius extending

through the center of the capitellum

Method 3   This method is termed as "Reduction through Rocking and Sudden Pulling ", particularly applicable for cases of children. The operation is performed under general anesthesia or brachial plexus anesthesia. The affected limb is abducted. The operator supports the patient's affected arm with one hand (thumb pressing the resupinate fragment to push it toward the joint space and the other fingers carrying the elbow) in case of over–inversion or over–eversion of the elbow during performance of rocking and has the carpometacarpal part of the child's affected limb in the other hand, extending and flexing the affected elbow alternately, rocking the arm from side to side with intervention of sudden mild pulling in times. The rocking is initiated first to the ulnar side (that is, to make inversion of the elbow) and the rocking magnitude can be gradually increased. The performance must be done harmoniously, mildly and evenly. No violence or rudeness is allowed. When sharp sounds are heard with disappearance of the bony crepitus during performance of the maneuvers, the fragment has been reposited. In case the reduction is not well achieved, additional supination or pronation of the elbow plus rapid extending—rocking with inversion of the elbow joint may be needed. These extra maneuvers will bring about satisfactory reposition.

Immobilization

1. Apply a square compress to the lateral condyle and a cotton pad to the elbow. Cover the compress and pad with four arch—shaped cardboard pieces and bind them firmly. Support the forearm with a sling with the elbow half—flexed(about 135 degrees).

2. Apply a square compress to the lateral condyle. The elbow is kept stretching straight with the forearm in full pronation. Fix the arm with four splints stretching from the middle part of the upper arm to the lower part of the forearm by tying the splints with laces. The elbow should be flexed at 90 degrees two weeks later.

Medication

See 1.3 Administration of Chinese Medicines on the Basis of Overall Analysis and Differentiation of Symptoms and Signs.

Exercises

At the initial stage, flexion—extension exericses of the fingers are recommended. Half a month later, all—direction movements of the shoulder joint and flexion—extension exercises of the wrist joint may be suitable. After the fracture has healed and external fixation is removed, active exercises to restore the functions of flexion, extension and rotation of the elbow joint are advisable.

2.6 Fractures of Medial Epicondyle of the Humerus

Pathagenesis

Fractures of medial epicondyle mostly occur in juveniles. These fractures are frequently caused by combined traction of an eversive force to the elbow and contraction of the flexors of the forearm, as in a fall. There are four types of medial epicondylar fractures. The classification depends upon the displacement of the fragments and the intensity of the force that causes the injury. Fractures with minimal displacement fall into Type I, fractures with gross displacement into Type II, jointimpacting fractures into Type III and joint—impacting fractures with displacement into Type IV.

Essentials for Diagnosis

1. A definite history of trauma.

2. Swelling, pain, tenderness and bony crepitus on the medial aspect of the elbow with a change of the normal triangle of the elbow.

3. "Disappearance" of the fragment as a result of impaction of it into the joint.

4. X—ray films in anteroposterior and lateral views may reveal the displacement (and its extent) of the fragment.

5. There may be symptoms and signs of injuries to the ulnar nerve that should not be neglected.

Treatment

Reduction

For a fracture of Type I, apply an 8-shape bandaging Cardboard fixation to the posteriority of the elbow which is kept in flexion of 90 degrees, The forearm should be supinated and supported with a triangular sling, and the wrist in a flexive position.

For a fracture of Type II. for instance, of the right hand, the reduction should be performed under local anesthesia. The assistant fixes the affected forearm and the wrist, keeping the elbow flexing at 90 degrees and the forearm pronated with the wrist in flexion so as to relax the flexors of the forearm. The operator then fixes the patient's affected elbow with the left hand and pushes and presses with the right thumb the fragment toward the posterosuperior direction to reduce it .

For a fracture of Type III, there are two ways of reduction.

1. The assistant fixes the patient's affected forearm and wrist in the same way as for a fracture of Type II. The operator holds with the left hand the lateral aspect of the upper segment of the affected forearm and pushes with the right thumb and forefinger the flexors of the jnjured forearm toward the distal end, and, simultaneously, the assistant quickly supinates the patient's forearm while everting and straightly extending the elbow joint and stretching the wrist joint dorsally. The same performance can be repeated a few times and the fragment will usually come out of the articular cavity. The fracture can then be managed in the same way as for a fracture of Type II.

2. Keep the patient's affected elbow flexing at 40 degrees and the shoulder joint abducting at 90 degrees. The assistant fixes the patient's affected forearm and hand and makes the affected forearm extremely pronate and abduct to obtain an enlarged space in the medial aspect of the elbow. With one hand fixing the

patient's lateral upper part of the affected elbow and the other hand fixing the medial lower part of it , the operator can produce a lateral semi--luxation of the affected elbow joint so as to release the fastening of the fragment by the semilunal incisure. This will enable the operator to palpate the boundary edges of the fragment at the medial lower part of the elbow. Then the assistant makes extreme dorsal extension of the patient's affected wrist joint for a few times and the fragment will withdraw from the articular cavity. In case the above maneuvers prove not enough to bring the fragment out, extreme supination of the affected forearm may be necessary to let the fragment be tracted away from the ulnar semilunal incisure. The operator then begins to push and press the lower end of the patient's affected condyle to the lateral side with one hand and to force the upper ends of the radius and ulna to the medial side with the other hand while the assistant forcibly extending the wrist joint of the patient dorsally, and this will lead to reposition of the elbow joint along with release of the fragment from the cavity. The fracture can then be managed in the same way as for a fracture of Type II (Fig. 36).

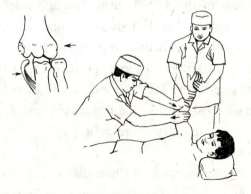

— 36-1 Method I

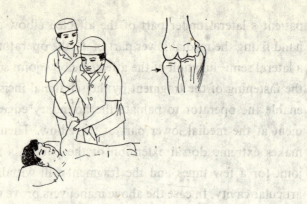

36-2 Method Ⅱ

Fig. 36 Reduction of an epicondylar fracture (Type III, originally

from Type Ⅳ) of the Humerus

Immobilization

1. Cardboard Fixation   Apply a square cloth compress to the medial epicondyle and cover it with a cotton pad. Fix the compress and pad with four arch—shaped cardboard slabs, keeping the elbow flexing at 90 degrees and the forearm pronating. Support the forearm with a sling with a flexed wrist.

2. Splint Fixation   Apply a flight—shaped compress to the lower part of the medial epicondyle and a terrace—shaped compress to the lateral upper part of the condyle. Cover the compresses with cotton pads and fix them with four splints, each respectively placed at the anterior, posterior, medial and lateral sides of the upper arm. Bind the splints with three laces. The elbow is flexed at 90 degrees, the forearm pronated. Support the forearm with a sling with a flexed wrist.

Medication

See 1.3:Administration of Chinese Medicines on the Basis of Overall Analysis and Differentiation of Symptoms and Signs.

Exercises

At the initial stage, fist—making attempt and movement of the wrist joint should be avoided though there is no need to restrict movement of the shoulder. At the intermediate stage, extension—flexion exercises of the fingers and the wrist, and rotatory movment of the forearm are recommended, Flexion and extension of the elbow can gradually be exercised at the natural cure stage.

2.7 Fractures of the Olecranon

Pathogenesis

These fractures are not clinically common. Adults are more susceptible to olecranon fractures than children. In most instances, the injury is produced by an indirect force though a direct force may also cause the fracture in times. In the former case, the result will be a transverse fracture while in the latter case a comminuted fracture, or, likely, a bone fissure in children.

Essentials for Diagnosis

1. A history of trauma, as caused in a fall, or occasionally produced by a violent impact.

2. Pain, swelling and distention around the elbow, and a change of the normal elbow triangle.

3. Restricted extension of the elbow joint, tenderness at the posterior cubital region, sometimes plus bony crepitus or palpable gap between the fragments.

4. X—ray films in anteroposterior and lateral views can help determine the fracture type.

Treatment

Reduction

As the injury is an intra—articular fracture, anatomical reposition must be attempted as hard as possible.

1. A bone fissure or comminuted fracture without evident displacement needs no reduction though it is necessary to immobilize the elbow joint with cardboard fixation, with the joint slightly flexed, for 3—4 weeks.

2. A displaced fracture must be reduced. The operation is performed under local anesthesia. The patient lies in dorsal position with the affected elbow in mild flexion. The assistant fixes the patient's affected forearm and wrist. The operator stands by the patient on his / her wounded side, presses with thumbs both the medial and lateral sides of the upper end of the olecranon and pushes the bone to the distal terminal. Then the assistant straightens the affected elbow joint so as to bring the fracture surfaces into close contact with each other. The operator fixes firmly the fragments and lets the assistant slightly extend and flex the patient's elbow a few times, as is beneficial to moulding of the fracture site by the trochlear of the humerus.

Immobilization

1. Superarticular Splint Fixation of the Forearm   Apply a flight—shaped compress to the olecranon area. Prepare four splints. The longer posterior one should have a moulded arc shape at the upper end which will be put over the elbow, stretching beyond the elbow joint by 7 cm and the other ones to be placed respectively on the medial, lateral and anterior sides, just reaching the joint. Apply the splints rightly to the forearm and bind them with three laces. Flex the elbow at 20—30 degrees and bandage it.

2. Closed   Fixation   with   Kirschner   Pins   The

immobilization is performed under local anesthesia. Two Kirschner pins are respectively brought through the upper and lower ends, parallel to the fracture line, from the medial side to the lateral side. The ways for the pins to get through must be kept away from the ulnar nerve. Fix the pins tight by fastening their ends together with certain devices such as holed wooden blocks or pieces of steel wire so as to apply an additional pressure to the fracture surfaces to reinforce the fixation. This method is particularly applicable to transverse fractures with gross displacement.

Medication

See 1.3:Administration of Chinese medicines on the Basis of Overall Analysis and Differentiation of Symptoms and Signs.

Exercises

At the initial stage, extension–flexion exercises of the wrist and all–direction movements of the shoulder joint can be performed. Extension and flexion of the elbow joint and rotatory movement of the forearm can be gradually initiated after the immobilization is discarded.

2.8   Fractures of the Radial Head

Pathogenesis

Fractures of the radial head are common. The injury is mostly produced by an indirect force. In children, the fracture is known as epiphysiolysis of the radius. According to where the fracture occurs and how the displacement is like, fractures of the radial head can be classified into such types as oblique fractures, resupinate fractures, greenstick fractures, fissure fractures, crack fractures, comminuted fractures, etc.

Essentials for Diagnosis

1. A definite history of trauma as caused in a fall.

2. Swelling, pain, and ecchymosis at the lateral lower part of the elbow.

3. Local tenderness. In oblique fractures and resupinate fractures, the displaced radial head can be palpated.

4. Restricted flexion and rotatory movement of the forearm.

5. The type of the fracture can be determined in X—ray films.

Treatment

Reduction: There is no need of reduction for such fractures as greenstick fractures, fissure fractures, crack fractures and impact fractures.

1. Oblique Fractures   These fractures must be reduced. The operation is performed under local anesthesia or brachial plexus anesthesia. The patient sits on a stool or lies in dorsal position with the affected forearm supinated and the elbow mildly flexed. Two assistants respectively fix the patient's upper arm and forearm for stretching traction. The operator supports with thumbs the lower part of the fragment from the lateral—posterior aspect of the radial head, and pushes and presses upwardly, anteriorly and medially while the assistants rotate the patient's forearm and flex and extend the elbow joint alternately. After good reduction has been achieved, the affected elbow should be kept in flexion at 90 degrees and the forearm at a neutral position (Fig. 37).

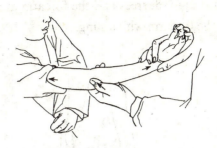

Fig. 37   Reduction of a fracture of the radial head

2. Resupinate Fractures   The pre—operative preparations are the same as for oblique fractures. The operator places a
thumb at the upper edge of the fragment, pushing medially and
forwardly, and supports with the other thumb the lower edge of
the fragment, pushing upwardly and forwardly. These maneuvers
will change the injury into an oblique fracture. Then do every-
thing the same as in 1. and the reduction will be completed. In
case the above—mentioned processes fail to bring about good apposition, an alternative method is available:Reduction through
Pin—driving. This requires sterilized operation. A Kirschner pin is
inserted from the lateral—posterior aspect of the elbow into the
limb until it reaches the fragment. Then forceful pushes through
the pin are made anterosuperiorly and medially so as to reduce
the fragment (Fig. 38).

Immobilization

Superarticular fixation of the forearm is usually employed.
Apply a rectangular compress to the posterolateral aspect of the
capilulum radii and four splints, the anterior one being in a concave shape at the proximal end and the posterior one stretching
over the elbow, to the forearm and fix them with laces. The elbow

should be flexed at 90 degrees and the forearm at a neutral position. Support the forearm with a sling.

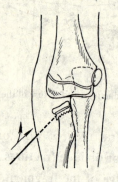

Fig. 38 Reduction of a fracture of the radial head
with the help of a steel pin

Medication

See 1.3:Administration of Chinese Medicines on the Basis of Overall Analysis and Differentiation of Symptoms and Signs.

Exercises

At the initial stage, flexion—extension exercises of the wrist and all—direction movement of the shoulder joint are recommended. Functional rotatory exercises of the forearm can be gradually practised at the intermediate stage. The patient is encouraged to do flexion—extension exercises of the elbow joint and increase the range of rotatory movement of the forearm at the natural cure stage.

2.9 Fractures of the Proximal 3rd of the Ulna Associated with Dislocation of the Radial Head (Monteggia Fractures)

Pathogenesis

Fractures of the proximal 3rd of the ulna associated with dislocation of the radial head are generally known as Monteggia Fractures. They mostly occur in children and youngsters. The injury is frequently produced by an indirect force and seldom by direct trauma. According to the direction of the causative force and the condition of displacement, these fractures can be clinically classified as Extension Type, Flexion Type and Adduction Type (Fig. 39). The Extension Type is the commonest.

Essentials for Diagnosis

1. A definite history of trauma, especially a trauma caused in a fall.

2. Swelling and pain at the upper part of the forearm and on the lateral side of the elbow, sometimes plus ecchymosis and tenderness.

3. Perceivable bony crepitus and notable pseudo–activities in the upper part of the forearm and palpable protrusion of the radial head at the lateral aspect of the elbow.

4. Dysfunction in forearm rotation and elbow flexion.

5. X–ray films of the upper part of the forearm and the elbow joint in anteroposterior and lateral views can help determine the type of the fracture.

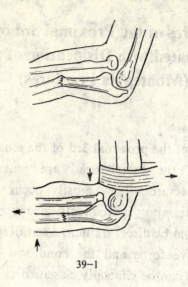

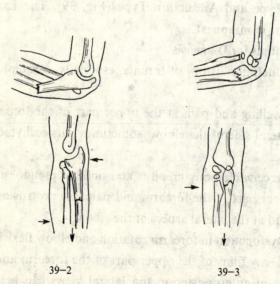

39–1

39–2   39–3

Fig. 39   A fracture of the proximal 3rd of the ulna associated

with a dislocation of the radial head

6. If the deep branch of the radial nerve is pressed or contused by the dislocated radial head, there will be difficulty in extending the wrist and such phenomena as hypoesthesia or even anesthesia at the part between the thumb and the forefinger on the dorsum of the hand. Electromyography can help determine the nature of the injury to the radial nerve.

Treatment

Reduction

1. Extension Type   The operation is performed under local anesthesia or brachial plexus anesthesia. The patient lies in dorsal position with the affected limb abducting at about 80 degrees, the elbow extending straight, and the forearm supinating. Two assistants perform stretching countertraction by fixing the patient's upper arm and wrist of the affected limb respectively. The operator supports with thumbs the lateral and palmar aspects of the affected radial head and pushes and presses the radial head towards the ulnar and dorsal sides so as to reposit it. Then the assistant fixing the patient's wrist proceeds to flex the involved elbow joint as hard as possible. As a rule, this will reduce the ends of the fractured ulna. If there is still some angular or lateral displacement of the ulna to the radius or the palm, certain extra maneuvers must be performed to correct it:(1) The assistants keep the patient's affected forearm in supination, the elbow joint in extreme flexion as well as in extroversion. (2) the operator fixes both the distal and proximal fractured ends of the ulna with the thumbs and forefingers, thumbs on the palmar side and forefingers on the dorsal side, pushes the distal end to the ulnardorsal side while increasing gradually the angular degree to

the palmar side, and, then, counterflexes the distal end in the dorsal direction to bring about satisfactory apposition (Fig. 40).

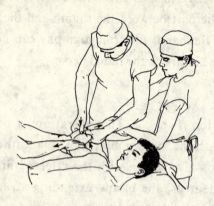

Correction of radius—inclining displacement of the ulna

Fig. 40   Reduction of a Monteggia fracture (Extension Type)

2. Flexion Type   The pre—operative preparations are all the same as for Extension Type. The patient's affected elbow is kept in a semi—flexion position and the forearm is pronated. The operation begins with stretching countertraction. The operator presses with thumbs the patient's dislocated radial head to the medial—anterior aspect and the assistants keep the patient's affected limb extending straight and supinate the forearm. This will normally reduce the radial head. If there is still displacement of the fractured ulna toward the radial side, the operator has to perform radius—ulna separation by applying the thumbs and forefingers to the space between the two bones to press them apart and push the dislocated distal end to its normal position, or he can resort to counterflexion process to reduce the displaced ulnar fracture.

3. Adduction Type   Again, all the pre—operative prepa-

rations are the same as for Extension Type. The patient's affected limb is kept extending straight and stretching countertraction is performed first. The operator presses with a thumb the dislocated radial head towards the medial side and simultaneously raises the medial aspect of the elbow with the other four fingers while holding the patient's forearm with the other hand and abducting it forcibly so as to reduce the dislocation of the radial head and the radius—inclining angular fracture of the ulna (Fig. 41).

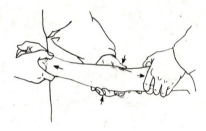

Fig. 41　Reduction of a Monteggia fracture (Adduction Type)

Immobilization

1. Extension Type　　　After reduction, a rectangular compress is applied to the anterolateral aspect of the radial head and is made in an arch shape to exercise a pressure on the radial head. A bone—separating compress is placed on the fracture site. Cover the compresses with cotton padding. Arrange four splints well; the proximal end of the lateral one must override the compress on the radial head. Bind the splints with three laces. The elbow is in flexion at degrees slightly smaller than a right angle and the forearm is supinated and supported with a sling (Fig. 42).

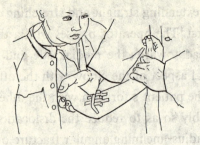

42-1　Placement of the small compress in the fixation

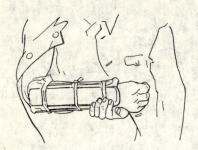

42-2　After the fixation

Fig. 42　Splint fixation for a Monteggia fracture (Extension Type)

2. Flexion Type　　After reduction, the patient's affected elbow is kept extending straight with a supinated forearm. Apply a rectangular compress to the posterolateral aspect of the radial head and cover it with cotton padding. Immobilize the forearm and elbow with superarticular splint / cardboard slab fixation for 2—3 weeks before changing to fixation with the elbow in semi—flexion (Fig. 43).

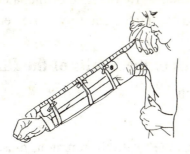

Fig. 43. Reduction of a Monteggia fracture (Flexion Type)

3. Adduction Type　　The immobilization is all the same as for Flexion Type except that the compress is applied to the lateral aspect of the radial head.

4. Closed Osseous—pin Fixation　　This fixation requires pre—operative local anesthesia or brachial plexus anesthesia and routine pre—operative sterilization. After the fractured ulna has been manipulatively reduced, the osseous pin that was previously inserted from the olecranal terminal into the proximal ulnar end at the beginning of the operation is further driven into the distal end. Then splint fixation or plaster support fixation is applied with the elbow flexing at 90 degrees. Keep the forearm in supination and support it with a sling.

Medication

See 1.3:Administration of Chinese Medicines on the Basis of Overall Analysis and Differentiation of Symptoms and Signs.

Exercises

At the initial stage, the suitable exercises are fist—making and all—direction movement of the wrist joint and the shoulder joint. Extention—flexion exercises of the elbow joint are helpful at the intermediate stage. By the time of the late stage, the patient is encouraged to practise rotatory movement of the forearm.

2.10   Fractures of the Shafts of the Radius and Ulna

Pathogenesis

These fractures are relatively common, mostly in children and in adults at the age of 20—50. In most instances, the injury is produced by an indirect force, usually with an upper radial fracture line and a lower ulnar fracture line. The most common forms are transvers or oblique fractures. Fractures caused by torsional forces often present upper ulnar fracture lines , mostly in a twisted appearance, but those caused by direct forces will show fracture lines at the same level, mostly in communited or transverse forms. If the fracture of the radius occurs at the upper—middle 3rd, the proximal end will be in a supinated and abducent state as a result of the traction of the supinator and the distal end in a pronated state as a result of the traction of the pronator.

Essentials for Diagnosis

1. A definite history of trauma.

2. Pain and swelling at the forearm with ecchymosis, angular / shortening deformity and dysfunction in rotation.

3. Local tenderness, impact pain with pseudo—activities and bony crepitus.

4. X—ray films in anteroposterior and lateral views can reveal the actual fracture position and the condition of the displacement.

Treatment

Reduction

In radioulnar fractures , the main problem is rotatory displacement. The maneuver "separating the bones by pinching" can effectively correct the displacement, making stable the ends of the radius and ulna, like those of a sigle bone, so as to assure good apposition.

The patient sits on a stool or lies in dorsal position. Two assistants respectively fix the upper aspect of the patient's affected elbow and wrist. For fractures of the lower—middle 3rd, the forearm should be in a neutral position. For fractures of the upper—middle 3rd, the forearm should be supinated. Stretching countertraction is necessary for correction of angular and overriding displacement. The operator pinches the dorsal and palmar aspects of the fracture part respectively with thumbs and the other fingers to make as apart as possible the fracture ends which have been brought close to each other since the injury. Meanwhile, the doctor should push the angularly displaced ends from the dorsal aspect with thumbs, raise with the rest of the fingers the other ends that are displaced to the palmar side, and gradually perform contraangular flexion (Fig. 44) to give replacement of the fracture ends. After reduction, in order to produce close contact between the ends, it is highly necessary to add such extra maneuvers as rocking or swaying the forearm from the palmar side to the dorsal side as well as from the radial side to the ulnar side, and vice versa, by the operator (who performs these maneuvers by fixing the fracture part with both hands). In the case of a fracture at the upper 3rd of the radius, the proximal end tends to be in rotatory displacement to radiodorsal aspect and the distal end to the ulnar—palmar aspect. This requires the operator to press and push the distal end to the dorsal aspect of the radius and the proximal end to the ulnar—palmar aspect so as to correct the displacement.

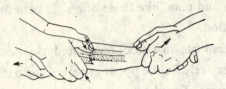

44—1 Increasing the degrees of the angular deformity

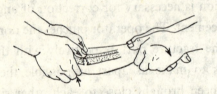

44—2 Pushing the ends back to the normal position

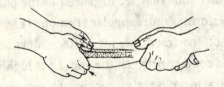

44—3 Restoring good apposition

Fig. 44 Reduction of radial—ulnar fractures

by contra angular bending maneuver

Immobilization

Two bone—separating compresses are applied respectively

to the palmar and dorsal aspects of the fracture ends and over them are placed two square compresses. Four splints are used on the palmar, dorsal, ulnar and radial aspects of the forearm respectively and fixed with three laces. Support the forearm with a sling. For fractures of the upper 3rd of the bones, the forearm is kept in supination; and for fractures of the lower—middle 3rd , the forearm is placed in a neutral position (Fig. 45).

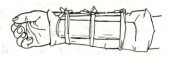

45—1   The anteroposterior view

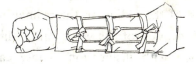

45—2   The lateral view

Fig. 45   Splint fixation for radial—ulnar fractures

Medication

See 1.3:Administration of Chinese Medicines on the Basis of Overall Analysis and Differentiation of Symptoms and Signs. If the forearm swells severely at the initial stage, modified *Fuyuan Huoxue Tang* (1) can be prescribed for oral administration.

Exercises

Attention must be paid to tightness of the splint fixation in case ischemic contracture or necrosis of the forearm occurs due to over—tightening. At the initial stage, the appropriate exercises are flexion—extension and fist—making of the fingers. Exercises of movement of the elbow joint and shoulder joint can be practised at the intermediate stage. At the natural cure stage, the patient is encouraged to do exercises of rotatory movement of the forearm.

2.11　Fractures of the Distal End of the Radius

Pathogenesis

These fractures are common, mostly in the elders. When they occur in young people, the result will be epiphysiosis, caused by an indirect force in most cases. The fractures can be divided into Extension Type and Flexion Type, dependent upon the posture in the fall(Fig. 46). A Barton's fracture is a fracture of the distal end of the radius on the palmar aspect associated with upward dislocation of the wrist joint, falling into Flexion Type complicated with dislocation. Those caused by direct forces are mostly comminuted fractures.

Essentials for Diagnosis

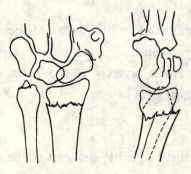

46—1　Angular displacement of the fragment, the fracture line away from the joint

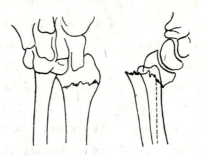

46-2 Dorsal displacement of the distal fragment, the fracture

line away from the joint

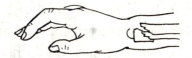

46-3   Displacemeht in a case with a Smith's fracture

Fig. 46   Fractures of the Distal segment of the radius (Extension Type)

1. A definite history of trauma, especially a trauma caused in a fall.

2. Pain and swelling at the wrist and a " fork-shape" deformity in ExtensionType.

3. Local crushing pain with crepitus and pseudo-activities and complete loss of the wrist functions.

4. X-ray films in anteroposterior and lateral views can help determine the fracture type.

Treatment

Reduction (for Extension Type)

1. The operation is performed under local anesthesia. The patient sits on a stool or lies in dorsal position, and the affected

forearm is kept in neutral position. The assistant fixes with both hands the middle portion of the patient's affected forearm and the operator fixes the wrist, thumb on the dorsal aspect of the distal fracture end and the other fingers supporting the proximal fracture end from the palmar aspect. Then the operator and the assistant perform stretching traction to correct rotatory or overriding displacement. Under the traction, the operator begins to press the distal end toward the palmar aspect with thumbs and raise the proximal end toward the dorsal direction with the other fingers and then makes the affected wrist abruptly flex to the palmar side and simultaneously incline to the ulna, and the displacement toward the radius and the dorsal aspect can be reduced. While keeping the affected wrist palmarly flexing as well as ulnarly inclining with one hand, the operator can correct the remaining displacement by pressing with the thumb of the other hand the dorsal aspect of the injured radius from the proximal end toward the distal end (Fig. 47).

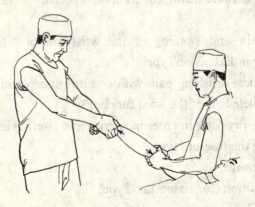

47-1   Correction of overriding and rotatory displacement under traction

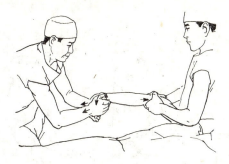

47—2　Abrupt forcible traction with simultaneous flexion of the wrist towards
the palmar side and inclination to the ulna

Fig. 47

2.　This is an alterative method. It requires the same preparations as for 1. Two assistants, one fixing the patient's affected
hand, and the other fixing the forearm, perform countertraction.
As the distal end of the fracture tends to pronate, the wrist
should be supinated slightly (about 10—15 degrees) during the
traction. The operator stands by the patient's affected side, but
slightly farther away than the assistants, supports and raises
with one hand the lower portion of the patient's affected forearm towards the radial side while pushing and pressing the affected wrist towards the ulnar direction with the other hand.
This will correct the displacement inclining to the radial aspect.
Now the operator pushes and presses the dorsal aspect of the
distal end towards the palmar aspect with both thumbs and supports and raises the palmar aspect of the proximal end with the
other fingers so as to reduce displacement inclining to the dorsal
side. Generally, it is necessary for the operator to press with
thumbs 1—2 times more the dorsum of the radius from the
proximal part to the distal part to complete the reduction

(Fig. 48).

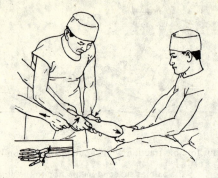

48-1　Correction of displacement inclining to the radial side

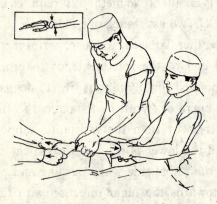

48-2　Reduction of palmar / dorsal displacement

Fig. 48　Reduction of a fracture at the distal end of the radius (ExtensionType)

It must be noted that when the traction is initiated, the distal end needs several minutes' traction in favourable direction towards the dorsal aspect of the radius until the impaction is released and, then, further traction along the vertical axis of the forearm can be done. When the traction is finished, the operator should place his hands respectively on the radial and ulnar aspects of the patient's forearm for relative compression as will reposit the distal radioulnar joint.

Immobilization

Splint Fixation   Wrap the affected forearm along with the wrist joint with cotton padding. Four splints are needed;the ones on the radial and dorsal aspects extend beyond the wrist joint and the other ones on the ulnar and palmar aspects just reach the joint. This design will inhibit the wrist joint from extending dorsally and inclining to the radius. Fasten the splints with laces. The forearm is kept in neutral position and supported with a sling (Fig. 49).

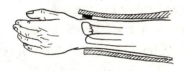

(1) The anteroposterior view

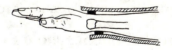

(2) The lateral view

49-1   Placement of the small compresses and splints

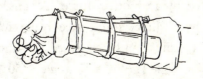

(1) The anteroposterior view

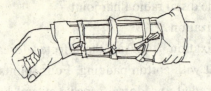

(2) The lateral view

49—2　External appearance of the fixation

Fig. 49　Fixation for a Colles' fracture

Medication　　See 1.3: Administration of Chinese Medicines on the Basis of Overall Analysis and Differentiation of Symptoms and Signs.

Exercises (for Extension Type)

Flexion—extension exercises of the fingers and flexion to the palmar side and inclination to the ulnar aspect of the wrist joint can be practised after immobilization. There is no restriction of movement of the elbow joint and shoulder joint. Flexion—extension of the wrist and rotatory movement of the forearm can be performed only after the immobiliozation is removed.

2.12　Fractures of the Scaphoid Bone

Pathogenesis

These fractures are relatively common in carpal injuries. They mostly occur in people at the age of 20—50. The injury is usually produced by an indirect force, as caused in a fall. It is rarely caused by a direct force. According to the " fracture angle", these fractures can be classified into three types: Type I (F angle $< 30°$), Type II ($30° \leqslant$ F angle $\leqslant 50°$) and Type III (F angle $> 50°$). With regard to the location of the fracture, these fractures can also be grouped in a different way:tubercle fractures, waist fractures and proximal fractures.

Essentials for Diagnosis

1. A definite history of trauma.

2. Swelling and pain in the snuffpot and impact pain in the 1st and 2nd metacarpal bones.

3. X−ray films of the affected wrist in anteroposterror and lateral views, plus a film of the hand in fist in oblique view, are helpful. If clinical signs suggest a fracture but the X−ray films present a negative result, it is necessary to restrict movement of the wrist for two weeks for another roentgenographic examination, for , by then, if there is a fracture, the bone substance will have been absorbed and the fracture line will be distinctly obvious in the films.

Treatment

Reduction

As a rule, navicular fractures do not need reduction at all as there can be but little displacement. Only really displaced fractures need bone setting. The reduction is performed as described below:(1) The patient lies in dorsal position. (2) An assistant fixes the forearm of the patient's affected limb, flexing the elbow at 90 degrees. (3) Another assistant fixes with a hand the thumb of the patient's affected hand and holds the other fingers with the other hand, performing stretching traction along the vertical axis of the patient's forearm. (This will place the patient's forearm at a slight pronated position and the wrist at a level stretching position tending to the ulnar aspect.). (4) The operator, standing on the lateral side and facing the distal extremity, presses the snuffpot with both thumbs and fixes the ulnar and palmar aspects of the affected wrist with the other fingers. (5) The 2nd assistant makes the patient's wrist mildly extend dorsally and incline to the radial side. (6) The operator presses the snuffpot toward the palmar—ulnar side. (7) The 2nd assistant makes sure that the patient's wrist is flexed palmarly toward the ulnar side slightly / moderately / intensely—dependent upon the "fracture angle".

Immobilization

Cardboard Fixation   After reduction, apply a small compress to the area of the snuffpot and cover it with a plate of cardboard. Fix the plate with adhesive tapes and override it with cotton padding. A specially prepared piece of cardboard is placed closely around the radius on the radial, dorsal and palmar aspects. On the ulnar aspect, a moulded splint is used. Bind the cardboard pieces and splint with 8—shape bandaging. This fixation will ensure a particular position of palmar—flexion and ulnar—inclination of the wrist to fit the "fracture angle" and benefit the stability of the fracture ends. Keep the forearm in neutral position and support it with a sling for 1—3 months (Fig. 50).

Medication

See 1.3:Administration of Chinese Medicines on the Basis of Overall Analysis and Differentiation of Symptoms and Signs. As the healing is generally slow, the course of oral administration of *Jiegu Dan* (11) should be correspondingly prolonged.

Exercises

There is no restriction of movement of the shoulder and elbow even at the initial stage. When the injury enters the intermediate stage, mild flexion—extension exercises of the fingers can be gradually started. Fist—making and wrist flexion—extension exercises can be practised only after the fracture has healed and the immobilization has thus been removed.

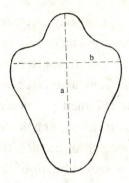

a   The median line, reaching the middle part of the forearm at the proximal end and extending to the interphalangeal joint of the thumb at the distal end

b   The largest width, allowing this part to cover the dorsum of the hand

Fig. 50   A specially designed cardboard splint

Notes:1.   "Fracture angle" refers to the angle between the fracture line and the ulnar deviation articulation at the lower end of the radius.

2.   "Degrees of palmar flexion" refers to the degrees of the flexional angle of the dorsal aspect of the wrist from the dorsal aspect of the forearm to the palmar direction, normally being 30 degrees.

3.   "Degrees of ulnar deviation" refers to the angular degrees between the 3rd metacarpal bone and ulnar deviation of the vertical axis of the forearm. Mild ulnar deviation means an angle smaller than 10 degrees, moderate ulnar deviation between 10— 15 degrees, and intense ulnar deviation about 20 degrees.

2.13 Fractures at the Base of the First Metacarpal Bone

Pathogenesis

These fractures are mostly incurred in a fall or by impaction. The injuries are clinically classified as simple fractures at the base of the metacarpal bone and fractures at the base of the metacarpal bone associated with dislocation of the carpometacarpal joint (Bonnett's fractures). The former are mostly transverse fractures with angular deformity toward the radiodorsal aspect as a result of traction to the distal end by the long flexor, short flexor and adductor of the thumb and traction to the proximal end by the long adductor of the thumb (Fig. 51), and the latter are actually avulsive fractures in which the medial triangular ossicle remains in its normal anatomical relation to the trapezium and the lateral fracture end is dorsally displaced from the trapezium joint to the lateral side with flexion—inclination to the palmar aspect due to traction of the long abductor of the thumb and contraction of the flexor of the thumb.

Essentials for Diagnosis

1. A history of trauma.

2. Local swelling and pain with angular deformity toward the radiodorsal aspect and complete loss of functions of the thumb.

3. Local tenderness with pseudo—activities and bony crepitus.

4. X—ray films in anteroposterior and lateral views can help determine the fracture type.

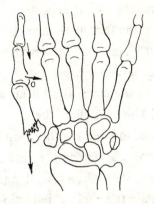

Fig. 51   A fracture at the base of the 1st metacarpal bone

(the arrows respectively showing the direction of the muscular

contraction and the direction of the displacement)

Treatment

Reduction

The patient sits on a stool. The operator fixes the patient's affected wrist with one hand, the thumb pressing at the protruding part on the dorsal aspect of the fracture area, takes the patient's injured thumb in the other hand with the involved metacarpalphylangeal joint flexing, performs countertraction and tries to abduct the head of the affected metacarpal as much as possible (but no abduction at all for the phylangeal bone). These maneuvers will reduce the ends well.

Immobilization

Abducent–splint Fixation   A splint moulded in an abducent shape at about 30degrees is prepared before hand. Apply a small compress to the protruding part and another to the palmar aspect of the metacarpal head. Before applying it to the affected part, give cotton padding to the moulded splint which should extend from the radial aspect of the forearm to the radiodorsal aspect of the first metacarpal bone, the summit of it precisely at the wrist joint. Fix the proximal end of the splint with a wide piece of adhesive tape and the distal end together with the compress on the metacarpal head with a narrow piece of adhesive plaster. This will allow the first metacarpal bone to be in an abducent position and the thumb in flexion (Fig. 52). In the case of a fracture associated with dislocation, the fixation may be unstable, and, then, thumb phalangette traction can be added so as to maintain the effect of reduction (Fig. 53).

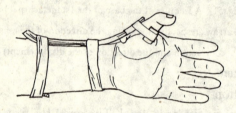

Fig. 52   Splint fixation for a fracture at the base of the 1st metacarpal bone

Medication

See 1.3:Administration of Chinese Medicines on the Basis of Overall Analysis and Differentiation of Symptoms and Signs.

Exercises

At the initial stage, flexion—extension exercises of the fingers except the thumb and functional movement of the elbow joint and shoulder joint are allowed. Flexion exercises of the thumb can be started from the intermediate stage on. The natural cure stage is the proper time for the patient to do exercises of flexion—extension and abduction—adduction of the thumb and to practise flexion—extension and rotatory movement of the carpal joint.

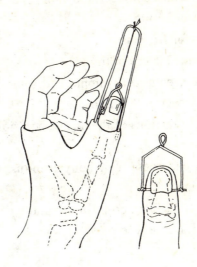

Fig. 53   Bone traction for an oblique fracture of the shaft
of the 1st metacarpal bone

2.14   Fractures of the Metacarpal Bones

Pathogenesis

These fractures are clinically common, mostly in individuals at the age of 20—50. The injury is usually produced by a transmitted force such as in a fall or when giving a punch in a boxing match. Occasionally, the fracture can also be caused by a direct force. The cervixes of the metacarpal bones, especially those of the 4th and 5th metacarpals are the most vulnerable areas to the injury. Transverse fractures are the most common. Less common than these are fractures of the metacarpal shafts. Fractures at the base parts are comparatively rare. As a result of traction by the flexor of the injured finger, the injury is often associated with dorsal angular deformity.

Essentials for Diagnosis

1. A definite history of trauma.

2. Swelling, pain, ecchymoma and a local protruding part on the dorsal aspect of the hand.

3. Loss of functions of the fingers occasionally with shorter metacarpal bones.

4. Local tenderness with bony crepitus, pseudo—activities and impact pain.

5. X—ray films in anteroposterior and lateral views can help determine the fracture type.

Treatment

Reduction

1. A Cervical Metacarpal Fracture   The patient sits on a stool. The operator fixes the patient's affected palm with one hand and the injured finger with the other hand and makes the involved metacarpalphalangeal joint flex at 90 degrees under traction. This will move the proximal articular surface of the adjacent phalangeal bone to the palmar aspect of the metacarpal head, hence leaving the lateral paraligament in tonicity, a condition beneficial to stability of the fractured metacarpal head. Then the operator can reduce the fracture by pushing the adjacent phalangeal head toward the dorsal side with a hand fixing the patient's injured finger and pressing the proximal end with the other hand (Fig. 54).

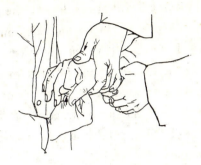

54-1　Maneuvers used in reduction of a cervix metacarpal fracture

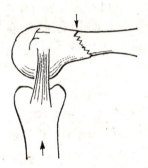

54-2　Direction of the force for the reduction

Fig. 54　Reduction of a cervix metacarpal fracture

2. A Fracture of the Metacarpal Shaft　　The operation is perdormed under local anesthesia. The patient sits on a stool. The operator fixes the patient's affected palm with one hand and the injured finger with the other hand and performs countertraction. He can then correct the angular deformity by pressing the protruding part of the dorsum of the patient's affected hand with thumbs and set right the lateral deformity by compressing the interosseous metacarpal space from both the palmar and dorsal sides with thumbs and forefingers. In the case of multiple fractures of the metacarpal bones, the routine pro-

cess includes: (1) placing a roll of bandage in the patien's affected palm so that it is kept in a functioning position and fixing the roll with adhesive plaster, and (2) reducing the ends of each fracture one after the other through manipulative maneuvers, fixing each of the distal terminals with adhesive tapes on the dorsal aspect of the fingers as a means of traction. Be sure that the verticle alignments of the fingers should all be kept directing to the navicular tubercle.

3. Fractures at the Bases of the Metacarpal Bones Fractures at this part with mild displacement do not need any reduction at all. Reduce those with severe angulation and displacement in the same way as described in 2. for fractures of the metacarpal shaft.

Immobilization

1. Cervix Metacarpal Fracutres   After reduction, a bamboo splint or a narrow piece of aluminum sheet, moulded in the shape of channel iron, is lined with cotton padding and applied to the hand on the dorsum, extending from the dorsal aspect of the palm to the dorsal aspect of the fingers, to keep the metacarpalphalangeal articulation in a position of a right angle. Fix the splint with adhesive tapes (Fig. 55).

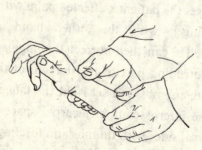

Fig. 55 Placement of the rectangular splint

2. Fractures of Shafts of the Metacarpal Bones
Wood—board Fixation   After reduction, two bone—separating compresses should be applied to the areas corresponding to the interosseous spaces on the dorsal aspect of the fractured part. Cotton padding is needed on both the dorsal aspect and the palmar aspect of the hand before two wood boards are used which are first fixed with adhesive tapes and then well bandaged (Fig. 56).

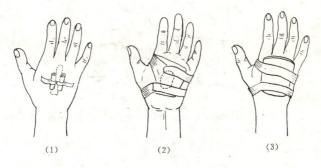

(1)   (2)   (3)

(1) Placement of the bonse—separating compresses and its fixation
   with adhesive plaster

(2) The palmar felt compress, the pad over it and their fixation
   with adhesive tapes

(3) The dorsal board splint and its fixation with adhesive tapes

Fig. 56 A blunt oblique fracture of the 3rd metacarpal bone

For an unstable fracture (in oblique or spiral form), a moulded bamboo or aluminum block should be applied to the hand on the palmar aspect, the moulded arch surface in firm and close contact with the skin to keep the fingers in a functioning position. Fix the blocks with adhesive tapes and cover the fixation with bandaging. Affix another piece of plaster tape alignmentally to the dorsal aspect of the injured finger, the distal end of the tape extending around the distal end of the palmar block where it is stuck firmly. On the dorsal aspect of the fracture area, bone separating compresses should be used in the interosseous spaces to set the injured bone apart from the adjacent bones. A cotton pad is needed to protect the compresses and the skin. Cover the pad with a piece of cardboard before bandaging (Fig. 57).

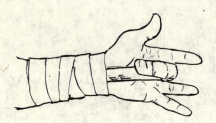

57-1   Adhesive-tape traction for the injured finger

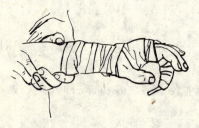

57-2   Bandaging of the fixation (the lateral view)

Fig. 57   Fixation for a fracture of the metacarpal shaft with hook-shaped

aluminum splint plus adhesivetape traction

3. Fractures at the Bases of the Metacarpal Bones   The fixation is the same as for fractures of shafts of the metacarpal bones.

Medication

See 1.3: Administration of Chinese Medicines on the Basis of Overall Analysis and Differentiation of Symptoms and Signs.

Exercises

At the initial stage, flexion—extension exercises of the affected finger and the wrist must not be attempted. 3—4 weeks later when the immobilization is discarded, gradual functional exercises of the fingers and the wrist can be actively practised, but passive pulling or stretching by force is not allowed, or stiff interphalangeal articulation may be the result.

2.15   Fractures of the Phalanges

Pathogenesis

Fractures of the phalanges are comparatively common. If the fracture is produced by a direct force, it is usually a transverse or comminuted fracture. The fracture may also be oblique or spiral when it is produced by a transmitted force as a result of impact against the distal extremity. Based on the location of the injury, these fractures can be sorted as fractures of the proximal phalanx, fractures of the middle phalanx and fractures of the distal phalanx.

Essentials for Diagnosis

1. A definite history of trauma.

2. Swelling and pain of the injured finger, with possible lateral process deformity and restricted flexion—extension of the affected finger in the case of a displaced fracture.

3. Local crush pain with pseudo—activities, bony crepitus and impact anguish.

4. X—ray films in anteroposterior and lateral views will help determine the fracture type. Fractures of the proximal phalangeal shaft may present angulation to the palmar aspect due to traction by the interosseous and lumbrical muscles. Frac-

tures of the phalangeal cervix may have dorsal rotation of the distal end at 90 degrees. In fractures of the middle phalanx, if the injury happens to be on the proximal side of the shallow flexor terminal, there will be dorsal angulation, and if the injury happens to be on distal side, there will be palmar angulation. In avulsion fractures at the dorsal base of the distal phalanx, a "hammer finger" deformity may be observed (Fig. 58).

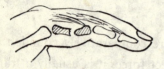

58–1 Palmar angulation of the
fragment in a fracture of
the proximal phalanx

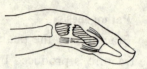

58–2 Dorsal angulation of the
fragment in a fracture of
the proximal segment of
the middle phalanx

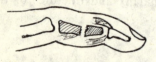

58–3 Palmar angulation of the
fragment in a fracture of
the mid–segment of
the middle phaianx

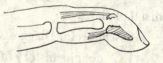

58–4 "Hammer finger"
deformity in an avulsion
fracture (from the
dorsal–base) of the
distal phalanx

Fig. 58 Displacement of ends in fractures at different parts of the finger

Treatment

Reduction

As the fingers have to perform exquisite, precise and dexterous functions, fractures of the fingers must be accurately reduced. Any remaining deformity will impair their conture and functions.

1. Fractures of the Proximal Phalanx   To reduce a fracture of the proximal phalangeal shaft, the operation is performed under phalangeal block anesthesia. The patient sits on a stool. The operator (1) fixes the proximal end with the left thumb and holds the distal end with three or all the other fingers of the right hand, performing countertraction; (2) fixes the fracture site by pinching the palmar and dorsal aspects with the left thumb and forefinger, making the proximal phalanx flex, and simultaneously pushes with the thumb the fracture ends toward the dorsal aspect. These maneuvers will correct the palmar angulation. If the fracture is complicated with lateral displacement, the operator needs, in addition, to lay his right thumb and forefinger on either side of the fractured bone and presses the ends from both sides so as to set right the displacement. However, in reducing a cervix fracture of the proximal phalanx, the proper manipulative maneuvers should be contra—angular flexing. The distal end should be tracted toward the dorsal aspect. The operator fixes both the dorsal and palmar aspects of both the distal and proximal ends by pinching them with the thumb and forefinger of each hand respectively and then quickly flexes the patient's affected finger while pushing the proximal end from the palmar aspect toward the dorsal aspect. This will produce good reduction (Fig. 59).

2. Fractures of the Middle Phalanx   The maneuvers for reduction of fractures of the middle phalanx are similar to those for fractures of the proximal phalangeal shaft though the operator has to take into account the location of the fracture and the

angulatory displacement that decides the specific maneuvers to be employed.

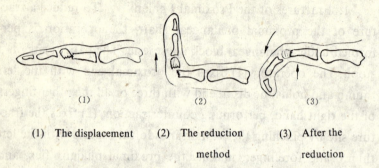

(1) The displacement   (2) The reduction   (3) After the

method   reduction

Fig. 59 A cervix fracture of the phalanx

3. Fractures of the Distal Phalanx   Fractures of the distal phalanx with little displacement hardly need any reduction. For a fracture with crack or lateral displacement, the operator can pinch the palmar and dorsal (or medial and lateral)aspects with the thumb and forefinger of a hand to correct it. In case the fracture occurs at the base, the operator should fix the proximal and middle phalanges of the injured finger with one hand, making the proximal interphalangeal articulation flex at 90 degrees, and pinch the distal phalanx with the thumb and forefinger of the other hand, making the distal interphalangeal joint overstretch. This will reduce the avulsed ends.

Immobilization

1. Fractures of the Proximal and Middle Phalanges

(1) Non-superarticular Fixation   Dependent upon the direction of the angulatory displacement, small compresses can be applied to either the palmar and dorsal aspects or the medial and lateral aspects of the fracture site and fixed with adhesive

tapes. Cover and wrap the compresses with a cotton pad, place two arch—shaped cardboard pieces (or four small splints) around the finger, not extending beyond the joint, and firmly fix them with adhesive tapes (Fig. 60).

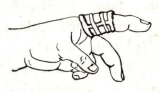

Fig. 60   Non—superarticular fixation with cardboard splints

(2) Functional—position Fixation   A piece of aluminus or bamboo sheet, short and moulded to fit the functional position of the injured finger, is needed for the fixation. According to the direction of the angulatory displacement, necessary compresses are applied to proper parts. Cover the compresses with cotton pads and apply two short small splints on either the medial and lateral sides. Arrange the aluminus or bamboo sheet appropriately and fix it with adhesive tapes before bandaging the fixation . For an unstable fracture, apart from the external fixation, phalangeal traction is necessary to maintain stability of the fracture ends(Fig. 61).

2. Fractures of the Distal Phalanx

(1) Fractures with Crack or Displacement   After reduction, the fixation is done simply with two small splints or cardboard pieces and some adhesive tapes.

(2) Fractures at the Base   A moulded aluminus or bamboo splint is prepared beforehand. Apply this splint to the fracture site and firmly fix it with adhesive tapes. Be sure that the fixation is done with the proximal interphalangeal joint flexing

at 90 degrees and the distal interphalangeal joint at an over—stretching position (Fig. 62). Three weeks later, replace the splint with a straight one which has a proximal end not exceeding the proximal interphalangeal joint and a distal end just up to the finger tip. A flight—shaped cotton compress is placed at the fore—half of the finger on the palmar side and overridden by the splint. Fix the compress and the splint with adhesive tapes, keeping the distal phalanx at a dorsal—extension position. During the period of immobilization, flexion—extension movement of the distal phalanx is not restricted. The fixation should be removed in three weeks.

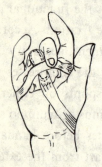

Fig. 61 Fixation for a fracture of the   Fig. 62 Fixation for a dorsal avulsion
proximal phalanx after   fracture at the distal phalanx
reduction

Medication

See 1.3: Administration of Chinese Medicines on the Basis of Overall Anlysis and Differentiation of Symptoms and Signs.

Exercises

At the initial stage, movement of the fingers except the injured one is not restricted. Unless for "hammer finger", fixation with the injured finger extending straight can at most last 2—3 weeks before it is changed to fixation with the injured finger at a functional position. When immobilization is removed, active exercises of functional flexion—extension of the affected finger are recommended, but forcible pulling or flexing by maneuvers must be avoided in case of avulsion of the adhesive articular sac which may worsen adhesive contracture of the interphalangeal joint.

2.16   Fractures of the Ribs

Pathogenesis

Rib fractures occur mostly in adults, especially in elderly people. The cause of the injury may be a direct force, an indirect force, a combined force or contracting forces of the muscles. The fractures are closed injuries in most instances. The injury may occur at one or more places in one or more ribs. In the latter case, there will be a number of ribs fractured, forming a "floating wall" of the thoracic cavity which may lead to paradoxical respiratory problems, a serious condition involving both the respiratory and circulatory systems. Open pneumothorax is clinically seen at times, mostly in injuries by sharp instruments or bullets, and should arouse careful attention of the clinicians as it is actually a severe trauma.

Essentials for Diagnosis

1. Local pain and swelling after trauma, sometimes plus presence of ecchymosis. The pain may be aggravated by deep breathing, coughing, sneezing or by turning the upper body.

2. Local tenderness, sometimes plus bony crepitus. The patient may feel suffering severe pains when the doctor compresses his / her thorax anteroposteriorly or bilaterally with hands or

presses the fracture site with one hand, or when the patient coughs as is told to by the doctor.

3. In cases with severe injuries, careful attention must be paid to the patient's blood pressure and to examination of the heart so as to ascertain how the internal organs have been damaged. The doctor must also be highly cautious not to neglect the possibility of subcutaneous emphysema or paradoxical breathing.

4. X—ray films of the thorax may help determine the fracture type and observe complications in the thoracic cavity.

Treatment

Reduction

Displaced fractures of the ribs require proper reduction. The patient sits on a stool. An assistant presses with hands the patient's upper abdomen and the lumbar region from the anterior and posterior aspects. The operator pushes the fracture ends with both hands, one hand on the fracture site and the other on the opposite aspect of the thorax, and tells the patient first to do deep breathing so as to expand the thoracic circumsference as much as possible and then to cough energetically while the assistant forcibly presses the patient's upper abdomen, and the fracture will be well reduced. In the case of a depressed fracture, the operator should lay his hands on either side of the fracture site for performance of bilateral compression so as to bring about reduction of the ends (Fig. 63).

Immobilization

1. Cardboard—bandage Fixation   A sheet of cardboard of proper size lined with cotton padding is applied to the fracture site and fixed with adhesive tapes. Encircle the thorax a few

rounds with a bandage so as to fix the fracture site along with the upper and lower neighbouring ribs (Fig. 64).

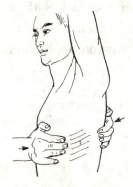

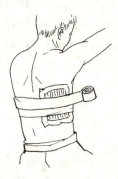

Fig. 63   Reduction of a depressed
fracture of a rib by
anteroposterior compression

Fig. 64   Cardboard—bandage
fixation for a rib fracture

2. Adhesive—plaster Fixation   This fixation is applicable to fractures of the 5th—9th ribs. 5—7 adhesive tapes, 5 cm in width and longer by 10 cm than half of the patient's thoracic circumsference, are prepared beforehand. The patient sits on a stool with both arms raising up and the hands crossing each other over the head. When the patient nearly completes a deep exhalation, that is, when the thoracic circumference is the smallest, the operator begins the fixation. Starting from the dorsal aspect of the fracture site at a point between the dorsal median line (on the median line of the unaffected scapula), the firmly stuck adhesive tape extends around the fracture site across the front median line by 5 cm (beyond the median line of the clavicle). Then apply the other tapes to the thorax the same way, one overriding another by 1 / 3—1 / 2 width, on both the upward and downward directions until the fracture site as well as the

upper and lower neighbouring ribs are all well fixed (Fig. 65). However, the doctor must be highly cautious not to prescribe immobilization of the thorax for aged cases or cases with serious injuries in case pulmonary dysfunction or peumonia occurs. Instead, *Shenjin Gao* (31) can be given for external application.

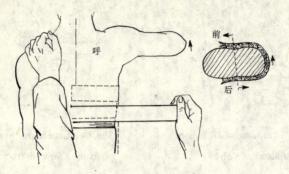

Fig. 65   Adhesive–plaster fixation for a rib fracture

Medication

At the initial stage, the principle for prescription is to activate circulation of the blood to remove blood stasis, promote the flow of *Qi* to relieve chest stiffness and pain. The usual recipe is modified *Fuyuan Huoxue Tang* (1) . To the recipe the following drugs can be added, Radix Platycodi, Semen pruni Armeniacae, Bulbus Fritillariae Thunbergii, Fructus Trichosanthis and Fructus Perillae. If the patient has hemoptysis, add Radix Notoginseng, Rhizoma Bletillae, Herba Agrimoniae pilosa and Nodus Nelumbinis Rhizomatis. The best prescription for patients at the intermediate stage is *Jiegu Dan* (11). At the natural cure stage when the fracture has healed and immobilization is removed, *Shenjin Gao* (31) can be externally applied to the injured part and *Shenjin Pian* (50) tablets orally administered.

Exercises

Patients with simple fractures of the rib(s) can walk on foot directly after immobilization is given, but movement of the upper limbs should be restricted to a resonable extent in case the fixation falls. In severe cases, the medical order must be given that the patient has to take bed rest until the condition becomes stable and allows him / her to walk on foot.

2.17 Fractures and Dislocations of the Cervical Spine

Pathogenesis

The injury is primarily produced by an indirect force such as a heavy blow on the top of the head, by impaction or collision, or in a fall from a height. The disease can be calssified into Flexion Type and Extension Type with regard to the direction of the force and the posture of the neck at the time when the injury occurs. The part that is frequently injured are atlas and axis. Severe injuries may cause spinal compression and nerve compression or even spinal fragmentation that will result in high paraplegia, a refractory sequela with unfavourable prognosis.

Essentials for Diagnosis

1. A typical history of trauma.

2. Neck pain that, frequently, forces the patient to support the head with both hands.

3. A stiff neck with restricted functions of flexion—extension and rotatory movement.

4. Symptoms of stimulated spinal cord in some cases.

5. X—ray films in anteroposterior and lateral views (or mouth—open film in anteroposterior view) can help determine

the position and severity of the injury.

Treatment

Reduction and Immobilization

1. Fractures of the Atlas　Un—displaced or mildly displaced fractures without evident symptoms of spinal / nerve compression can be managed with cervical traction in a cervical traction frame or with halo immobilization for 3—4 months. If the fracture is evidently displaced, skull traction can be used to reduce it.

2. Dislocation of the Atlas　Subluxation without neurological symptoms requires manipulative reduction:

(1) Uni—lateral Subluxation of the Atlas　It is necessary to apply manipulative massage to the neck to relax the stiff muscles before reduction. The patient lies in prone position. An assistant supports the lower side of the patient's occipital bone with the right hand and raises the jaw from beneath with the left hand. Another assistant fixes the patient's shoulders with both hands and pulls them downward, performing countertraction in cooperation with the first assistant. The operator stands on the patient's affected side, lays thumbs respectively on the axis spinous process and the posterior palatine arch of the patient. The first assistant then starts to set right gradually the patient's neck from the inclination to the normal position and makes it over—extend dorsally. The operator simultaneously depresses forward the axis spinous process and the posterior palatine arch with both thumbs and the reduction will be achieved with a characteristic sound. Now the first assistant can mildly brings the patient's neck back to the normal position, ensuring the lower jaw to be just on the median line. The reduction must be followed by post—operative cervical traction with a cervical trac-

tion frame or with a jaw—occiput strape (Fig. 66).

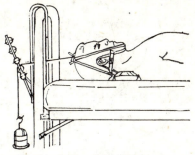

Fig. 66   Jaw—occiput strap traction

(2)   Bilateral Subluxation of the Atlas   The preparations are all the same as described above in (1). As bilateral dislocation will cause anteverted deformity of the neck, the reduction must begin with countertraction along the vertical axis of
the body trunk. The operator stands on the Right side of the patient and places thumbs respectively on the patient's axis spinous
process and the posterior palatine arch. The first assistant makes
the patient's head passively turn dual—directionally and then
gradually overextend dorsally. Now the operator depresses
steadily with both thumbs the patient's axis spinous process and
the posterior palatine arch and the reduction will be achieved
with a characteristic sound (Fig. 67).

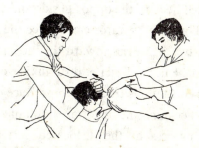

67—1   Countertraction by the assistants

· *139* ·

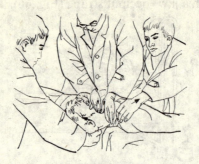

67-2   Pressing the dorsally protruding spinous process with the

patient's neck extending posteriorly

Fig. 67   Reduction of bilateral subluxation of the atlas

(3)   Subluxation or Temporary Dislocation of the Cervical Vertebral Joint   The injury is primarily produced by a force at a time when the neck is in flexion or by hyperflexion of the neck as during sudden halt of a car. The preparations for the reduction are all the same as previously described in (1). For uni-lateral cervical subluxation that diverts the spinous process away from the median line, the operator lays a thumb on the diverted spinous process and the other thumb on the spinous process of the next dislocated vertebrae. The first assistant tries, under continuous traction, to produce flexion and rotation of the patient's deviated neck to the opposite side and make it over-extend dorsally. Then the operator can reduce the spinous process by pressing the two processes toward the median line with both thumbs. In management of bilateral subluxation, the first assistant tries, under continuous traction, to produce dorsal extension of the patient's neck and the operator simultaneously presses the lower spinous process of the dislocated vertebrae with both thumbs. This will bring about good reduction.

(4) Compression Fractures of the Cervical Vertebral Body   Manipulative reduction is applicable for cases without symptoms of spinal nerve compression. The patient lies in dorsal position with the head and neck extending beyond the bed. An assistant fixes the patient's shoulders. The operator supports the occiput of the patient with one hand and fixes the lower jaw with the other hand. They then perform countertraction and gradually make the patient's neck extend dorsally and the fragments will be reduced. The operation must be followed by immobilization through traction with a cervical traction frame.

(5) Flexion Dislocation of the Cervical Joints   This disorder mostly occurs in the joints between C4 and C5 or between C5 and C6. It may be an instantaneous dislocation or an interlace of minor articular processes. However, either case will be complicated with severe injury of the spinal cord or nerve root. Patients with instantaneous dislocation can be managed with traction through a neutral–position occiput–jaw strape or through a cervical traction frame as will prevent recurrence of dislocation. Patients with interlaced minor articular processes should be carefully tended. The management requires to reduce the interlaced minor processes through traction so as to release the nerves from compression. Reduction by simple hyperextension will aggravate the injuries to the spinal nerves and should therefore be discarded. It is recommended first to apply skull traction with a weight of about 10 kg in favourable direction and, after reduction with a weight of 2—3 kg, in neutral position. The traction can be kept for 4—6 weeks.

Medication

See 1.3: Administration of Chinese Medicines on the Basis

of Overall Analysis and Differentiation of Symptoms and Signs.

Exercises

At the initial stage, the patient must lie dorsally on a wooden board bed. The limbs can move freely, but the head and neck are strictly restricted in movement. After the traction or immobilization is removed, the patient can walk on foot and perform flexion—extension and rotatory exercises of the head and neck.

2.18 Compression Fractures of the Thoracolumbar Vertebrae

Pathogenesis

These fractures are common in spinal injuries. They are mostly produced in a fall from a height or through direct hit by a heavy object when the patient happens to be in a bending posture. Most of the victims are adults at the age of 20—50. Elderly people often have osteoporosis and this makes them vulnerable to these fractures even in a mild trauma as caused in a fall. Thoracolumbar fractures usually occur in T11—T12 or L1—L2, with one or, occasionally, two vertebral bodies impaired. Considering the force causing the fracture, posture of the patient at the time of the injury, age and constitution of the victim, we can classify these fractures as Flexion Type and Extension Type, Stable Type and Unstable Type, or Type with Spinal neurological impairment and Type without Spinal Neurological Impairment.

Essentials for Diagnosis

1. A history of trauma, such as injuries caused in a fall or

through direct hit by a heavy object.

2. Pain and slight swelling in the lumbodorsal region, with deformity of dorsal protrusion and widened space between the spinous processes in the case of Flexion Type.

3. Local tenderness and percussion pain which will be aggravated during coughing or sneezing. The patient is unable to stand, nor to sit upright.

4. In cases with spinal neurological impairment, there will be changes below the affected vertebae in sensation, muscular tension, myokinesis, physiological and pathological reflexion. Normal urination and defecation will also be changed.

5. Enteroparalysis may occur due to rectroperitoneal hemotoma with symptoms of stagnancy of *Qi* and blood stasis of the stomach and intestines such as abdominal pain, nausea, vomiting and difficulty in urination and defecation.

6. X−ray examination helps determine the fracture type and its nature.

Treatment

Reduction and Immobilization

1. Stable Thoracolumbar Fractures

(1) Method of Functional Exercises   This method is safe, simple and effective. The patient lies dorsally on a board bed with the fractured part supported by a soft cushion. When the pain has certainly subsided, the patient can initiate exercises of the lumbodorsal muscles. Step 1, Five Fulcra Exercise:The patient fisrt flexes the elbows and raises the shoulders, and, then, flexes the knees and extends the coxae, that is, supports the body with the elbows, feet and head, lifting the lumbar region and buttocks so as to make hyperextension of the spine. Step 2,

Three Fulcra Exercise:This is similar to Step1 except that the elbows are no longer used as two fulcra. Instead, the forearms cross each other in front of the chest. Step 3, Four Fulcra Exercise:The patient supports the body with the hands and feet, lifting the body trunk to form a bridge—like arch. Step 4, " Flying—swallow" —like Posture Exercise:The patient lies in prone position, raises the head and throws out the chest, extends the shoulders dorsally with the upper limbs stretching upward, bringing both the head and chest off the bed, and, then, extends the knees straight, lifting the lower limbs up from the bed. The posture now looks like a flying swallow. These exercises should be practised by following the steps one by one in the order they are given. Generally, the patient can stop bed rest and perform dorsal extension exercises of the lumbodorsal muscles in 4 weeks (Fig. 68).

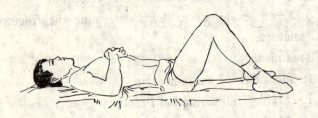

68—1   The patient lying dorsally on a board bed

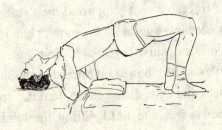

68—2   5—fulcra exercise

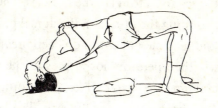

68-3   3-fulcra exercise

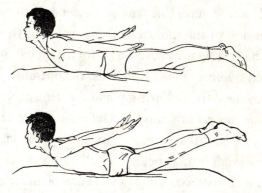

68-4, 5   "Flying-swallow-like" posture exercise

Fig. 68   Functional exercises for reduction of a compressed fracture

of the thoracolumbar vertebra

(2) Method of Manipulative Reduction   This method is applicable for adults at the age of 20— 50 and for manual labourers.

① Reduction with the Patient Lying in Prone Position
The patient lies in prone position and is given some analgesic medicine. Two assistants perform coutertraction, one standing near the patient's head and fixing with hands the patient's subaxillary parts, the other standing near the patient's feet and fixing the patient's ankles. The operator stands besides the patient and begins the reduction with massaging the patient's

lumbar soft tissues so as to relax the muscles. Then, he lays both palms, one overriding the other, on the dorsal protruding part of the fracture and tells the patient to do deep breathing. When the patient inhales, the operator slowly presses the protrusion. Repeat this several times so as to correct the deformity.

② Ankles—suspending Traction   The patient lies in pronation on a bed. Protect the patient's ankles with cotton pads and slowly have the ankles suspended so as to make hyperextension of the thoracolumbar portion of the body. The patient's body weight now acts as a force that can separate the compressed fracture ends. Meanwhile, the operator presses with both hands the dorsal protrusion and the deformity will be corrected. The operation must be followed by external splint fixation of the spine or by fixation with an I—shaped lumbodorsal supporting apparatus.

2. Fracture—dislocation of the Thoracolumbar Spine   It is difficult to reduce the injury simply by manipulative maneuvers. To release articular interlace simply by passive hyperextension of the spine will prove an attempt too ambitious to be realistic. Moreover, it may even result in epiphysiolysis of the vertebral body, causing impairment of the spinal nerves. So the reduction must be performed carefully. The patient lies in prone position. Forcible stretching traction is initially made and subsequently followed by pressing so as to correct the deformity of dorsal protrusion. Be cautious not to exercise violent force though the lumbar portion must be overextended for reduction of the dislocation. A post—operative bed rest must be prescribed as medical order for the patient, who should lie dorsally in a posterior extension position.

Medication

At the initial stage, modified *Shunqi Huoxue Tang* (6) can be prescribed for cases with complication of stagnacy of *Qi* of the stomach and intestines, and modified *Dacheng Tang* (7) for cases with complication of stagancy of *Qi* and blood stasis (or Folium Cassiae as a substitution for tea in daily drink). At the intermediate stage, the beneficial prescription is *Jiegu Dan* (11). *Shenjin Pian* (50) is constructive in rehabilitation at the natural cure stage. In addition, for patients enfeebled due to delayed disease or injury, oral administration of *Zhuangyao Jianshen Tang* (51) plus external application of *Shenjin Gao* (31) or *Refu Ling* is necessary.

Exercises

At the intial stage, the proper medical order is to advise the patient to take bed rest. When turning over, the patient has to keep a hyperextensive position of the thoracolumbar portion of the body. Exercises of posterior extension of the lumbardorsal muscles in bed, a few times a day, are recommended at the intermediate stage. One month after the fracture, the patient is allowed to terminate bed rest and do exercises of dorsal extension of the waist, but anterior bending must not be attempted. It is two months later that lumbar flexion—extension exercises can be gradually initiated.

2.19   Fractures of the Femoral Neck

Pathogenesis

This injury is a most common affliction to the aged. Elderly people often have osteoporosis, which makes them vulnerable to fractures even in a mild trauma. Fractures of the femoral neck are not frequently seen in people younger than 50, but if this injury should occur in them, the force causing the fracture would be more powerful. These fractures can be classified as Adduction Type and Abduction Type with reference to the mechanisms, Intracapsular Type and Extracapsular Type with reference to the location, and Transverse Type and Oblique Type with reference to the fracture line. They can also be divided into Stable Type and Unstable Type. As blood circulation in the femoral neck is poor, fractures at this area, especially intracapsular fractures, have a high proportion of nonunion.

Essentials for Diagnosis

1. A history of trauma, in the elderly, an injury caused in a fall, in people younger than 50, an injury caused in a fall from a height or in a vehicular accident.

2. Pain in the affected hip without distinct swelling. In most instances, the patient will refuse to stand or to walk. Occasionally, the patient will complain about pains in the anterior medial aspect of the knee joint.

3. Slight genuflex, hip—flexion and extorsion deformity of the affected limb. In cases with displaced fractures, the affected lower limb will appear shorter by 1—2 cm than the normal length.

4. Tenderness at the inguinal midpoint, and impact pain at the greater tuberosity or at the heel with restricted movement of the affected hip.

5. Lower value in osseosonometry than the normal (in a test with the ossiphone at the pubic symphysis during percussion of the medial malleolus).

6. X—ray films of the affectd hip in anteroposterior and lateral views can help determine the fracture type.

Treatment

Reduction

The patient lies in dorsal position and pre–operative injection of 10 ml of 0. 5% procaine into the affected articular capsule is necessary. An assistant pulls the patient's axillae with both hands and another assistant presses the anterosuperior spine of the hips with hands. The operator stands on the patient's affected side, fixes the ankle of the homolateral limb with one hand and supports the limb by the popliteal fossa with the elbow of the other hand, making the affected hip flex half way and the knee joint flex at 90 degrees. Then the operator can begin the actual reduction: (1) Elevate the fossa while pressing down the ankle with simultaneous mild rocking. (2) Turn the affected limb medially and stretch it straight, placing it in an abducent position of 30 degrees. If measuremant of the lower extremities shows a result of equal length, it suggests that the reduction has been achieved. Then the second assistant releases the fixation of the anterosuperior iliac spine and changes to fixing the opposite side of the pelvic and the operator begins to beat the greater tuberosity in the anatomical direction of the femoral neck with a fist or a heel to make the ends inlay each other (Fig. 69).

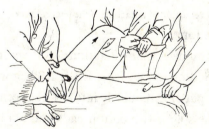

69–1   Pull traction of the hip joint at semi–flexion position

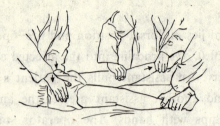

69-2　Turning inwardly, stretching straight and abducting the affected leg

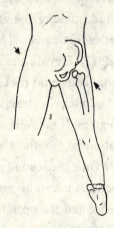

69-3　Percussion maneuver in reduction of a fracture of

the femoral neck: the direction of the force exerted

Fig. 69　Closed reduction of a fracture of the femoral neck (Adduction Type).

Immobilization

1. Long Moulded—splint Fixation　Prepare a splint with a length correspoding to that from R6 or R7 below the armpit to the heel of the patient, mould it into an abducent shape of 30 degrees. Line the splint with cotton pads and apply it to the lateral aspect of the affected hip, the padded surface inward, and make sure that the convexity of the splint rightly faces the great-

er tuberosity. Bandage the splint, keeping the affected limb in intorsion and abduction by 30 degrees (Fig. 70). After the operation, the patient must lie in a specially designed "leaking bed" with a pneumatic ring under the buttocks so that there is no need at all for the patient to move the clunis even during urination or defecation.

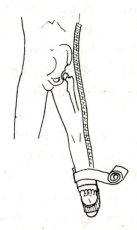

Fig. 70 Superarticular splint fixation for a fracture of the femoral neck

2. Internal Fixation with Osseous Pins   After reduction, the patient is given local anesthesia and routine pre–operative sterilization. A thick osseous pin is driven into the femur from the area 2 cm below the greater tuberosity towards the center of the femoral head (1 cm laterally below the central point in the crossing course of the femoral artery and the inguineal ligament) up to a depth of 8 cm or so, and two more pins into the femur, too, from the same place, but crossing each other with an upward or downward deviation of 10— 20 degrees. When the X–ray films in anteroposterior and lateral views show a satisfactory result of the fixation, cover the pin heads with disinfected

gauze. The patient should be given a T—shaped shoe for the affected foot with the whole limb at a neutral position in abduction of 30 degrees.

Medication

As the victims are mostly elderly people, or they are in most instances seriously injured if they happen to be under the age of being old, grave systemic responses are common. Management of this fracture at the initial stage in TCM includes administration of Chinese medicines to recuperate the body systematically. Modified *Dacheng Tang* (7) should be prescibrd for patients with stagnacy of *Qi* in the stomach and intestines and symptoms of constipation, modified *Suzhi Jiangqi Tang* (52) for those with obstruction of lung—*Qi* and the symptoms of coughing and gasping, and modified *Fuyuan Huoxue Tang* (1) for victims with severe pain and distention of the hip. At the intermediate stage, oral administration of *Jiegu Dan* (11) is routine. When the fracture has healed, further prescription of *Shenjin Pian* (50) for oral use and No. 2 Washing Recipe for external fumigation is necessary.

Exercises

After the reduction, though flexion—extension of the toes and the ankle joint and relaxation—contraction of the femoral quadriceps muscle can be performed, movement of the affected hip should be restricted. The patient must not turn over at will, nor sit with legs crossing each other. When the fracture has healed, the patient can begin flexion—extension exercises of the hips and the knee joints without any weight—bearing, but adduction or abduction of the affected coxa must be avoided. Later, he / she can gradually learn to practise crutch—walk on the ground, first with a pair of crutches, then, with a single one, and finally, with none at all or even with some weight–bearing. If signs of necrosis of the femoral head are found in a follow–up examination, the time for the patient to begin walking with weight bearing must be deferred.

2.20   Fractures of the Femoral Shaft

Pathogenesis

Fractures of the femoral shaft are common in orthopedic practice. They are mainly produced by a strong force, with remarkable displacement and severe soft tissue injuries. The force causing the fracture is mostly a dircet force and the fracture thus produced may be transverse, oblique or comminuted. Indirect forces can also produce fractures of the hemoral shaft and the fractures will be oblique or spiral in most instances, or, greenstick fractures in children. The part of the shaft that is injured may be the distal, the middle or the proximal segment, but the middle part is the most frequently afflicted. A fracture of the distal part usually presents a forward, lateral and rotatory displacement of the proximal end and a dorsal, medial and upward displacement of the distal end. A fracture of the middle segment mostly presents a medial and upward displacement of the distal end and a forward, lateral and angular deformity of the fracture ends. A fracture of the proximal segmant will present a dorsally oblique displacement or a dorsal angulation of the distal end. The popliteal arteries and veins, as well as the tibial nerve, may be pressed or even stabbed by the end in severe cases.

Essentials for Diagnosis

1. A definite history of trauma.

2. Swelling and pain of the affected limb associated with a shortening, angular or rotatory deformity.

3. Local crushing pain and impact pain at the heel with bony crepitus and pseudoactivities.

4. Gross loss of blood due to internal hemorrhage as a result of severe injury. If the blood loss amounts to 1 000 ml or more, shock may follow.

5. As fractures with gross displacement may cause injuries to the sciatic nerve, the femoral artey and vein, the condition of the foot dorsal artery, tibial artery and mobility of the toes must be carefully evaluated.

6. X—ray films of the affected thigh in anterioposterior and lateral views can help determine the fracture type and location of the injury. The fracture may quite probably be complicated with dislocation of the homolateral hip joint, so careful examination of the hip joint is of great importance.

Treatment

In management of fractures of the hemoral shaft , therapies are dependent on the age of the patient and the type of the fracture.

Reduction and Immobilization

1. Manipulative Reduction with Suspension Skin Traction of the Lower Extremities   This method is applicable for children under 5 years old with displaced unstable fractures. The operation is performed under local anesthesia. The child lies dorsally. The assistant fixes the child's pelvic with both hands pressing firmly on the anterior superior iliac spine. The operator fixes with one hand the knee of the child's affected limb, per-

forming stretching countertraction so as to correct overriding displacement, and properly compresses the fracture ends with the thumb and the other fingers of the other hand so as to correct the lateral displacement (Fig. 71). The child should be given post—operative splint fixation with suspension skin traction of the lower limbs (Fig. 72) or splint fixation with a long external wood stabilizer (Fig. 73) for 3 weeks.

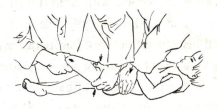

Fig. 71   Reduction of an infantile fracture of the femoral shaft

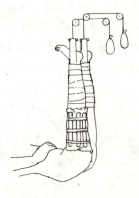

Fig. 72   Local splint fixation of the affected limb plus skin

suspension traction of both of the lower limbs

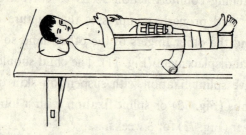

Fig. 73　Simple fixation with splints and a long external stabilizer

2. **Manipulative Reduction with Skin Traction and Local Splint Fixation**　This method is applicable for patients of 6—15 years old with displaced fractures. Preoperative preparations are all the same as in 1. but one more assistant is needed. In the operation, the new assistant fixes with hands the ankle and the part directly below the knee of the patient's affected limb and performs countertraction with the affected hip joint at a semiflexional position so as to correct overriding displacement. The operator, then, pushes and presses with both hands the displaced end to the opposite direction while propping the other side to set right lateral displacement (Fig. 74). The patient should be given postoperative splint fixation with level skin traction (Fig. 75) or flexed—knee skin traction (Fig. 76) for 4—6 weeks.

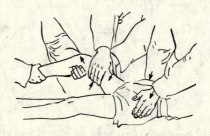

Fig. 74　Reduction of a fracture of the femoral shaft in a child

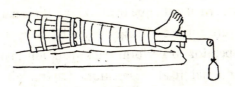

Fig. 75 Level skin traction of the affected limb

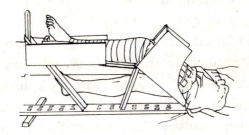

Fig. 76 Flexed—knee skin traction

3. Manipulative Reduction with Skeleton Traction and Local Splint Fixation   This method is applicable for adults with displaced fractures. The operation is performed under local anesthesia or general anesthesia. The patient lies dorsally with the affected hip joint flexing by 30—60 degrees and abducting by 20 —40 degrees and the knee joint flexing by 70—80 degrees. An assistant stretches a cloth strap round the patient's perineum with both terminals coming upward and extending till above the shoulder of the unaffected side where they are firmly fixed in hand by the assistant. Another assistant fixes the patient's pelvic with both hands pressing the anterior superior iliac spine. A third assistant now performs stretching countertraction by fixing the lower part of the knee joint of the affected limb with both hands so as to correct overriding displacement. In case this fails

to work, the operator can perform contra—angular flexing maneuver to set it right. Oblique or spiral fractures may occasionally have fracture surfaces facing each other's opposite. This requires the operator to perform back—rotation maneuver to restore their normal relative position. Lateral displacement of transverse fractures or of short oblique fractures can be reduced through appropriate maneuvers with palms or fingers by the operator. Some patients are stout and strong with powerful muscles, and the operator has to lay his forearms on either (the medial and lateral / the anterior and posterior) aspects of the fracture site and presses from both sides to reduce the ends. In reducing fractures of the proximal part of the shaft, the affected hip joint should be flexed in a position of a larger abducent angle with slight extorsion. The assistant fixes the proximal end and pushes medially and posteriorly while the operator fixes the distal end and raises it towards the anterior and lateral direction. Reduction of fractures of the middle 3rd requires a slightly flexed coxa joint in mild abduction and extorsion. The operator first pushes the fracture ends to the medial side with one hand and then compresses from both sides (the anterior and posterior / the medial and lateral) of the fracture site. In setting fractures of the distal 3rd of the hemoral shaft, the knee joint should be flexed as much as possible. The operator fixes the popliteal part with both hands and takes it as the bearing point and then pulls or raises the distal fracture end toward the anterior direction (Fig. 77). After reduction, according to need of the condition of the angular displacement, apply compresses to proper places and immobilize the fracture site with splint fixation. The affected limb should be rested on a traction frame and skeletal traction is provided (Fig. 78).

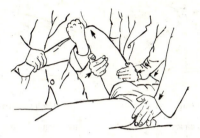

77−1   Reduction of a fracture at the proximal 3rd of the femur

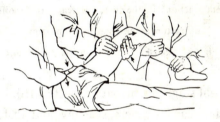

77−2   Reduction of a fracture at the distal 3rd of the femur

Fig. 77   Closed reduction of fractures of the femoral shaft in adults

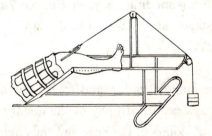

78−1   Supracondylar traction for a fracture at the middle or distal

3rd of the femur on the Brown's Frame

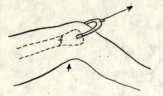 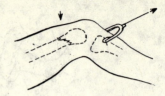

(1) The pin through the supracondyle in cases with Flexion Type of femoral fractures

(2) The pin through the fibular tuberosity in cases with Extension Type of femoral fractures

78−2 Skeletal traction with the pin at different parts for different types of fracture at the distal 3rd of the femur

Fig. 78 Skeletal traction for a femoral fracture

Medication

At the initial stage, as the patient suffers from gross internal hemohrrage that causes severe swelling and distention of the thigh, large doses of drugs that can promote blood circulation to remove blood stasis should be administered bacause these drugs will not only subdue the swelling but also prevent infections. The usual prescription is modified *Fuyuan Huoxue Tang* (1). At the intermediate stage and the natural cure stage, routine medication works.

Exercises

Long−term immobilization and traction is often followed by amyotrophy, especially atrophy of the quadriceps muscle of the thigh, and stiff joints of the knee and the ankle. This will interfere with functional rehabilitation of the limbs. Active exercises for restoration of functions should therefore be practised after reduction and immobilization. At the initial stage, there is no problem doing normal movement of the upper limbs, and flexion—extension exercises of the toes and the ankle of the affected lower limb are allowed. When the fracture becomes stable 2—3 weeks later, the patient can take a semi—reclining position and try to do, by lifting the clunis with arms propping it, extension—flexion exercises of the hip joint, making the lower part of the body ascend and descend together with the affected limb and moving the traction weight synchronously. From the 3rd or 4th week on, the patient is encouraged to elevate the clunis by bearing the upper part of the body with both hands through pulling a pair of suspending rings and supporting the body weight partially with the affected lower limbs. In the 4th or 5th week, he / she can try to stand on the healthy limb with the hands leaning against the bedstead to support the body. At the natural cure stage when the fracture has healed clinically, traction and the external stabilizer should be removed, but the splints are retained, and the patient can do functional movements of the affected limb without weight—bearing. In addition, proper massage and medicinal fumigation and / or bathing of the affected extremity will enhance functional rehabilitation. After bone union has been realized, the patient can begin to walk on foot without help of the crutches as a means of muscular exercise.

2.21 Fractures of the Patella

Pathogenesis

Fractures of the patella are intraarticular fractures. The most common victims are elderly people. The injuries can be produced by direct forces or by indirect forces, but those produced by indirect forces as caused in a fall are more frequently seen in orthopedic practice and the fractures are usually transverse fractures at the middle 3rd or the distal 3rd of the bone with gross displacement. Fractures produced by direct forces are mostly comminuted fractures with less displacement, as caused by a direct blow at the knee joint (Fig. 79).

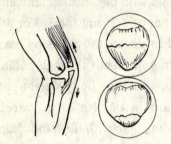 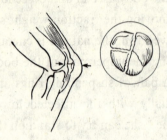

79-1　A fracture produced by an　　　79-2　A fracture produced by a

　　　　indirect force　　　　　　　　　　　direct force

Fig. 79　Pathogenesis and displacement of fractures of the patella

Essentials for Diagnosis

1. A definite history of trauma, such as an injury caused in a fall or by a direct blow.

2. Severe anterior swelling of the knee joint due to intraaricular hematocele, painful ecchymosis and loss of functions of the knee joint in flexion and extension.

3. Tenderness at the knee joint and fluctuation of the knee cap. In displaced fractures there will be a palpable fracture space or isolated fragments.

4. X-ray films of the knee joint in anteroposterior and lateral views will help determine the fracture type.

Treatment

As the injuries fall into intraarticular fractures, anatomical apposition is of great importance in reduction.

Reduction and Immobilization

1. Undisplaced fractures do not need any reduction. After thorough aspiration of hemotocele from the knee joint, strap the knee with thick cotton padding and bandage it. Apply a long wood slab to the lateral or posterior aspect of the affected knee joint and get it bandaged with the knee joint in a slightly flexing position.

2. Displaced fractures must be reduced.

(1) Reduction Followed by Knee—crown Fixation   This method is applicable to fractures with slight displacement. Before the operation, a well designed knee—crown must be made with bandage or soft vine, the diameter of which should agree with the size of the patella. Cover the crown with a few layers of bandage and fix on the crown four laces. Prepare a wood slab of a length extending from the middle of the thigh to the ankle with four nails in the middle part on the lateral edges. The patient lies in dorsal position with the affected knee joint extending straight. The reduction is performed under local anesthesia after all the intraarticular hematocle has been aspired. ① The operator stands on the patient's affected side, energetically presses the proximal fracture end downward with the thumb, forefinger and middle finger of a hand to bring it close to the distal end, and, then, makes the ends move relatively in the medial and lateral directions so as to force the broken fascia out of the fracture space. If this is followed by perceivable crepitus, it shows that the reduction has been achieved (Fig. 80). ② The operator lays the thumb, forefinger and middle finger of one hand on the upper and lower parts of the fragment and places the thumb of the

other hand on the anterior aspect of the patella. If the thumb percieves any ups and downs there, it suggests that there is some anteroposterior displacement between the fracture ends. This requires the operator to press with the thumb the anteriorly protruding fragment to replace it. ③ The operator firmly compresses the fracture ends with thumbs, forefingers and middle fingers of both hands, and ④ The assistant applies a cotton pad to the fracture site, covers it with a cardboard disc, and crowns the disc with the knee—crown to hold the patella.

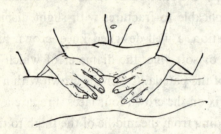

Fig. 80   Reduction of a fracture of the patella

The rest of the process for the fixation includes

——to apply and fix the long wood slab to the posterior aspect of the affected limb.

——to apply a cotton pad to the space between the popliteal fossa and the slab so as to keep the knee joint slightly flexing.

——to affix the crown with the laces attached to the nails on the slab.

——to encircle the limb and slab with bandages.

Position of the knee—crown and tensity of the fixation must be carefully observed at all times during the whole course of immobilization (Fig. 81).

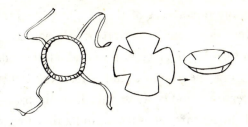

81-1　The knee-crown and the cardboard disc

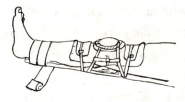

81-2　Fixation in the lateral view

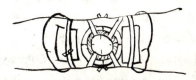

81-3　Fixation in the anteroposterior view

Fig. 81　Fixation of a fracture of the patella

(2) Closed Pin Fixation with Pressure　This method is applicable to fractures with gross displacement that negatively respond to manipulative reduction. Routine pre-operative sterilization and local anesthesia are necessary for the operation. Two Kirschner pins are respectively brought through the upper and lower ends from the medial aspect to the lateral aspect. The pins should be kept parallel to the fracture line and the pin holes

should be protected with disinfected gauze. When the operator presses the anterior aspect of the patella with thumbs, forefingers to reduce the anteroposteriorly displaced ends, an assistant should pull together the medial ends and lateral ends of the pins so as to bring the fracture ends close to each other. Two specially prepared wood blocks with holes in proper places for the pin ends to get through are used to fix the pin ends. The fracture ends can be made in close contact with each other by pressing the blocks together. When this is realized, the blocks should be fixed firmly with adhesive tapes. After the operation, the patient should be given long—wood—slab fixation with the affected knee joint in slight flexion for 2—3 weeks.

Medication

At the initial stage, in addition to drugs with the action of promoting blood circulation to remove blood stasis, diuretics with the effect of eliminating dampness such as Semen Coicis, Radix Stephaniae Tetrandrae, Caulis Akebiae and Semen Plantaginis should be prescribed as there is gross intraarticular hemotocele and aspiration of it is often followed by subsequent re—exudation. At the intermediate stage and the natural cure stage, routine medication works.

Exercises

At the initial stage, bed rest is necessary, but movement of the upper limbs and the unaffected lower extremity, as well as of the lumbodorsal part, is in no way restricted. Flexion—extension exercises of the toes and the ankle joint can be practised with the affected limb in an elevated position. Exercises of relaxation—contraction of the quadriceps muscle and flexion—extension of the knee joint can be initiated two weeks later, the range of the related movement, however, should be kept within 15 degrees. In three weeks after the fracture, the swelling will subside, and the patient can walk on crutches without weight—bearing. At the end of the 4th or 5th week, the external fixation should be discarded, the range of active flexion and extension of the knee joint can be expanded and the patient can then walk with a single crutch. Curative fumigation and bathing of the affected limb with the decoction of certain medicines will enhance the healing at this stage.

2.22   Fractures of the Tibia and Fibula

Pathogenesis

These fractures are clinically common, mostly in children and in adults at the age of 20—50. Poor blood circulation and osteodystrophy at the part between the middle 3rd and the distal 3rd of the tibia or fibula makes this area most vulnerable to fracture. Moreover, fractures at this part tend to delay in healing. An indirect force may produce an oblique or spiral fracture whereas a direct force will cause a transverse or comminuted fracture. If both bones are fractured, the injuries will in most cases be at the same level (Fig. 82). As the medial subcutaneous tissues anterior to the fibula are quite thin, the fracture end(s) may easily stab through the skin, forming open fractures. Muscular traction and certain specific posture often cause extorsion displacement of the distal fracture end and anteromedial angulation of the proximal end. Crush trauma tends to result in swelling of the shank or high pressure syndrome of the fascial space in severe cases.

Essentials for Diagnosis

1. A definite history of trauma or exhaustion.

2. Pain and swelling of the affected shank with loss of functions. In severe cases, there will also be shortening, angular and extorsion deformity.

3. Local tenderness, percussion pain at the heel, and bony crepitus and pseudoactivities in severe cases.

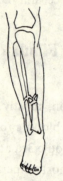

82—1 A comminuted fracture   82—2 A segmental fracture

Fig. 82   Common types of fractures of the shaft of the fibula and / or tibia

4. Examination of pulse beating of the dorsal artery of the foot and the poste rior artery of the tibula will help determine whether there is any injury to the popliteal artery or not. Examination of the flexion—extension functions of the toes will help determine whether there is any injury to the nerves or not.

5. X—ray films of the shank in anteroposterior and lateral views can help determine the fracture type.

Treatment

Management of fractures of the tibia and fibula aims primarily at restoration of the original length of the bones and their normal function of weight—bearing. Therefore, any angulatory, rotatory or overriding deformity must be corrected in case traumatic arthritis of the ankle joint follows.

Reduction

The operation is performed under local anesthesia. The patient lies in dorsal position. Two assistants respectively fix the patient's affected shank and ankle and perform countertraction to correct overriding and angulatory deformity. The operator fixes the proximal fracture end with one hand and the distal end with the other hand, tries to make the distal end precisely meet the proximal end, and performs pushing–pressing and elevating–up–supporting maneuvers to reduce lateral displacement (Fig. 83). Then the assistant fixing the ankle mildly rocks the distal end so as to make the ends in close contact with each other.

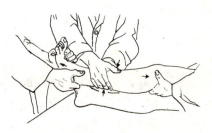

Fig. 83   Reduction of a fracture of the shaft of
the fibula and / or tibia

Immobilization

According to the need of the fixation that is dependent upon the location of the fracture and angulation and displacement of the ends, a compress is applied properly to the fracture site and fixed with adhesive tapes. Cover the compress with a cotton pad. Five splints are used and bound with laces. A long wood slab is applied to the lateral aspect of the shank. The actual position of the slab depends upon the location of the fracture. For a fracture of the proximal 3rd, the slab should extend beyond the knee, and for a fracture of the distal 3rd, the slab beyond the ankle. Bandage the slab firmly to complete the fixation.

Cautions for the Fixation:

1. The splints should be moulded to fit the anterolateral arc of the tibia.

2. Mind the danger of injuring the peroneal nerve by the upper end of the lateral splint.

3. Mind the danger of injuring the Achellus tendon and the heel by the posterior splint.

4. Necessary transcalcaneal traction should be applied to unstable fractures.

5. The tensity of the splint fixation must be adjusted timely in case high pressure syndrome of the fascial space occurs.

Medication

As blood circulation at the distal 3rd of the tibia is poor, the healing may be very slow. This requires due emphasis on tonification of the liver and kidney and on reinforcement of the bones, tendons and muscles. So, at the initial stage, apart from large doses of drugs to invigorate the flow of *Qi* and activate blood circulation to remove blood stasis, heat–clearing and detoxifying drugs such as a modified combined recipe of *Taoren Chengqi Tang* (8) and *Wuwei Xiaodu Yin* (5) should be prescribed for patients with severe swelling of the shank accompanied by blisters. *Zhuangyao Jianshen Wan* (51)or *Jiegu Dan* (11) for oral administration is helpful at the intermediate stage.

By the time when the natural cure begins, the patient can be given *Shenjin Pian* (50) for oral intake and No. 2 Washing Recipe for fumigation and / or bathing of the affected shank.

Exercises

At the initial stage, the patient can sit on the bed and do flexionextension exercises of the toes and contraction—relaxation exercises of the quadriceps muscle of the thigh. The slab and traction should be discarded after the fracture has become stable and the patient can begin to do flexion—extension exercises of the knee joint and the ankle joint. At the natural cure stage, the splint should be removed and the patient can begin crutch—walking. He / She can gradually learn to do the practice first with a pair of crutches, then with a single one, bearing a small weight, and finally with no crutch at all.

2.23   Fractures of the Ankle

Pathogenesis

Fractures of the ankle are intraarticular fractures frequently seen in orthopedic practice. These injuries primarily occur in young people, especially the teenagers. They are in most instances produced by indirect forces such as a torsion during walking or running. The ankle joint is vulnerable to inversion or eversion injuries due to instability when it is in planter flexion position; and so fractures, sometimes complicated with dislocation, are frequently produced. Considering the force and its direction and the posture of the patient at the time of injury, fractures of the ankle can be classified as Inversion Type, Eversion Type, Extorsion Type and Compression Type. Of the four types,

Inversion Type is the most common and Eversion Type comes next. When the fractures are produced by direct forces, they are generally open injuries.

Essentials for Diagnosis

1. A definite history of trauma, especially a history of a sprain.

2. Swelling, ecchymosis and pain in the ankle area, with blisters in severe cases.

3. Local tenderness with perceivable bony crepitus when palpated.

4. Inversion / Eversion deformity of the ankle.

5. X—ray films of the ankle in anteroposterior and lateral views, plus other signs, can help determine the fracture type. Roentgenographic examination should include the ankle area as well as the distal 3rd of the shank.

Treatment

As ankle fractures are intraarticular fractures, anatomic reposition is required. The injury frequently involves the adjacent soft tissues, and this determines the principle "paying equal attention to the fracture and the soft tissue injuries" in the treatment. The above principle of treatment will benefit later restoration of functions and weight—bearing ability.

Reduction

1. The patient lies in dorsal position and is given nerve block anesthesia. An assistant fixes the patient's affected shank with both hands while another assistant fixes the dorsum pedis with one hand and the heel with the other. The two assistants perform stretching countertraction in conformity with the displacement direction. For an inversion fracture, the traction

should gradually change from inversion to eversion (Fig. 84), and, for an eversion fracture, from eversion to inversion (Fig. 85). Meanwhile, the operator compresses the patient's ankle with both hands from both the medial and lateral sides so as to correct the displacement. In reduction of an inversion fracture, the orthopedicist should fix with one hand the part above the affected medial ankle and push and press the lateral malleolus inward. In reduction of an eversion fracture, the operator should fix the part above the lateral ankle and push and press outwardly. If the fracture is associated with tibiofibular diastasis, while an assistant fixes the patient's affected foot and slightly rotates it, the operator compresses with palms both the medial and lateral malleoli so as to eliminate the diastasis and to reduce lateral displacement of the talus. Then the first assistant presses the shin backward under traction and the second assistant raises and pulls the foot anteriorly and gradually flexes it dorsally in 90 degrees. This will correct posterior displacement of the talus and the forwardly fissured medial malleolus. When it is necessary to clear up any residual fissure, the operator may push and press with a thumb the posterior lower part of the affected medial malleolus.

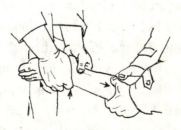

Fig. 84   Reduction of an eversion fracture of the ankle

After reduction, some auxiliary passive movement of the affected foot will be helpful. The patient's affected foot should be kept in a neutral position. The operator fixes the front part of the foot with one hand and the ankle with the other hand, and makes flexion and extension of the foot several times so as to restore the normal articular surface through the moulding effect of the talus on the ankle mortar.

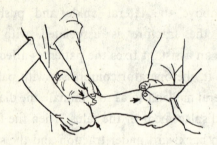

Fig. 85   Reduction of an inversion fracture of the ankle

2. Reduction of Trimalleolar Fractures   If the fracture fragment of the posterior malleolus is smaller than a 3rd of the distal tibial articular surface, it can be reduced simply through manipulative maneuvers. The steps are as follows: (1) Reduce fractures of the medial and lateral malleoli as described above. (2) Perform reduction of the fracture of the posterior malleolus. (3) After the above two steps have been finished, have both the medial and lateral malleoli of the affected foot compressed energetically by the second assistant, and (4) push backward the lower part of the affected leg with one hand, raise the foot and make it flex dorsally with the other hand. As a result of tension—traction of the posterior articular sac, the fracture of the posterior malleolus will be reduced along with the backward

subluxation of the talus. If the fragment of the posterior malleolus is larger than a 3rd of the distal tibial, articular surface, dorsal flexion of the ankle joint may in no case be tried as this will lead to further posterior translocation of the talus, which will deteriorate upward displacement of the fragment. Instead of manipulative reduction, suspension traction or transcalcaneal traction with stockinet should be applied, for suspension traction will gradually reposit the posterior malleolus (Fig. 86).

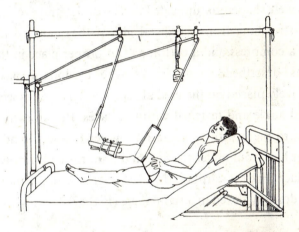

Fig. 86　Stockinet traction through overhead suspension

Immobilization

1. Splint Fixation　If there is no inversion or eversion deformity after reduction, the affected foot should be fixed at neutral position; if there exists inversion deformity, the fixation should be at the eversion position, and vice versa. (1) Apply a compress to the lower part of the lateral malleolus (for eversive fractures) or of the medial malleolus (for inversive fractures) and fix it with adhesive tapes. (2) Cover the compress with a cotton pad. (3) Properly arrange the splints (5 in all, all mould-

ed in arch shape but of different radius), 2 on the front aspect, that is, on either side of the tibia, and 3 on the lateral, medial and posterior aspects respectively. (4) Fasten the splints with three laces. (5) Fix the distal ends of the lateral and medial splints from under the heel with an extra lace and knot it on the lower lace so as to keep the foot in dorsal flexion of a right angle.

2. Cardboard Fixation   Prepare two pieces of cardboard well shaped as up—sidedown isosceles trapezoid, with a height stretching from the distal 3rd of the shank to the heel. Apply a compress and a cotton pad to proper place in the same way as described above in 1. The cardboard pieces are respectively placed on the medial aspect and lateral aspect of the affected ankle and fastened with two laces. Put an extra square cardboard piece with a cotton pad under the heel, bind it with another lace from under the heel and knot the ends firmly on the lower lace. Fix the cardboard pieces further with a bandage; the foot is dorsally flexed in a right angle (Fig. 87).

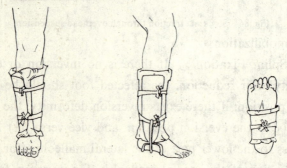

(1) The anteroposterior view   (2) The lateral view   (3) The sole—aspect view

Fig. 87   Cardboard fixation for an ankle fracture

Medication

See 1.3: Administration of Chinese Medicines on the Basis of Overall Analysis and Differentiation of Symptoms and Signs. For cases with severe swelling of the ankle joint at the initial stage, modified *Fuyuan Huoxue Tang* (1) can be prescribed.

Exercises

At the initial stage, the patient is encouraged to do flexion—extension exercises of the toes in a sitting position on the bed with the affected leg elevated. Movement of the knee joint is not restricted and exercises of the ankle joint for extension and flexion can be gradually introduced, but any risk of repeating the injury mechanism must be avoided. Four weeks after the fracture, external fixation can be discarded and active flexion—extension exercises of the ankle joint without weight—bearing are encouraged in case articular adhesion should occur. In addition, these exercises also prove beneficial to remoulding of the joint with a smooth articular surface.

2.24 Fractures of the Calcaneus

Pathogenesis

Fractures of the calcaneus are mostly found in adults. A fracture of the calcaneus is frequently incuured from a fall. The injury is in most cases at the calcaneus body and the tuberosity portion. The normal tuber—joint angle of the calcaneus is about 40 degrees. When the fracture occurs, as the injury is mostly a compression fracture, the angle will appear smaller, causing collapse of the planter arch and increased width of the calcaneus. Fractures of the calcaneus can generally be classified into two major types according to the position where the injury occurs:

Type A, isolated fractures of the calcaneus, and Type B, fractures with involvement of the subtalar joint, which falls into intraarticular fractures frequently resulting in traumatic arthritis.

Essentials for Diagnosis

1. A definite history of trauma, especially an injury caused in a fall.

2. Swelling and pain in the heel, and a shallower plantar arch and a broader heel, frequently with ecchymosis.

3. Crush pain at the heel that hurts so much that the patient is reluctant to stand bearing a weight.

4. X—ray films of the heel in lateral and axial views can help determine the fracture type.

Treatment

Reduction and Immobilization

1. Isolated Fractures of the Calcaneus

(1) Fractures of the Tuberosity of the Calcaneus

① Longitudinal Fractures   The patient lies in prone position. An assistant fixes the patient's affected shank and another assistant fixes the front portion of the foot to make the knee joint flex at 90 degrees and the ankle joint flex towards the metatarsal bones. The operator then inserts a Kirschner pin transversely into the tuberosity of the calcaneus and sets the pin on a traction arc for posterior traction to release the interlock of the fracture surfaces and then for downward traction to reduce the ends.

② Transverse Fractures   The preparations are all the same as for longitudinal fractures. The operator lays the thumb and forefinger of a hand on the patient's affected Achillus tendon and pushes energetically the fragment towards the distal terminal.

After reduction, the fragments must be fixed with splints. Four splints and a small wood block are needed. Apply two flight—shaped compresses to the lateral aspect and the medial aspect of the affected calcaneus respectively and cover them with two arch—shaped splints for superarticular fixtion of the ankle joint. A long bow—shaped splint stretching from the upper 3rd of the shin to the bases of the toes is placed on the anterior aspect. The posterior splint is shorter, reaching just above the calcaneus. The wood block in proper size is placed under the planter arc with sufficient cotton padding. Fix the splints firmly with laces. The affected foot is kept in extreme flexion towards the metatarsal bones and the knee joint in mild flexion (Fig. 88).

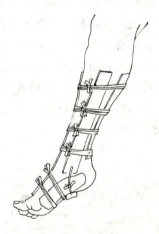

Fig. 88   Splint fixation for a fracture of the calcaneus

(2) Fractures of the Calcaneus Body Adjacent to the Subtalar Joint

As this type of fracture produces increase of compressed

width of the calcaneus body and causes upward displacement of the posterior upper half of the calcaneus body, the patient has to lie dorsally for the reduction with the knee of the involved limb raised by some means to produce flexion of the knee joint. An assistant fixes the shin. The operator compresses with both hands the part beneath the ankle from the lateral and medial sides so as to correct lateral displacement, and, then, begins stretching traction by fixing the front part of the foot with one hand and the tuber—joint part of the heel with the other hand. The traction can make extreme flexion of the foot towards the metatarsal bones and thus reposit the fragments and bring about restoration of the normal Böhler angle and the plantar arch (Fig. 89). Immobilization of this type of fractures may be the same as described in (1)for fractures of the tuberosity, or may be performed with Orthopedic Wood—shoe Fixation. Prepare a foot—shaped wood block that has a prominent center to fit the plantar arc well. Give sufficient padding before the "shoe" is applied to the plantar and fixed firmly with laces in a ∞—shape dressing (Fig. 90). The posterior melloilus should be supported and elevated to a proper height with a sand—bag so as to produce a slight flexion of the joint.

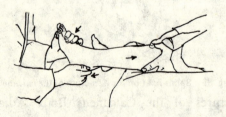

Fig. 89   Reduction of a fracture of the calcaneus

2. Fractures of the Calcaneus with Involvement of the Sub—talar Joint

This type of fractures are most common in fractures of the calcaneus. The injury may cause comminution and collapse of the calcaneus with increment of width and eversion of the calcaneus body. The tuberosity will rise and the sub—talar joint apperas depressed. A poor reduction may lead to severe traumatic arthritis. The way of reduction for these fractures is the same as described in (2) of 1. for fractures of the calcaneus body adjacent to the sub—talar joint, which aims at restoration of normal joint angle and original width of the calcaneus body.

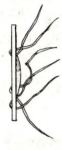

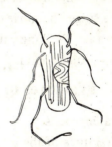

90—1   The orthopedic shoe in the   90—2   The orthopedic shoe in the
       lateral view   anteroposterior view

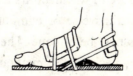

Fig. 90   Fixation for a fracture of the calcaneus with an orthopedic wood—shoe

Medication

See 1.3: Administration of Chinses Medicines on the Basis of Overall Analysis and Differentiation of Symptoms and Signs.

Exercises

Generally, the patient should start rehabilitation exercises possibly earlier but begin weight–bearing much later. At the initial stage, the affected limb should be raised high with the knee joint and ankle joint in flexion. Flexion–extension exercises of the toes and contraction and relaxation of the quadriceps femoris can be performed. The fracture ends will become stable at the intermediate stage. Walking without weight–bearing and metatarsal flexion of the foot can be initiated, but the splints must be maintained as a means of exercise control. At the natural cure stage, the range of movement of the foot can be gradually increased. Walking with a load can be tried only after the fracture has healed sound.

2.25　Fractures of the Metatarsus

Pathogenesis

Fractures of the metatarsus are most frequently seen in injuries of the foot. In most cases, the fracture is produced by a direct force such as a hit by a heavy object or a crush by a car or the like. An indirect force can also cause injuries such as a sprain that may result in a fracture of the metatarsus. Fractures caused by direct forces may be transverse or comminuted while those caused by indirect forces may be oblique. The injury may occur in the base, diaphysis or neck of the metatarsus. The fracture ends are liable to form an angle towards the metatarsal aspect with likely displacement of the distal end to the same side or to the lateral side. If the fracture happens to be in the base of the

5th metatarsus, it will mostly be an avulsion fracture with little displacement. It is common to find dislocation of the tarsometatarsal joint in association with the injury, especially the injury of the 1st and 5th metatarsi.

Essentials for Diagnosis

1. A definite history of trauma or exhaustion.

2. Swelling, edema, pain and ecchymosis on the dorsum of the affected foot. The patient strongly refuses to try any weight—bearing.

3. Local tenderness and impact pain of the metatarsus, sometimes with perceivable bony crepitus.

4. X—ray films of the foot in anteroposterior and lateral views will help determine the fracture type.

Treatment

The 1st and 5th metatarsal heads function as two of the three supporting points of the foot and the arrangement of the five metatarsi forms the transverse arch of the anterior part of the foot. Therefore, whenever a fracture happens in the metatarsi, every effort must be made to restore their original structural shape.

Reduction

1. Reduction by Two Performers   The operation is performed under local anesthesia. The patient lies in dorsal position. The assistant fixes the middle—lower part of the leg. The operator dresses the affected toe(s) of the patient with gauze and begins stretching traction, with one hand, in an angular direction to the dorsum by 20—30 degrees from the normal axial line of the foot so as to correct overriding displacement, and then, changes the traction direction to the metatarsal side with an an-

gle of 10—15 degrees from the foot axial line while simultaneously pushing and pressing the distal fracture end to the dorsal aspect with the thumb of the other hand so as to correct the angular deformity towards the metatarsal side. The operator can further correct the lateral displacement in the following steps: (1) Fix the patient's affected toes with one hand for stretching traction. (2) Lay the thumb of the other hand on the dorsal side at the proper bone gap between the toes and the other fingers on the planter side for relative compression from both sides so as to separate the bones. If the fracture is associated with dislocation of the tarsometatarsal joint, reduction of the dislocation must be performed first (Fig. 91).

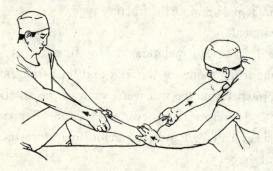

91-1   Pulling traction

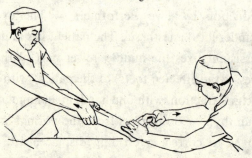

91-2   Correction of overriding and angulation to the metatarsal side

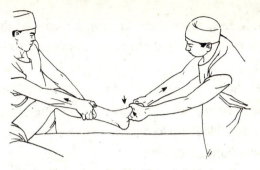

91-3 Correction of residual lateral displacement

Fig. 91 Reduction of a fracture of the metatarseus

2. Redcution by One Performer The operation is performed under local anesthesia. The patient lies in dorsal position. The operator stands on the medial side of the patient's affectd foot, and (1) fixes the distal and proximal fracture ends with thumbs and forefingers of the hands, the former on the dorsum and the latter on the plantar. (2) performs energetic traction to correct overriding displacement. (3) presses downward with the thumb fixing the proximal end and raises upward with the forefinger fixing the distal end so as to correct displacement to the metatarsal aspect. (4) pinches either gaps beside the affected bone with thumbs on the dorsum and forefingers on the plantar to separate the bones so as to reduce lateral displacement.

Immobilization

1. Splint fixation On the dorsal aspect, two bone—separating compresses are respectively applied to either of the bone gaps beside the affected metatarsus. Cover each of the compresses with a cotton pad and fix them with adhesive plaster. Prepare two splints, one of 8 cm length for application to the dorsal aspect, the other of 6 cm length for application to the

metatarsal aspect, place them at proper places of the foot and bandage them firmly. Elevate the heel of the affected foot with a sand bag.

2. Cardboard Fixation   Prepare two pieces of cardboard, one to be applied to the dorsal aspect and the other to the plantar aspect. Place them at the correct parts of the foot and get them well bandaged.

Medication

See 1.3: Administration of Chinese Medicines on the Basis of Overall Analysis and Differentiation of Symptoms and Signs. In case of subsequent severe swelling and distention, *Fuyuan Huoxue Tang* (1) can be prescribed for the patient. At the natural cure stage, fumigation and / or washing of the affected foot with decoction of *Huoxue Zhitong San* (45) is beneficial for functional restoration.

Exercises

After reduction and fixation, it is significant to elevate the affected limb to a certain height for exercises of dorsal flexion of the ankle joint and flexion—extension of the knee joint. When the fracture becomes stable, crutche—walking without any weight—bearing is encouraged. In case delayed or abnormal healing occurs, free walking can never be attempted until the fracture has completely healed though walking—drilling in wood—sole shoe with plantar—arch padding can be initiated 4 weeks after the injury.

3 Dislocations

3.1 Introduction

Pathogenesis

Dislocations are mostly produced by direct forces or indirect forces. They may also be caused by general asthenia, maldevelopment and relaxation of ligaments around an articular sac or around a joint.

If a dislocation is not completely cured or if the injured ligaments around a joint or the articular sac are not thoroughly repaired, the injury tends to recur repeatedly and will result in habitual dislocation. In addition, pathogenic changes such as tuberculosis or suppuration of a joint may lead to pathogenic dislocation.

Classification

There are Complete Dislocation and Semi—luxation with regard to the degree of displacement; Anterior Dislocation, Posterior Dislocation, Superior Dislocation, Inferior Dislocation and Central Dislocation with regard to the direction; Traumatic Dislocation, Pathologic Dislocation, Habitual Dislocation and Congenital Dislocation with regard to the cause; Fresh Dislocation (dislocations within 2—3 weeks after the injury) and Old Dislocation (dislocations that have not yet been reduced for over 2—3 weeks since the injury) with regard to the duration after the injury; and Open Dislocation and Closed Dislocation with regard to whether there is any open traumatic injury of the relevant dislocated joint.

Essentials for Diagnosis

1. General Symptoms Local pain and swelling with dysfunction of the affected joint.

2. Characteristic Signs

Deformity For instance, an anterior dislocation of the shoulder joint will be associated with deformity of a "square shoulder", and a posterior dislocation of the elbow will present a "boot—shape elbow". Different dislocations will produce their characteristic consequent deformities.

Empty Glenoid Cavity As dislocation may cause herniation of the caput articularis from the glenoid cavity, the cavity will become empty. For instance, there will be a perceivable excavation in the area anterior to the antilobium in a dislocation of the mandibular articulation.

Plastic Resistance As the affected part is fixed at a particular abnormal position by the spastic muscles and ligaments around the dislocated area, a plastic resistance can be felt when the part is moved passively even if there is still some faint active movement.

Complications

The common complications associated with dislocations are fractures, injuries to the vessels and nerves, traumatic arthritis, myositis ossificans, etc. Whenever necessary, Rontgenographic examination or other helpful examinations should be made to establish correct diagnosis.

Treatment

Manipulative Reduction

1. Traumatic Dislocations Fresh traumatic dislocations

should be reduced under proper anesthesia as early as possible though the operation can never be performed unless a definite diagnosis (concerning the mechanism, direction, etc.) has been established. It is recommended to do the reduction by making use of the lever principle as far as possible.

2. Old Traumatic Dislocation   As the injury is old, it is usually difficult to perform the reduction since there has been organization of hematoma in and outside the joint and adhesion of scars of the soft tissues. Curative effect, however, has been raised in recent years due to development of certain new therapies. Reduction of this type of dislocations requires prolonged duration of traction under anesthesia; the force for the traction should be exerted gradually from mild to strong. The reduction must be slow, steady but forceful enough and the dislocated joint should be moved, under traction, in various manners including flexion, extension adduction, abduction, rotation, etc. This may gradually release the adhesive scars, thus ensuring greater rate of successful reduction.

Immobilization

Fixation posterior to successful reduction is necessary for better repair of the soft tissues in case dislocation recurs. The immobilization should usually be kept for 2—3 weeks. In the case of old dislocations, the duration of immobilization needs to be slightly prolonged.

Proper functional exercises for rehabilitation and medicinal therapy can be prescribed after the dislocation has been well reduced and immobilized. For more detailed information, please refer to General Introduction of this volume.

3. 2 Dislocations of the Shoulder Joint

Pathogenesis

Anatomically, the shoulder joint is composed of the humeral head and the scapula glenoid cavity. The former seems to be a little too large for the latter to seat. As the range of movement of the shoulder joint is quite wide and the articular sac is considerably loose, without muscles in the lower front, the hemeral head is vulnerable to dislocation when this part is injured traumatically. The most common types are anterior dislocations and inferior dislocations (Fig. 92).

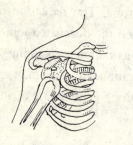 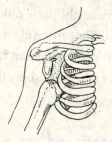

92-1   An anterior dislocation   92-2   An inferior dislocation

Fig. 92   Shoulder dislocations

Essentials for Diagnosis

1. A definite history of trauma, pain and swelling in the affected shoulder with restricted range of movement.

2. A "square shoulder" deformity (Fig. 93) with palpable dislocated humeral head in the armpit, subcoracoid or infraclavicular part.

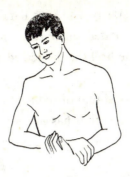

Fig. 93 "Square shoulder" deformity of the right shoulder joint

3. A positive result in Dugas'test (The elbow is unable to touch the chest when the palm of the affected limb is placed on the other shoulder or the palm of the affected limb is unable to rest on the other shoulder when the elbow joint is firmly pressing the chest).

4. Likely in association with an avulsion fracture of the greater humeral tuberosity, or with lesion of the axillary nerve which may require radiographic examination or other relevant examinations for detection of any neurological injuries.

Treatment

Reduction

Reduction of dislocation of the shoulder joint usually does not require any form of anesthesia.

1. Method of Sole—supporting   The patient lies dorsally on a bed. The operator sits on the patient's affected side, facing the patient, and, then, (1) fixes his / her wrist of the affected limb with both hands, (2) props the patient's affected armpit with a sole (left sole for dislocation of the left shoulder and right sole for dislocation of the right shoulder), (3) pulls the arm straight with simultaneous abduction of 30 degrees. (4) performs stretching

traction steadily and slowly with both hands, (5) gets the affected limb abducted and rotated outwardly under the traction, (6) slightly props with the heel the dislocated humeral head towards the lateral side.

When a click—like sound of reduction is perceived or heard, it suggests that the operation has already been completed. This method is applicable to inferior dislocations (Fig. 94).

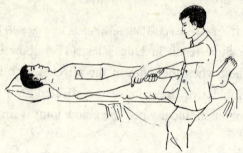

Fig. 94   Method of foot—supporting

2.   Method of Knee—supporting   The patient sits on a bench. The operator stands by his / her affected side (for instance, the left side) on the uni—lateral foot with the other foot on the bench, facing the same direction, and, then, (1) abducts the patient's affected limb by 80—90 degrees, placing it around the operator's lumbar portion, (2) seizes the wrist with the left hand and fixes it firmly against the operators left hip, (3) places the right palm on the patient's left acromion and props the affect- ed armpit with the right knee, (4) pushes with the right hand, pulls with the left hand and raises forcibly with the right knee, (5) slowly but energetically turns to the left and (6) supports the humeral head with the right knee and elevates it suddenly with great effort.

This method is applicable to inferior dislocations (Fig. 95).

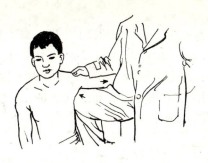

Fig. 95   Method of knee—supporting (the anterior view)

3. Method of Elevating with a Bar   A bar of a meter in length with a diameter of about 5 cm is needed. The middle portion of the bar should be wrapped with soft materials such as a towel or some cotton. The patient sits on a stool. An assistant carries the bar in hand by one end with middle portion under the patient's armpit. Another assistant fixes the patient's wrist of the affected limb and performs downward traction. The operator carries the bar by the other end and elevates it energetically with synchronous collaboration of the first assistant. This elvation plus the downward traction will form countertraction. Keep the countertraction until a sound of reduction is heard (Fig. 96).

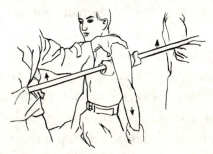

Fig. 96   Reduction of a shoulder dislocation through pole—lifting

Immobilization

When the dislocation has been reduced, immobilization of

the affected shoulder is significant. The affected upper arm should be firmly pressed against the chest in an adducent and intorsive position and the elbow joint should be kept in flexion by an angle less than 90 degrees. Bandage the limb along with the shoulder (Fig. 97).

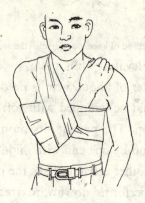

Fig. 97 Bandage—fixation for a dislocation of the shoulder joint

Management of Old Dislocations   If a dislocation of the shoulder joint remains unreduced for as long as 3 weeks after the injury, peripheral adhesion around the shoulder will occur. The longer the reduction is delayed, the more difficult it will be. However, if the shoulder has not yet become too rigid for manipulative reduction, proper maneuvers can be tried. In case this proves unsuccessful, operative surgery can be considered.

Certain Chinese medicines, particularly those with the property of activating blood circulation to remove blood stasis and those of softening hard masses, can help soften the adhesion and contracture of the soft tissues. Administration of these medicines a few days before manipulative reduction will raise the rate of successful operation. The usually prescribed recipe is as follows:

Radix Angelicae Sinensis	9 g
Radix Paeoniae Rubra	12 g
Eupolyphaga seu Steleophaga	9 g
Flos Carthami	6 g
Radix Clematidis	12 g
Squama Manitis	6 g
Radix Trichosanthis	12 g
Radix Aucklandiae	6 g
Pericarpium Citri Reticulatae	9 g
Resina Draconis	3 g
Ramulus Mori	15 g
Radix Glycyrrhizae	6 g

Administration: Decoct these drugs in a proper amount of water and drink the decoction. Use the same prescription in succession for 3—5 days and renew the drugs each day.

In addition, No. 2 Washing recipe can be used for hot decoction—soaking, or heated wine / vinegar dregs for hot compress, 1—2 hours before the reduction.

Adequate anesthesia should be given prior to the reduction. The patient lies dorsally. The operator fixes the patient's affected shoulder with both hands. An assistant makes passive movement of the patient's affected limb in all directions by fixing the wrist with hands, including circling the affected shoulder, and increases the range of movement gradually so as to release local adhesion as much as possible. Then the dislocation can be reduced by traction—supporting process in the following steps (Fig. 98). (1) Another assistant encircles the patient's bosom from the un—affected side with both hands (this can also be realized with a strap of cloth);(2) The two assistants perform countertraction; (3) The operator lays thumbs on the patinet's affected acromion while pulling the humeral head to the lateral side with the other fingers. When these performances have dispersed all the signs of dislocation and deformity, the reduction has been successfully completed. Sometimes it is unlikely to hear the sound of reduction, and X—ray films should be taken so as to affirm how the result is like. As described previously, fixation after reduction is indispensable. At the natural cure stage, functional exercises for rehabilitation is highly helpful in prevention of recurrence of adhesion.

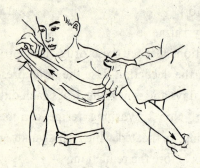

98—1   Reduction with the patient sitting on a stool

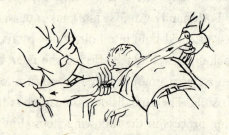

98—2   Reduction with the patiernt lying on a board bed

Fig. 98   Reduction of an old dislocation of the shoulder joint

3. 3   Dislocations of the Elbow Joint

Pathogenesis

The elbow joint is composed of the trochlea of the distal end of the humerus, the compitulum of the humerus, the semilunal insisure at the proximal ulnar end and the compitulum radii. Dislocations of the elbow joint can be classified as anterior dislocations, posterior dislocations and lateral dislocations with regard to the direction of the injury on the articular surface at the proximal ulnar and radial ends. Posterior dislocations of the elbow joint are far more common than anterior dislocations, therefore only the former is dealt with in this volume.

Essentials for Diagnosis

1. A history of trauma, especially a traumatic injury when the patient's affected arm is in an abducent position and the elbow joint is extending straight.

2. Swelling and pain at the elbow joint in association with restricted movement of it.

3. Fixed flexibility of the elbow joint at a semi—flexion position (about 130 degrees) and notable posterior protrusion of the tip of the olecranon with plumped cubital fossa. The smooth distal end of the humerus is palpable and the normal triangle in the posterior cubital region is absent.

4. If the dislocation is associated with lateral displacement, deviation of the olecranon to either of the lateral sides will be palpable. X—ray films of the elbow joint can help detect whether the dislocation is complicated with fractures or not.

Treatment

Manipulative Reduction

1. Tracting—pushing Method   The patient takes either sitting or dorsally lying position. An assistant firmly fixes the distal segment of the patient's affected arm. The operator stands on the patient's affected side and (1) fixes with one hand the distal portion of the affected forearm and performs downward traction along the direction of the longitudinal axis of the forearm, (2) fixes with the other hand the affected elbow joint of the patient and pushes superoposteriorly with the thumb the distal end of the humerus while pulling anteroinferiorly with the other fingers the olecranon from the posterior cubitus and (3) gradually flexes the patient's affected elbow joint until a sound of reduction is heard (Fig. 99).

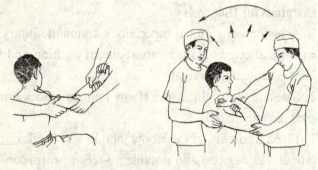

Fig. 99   Tracting—pushing Method

2. Pulling and Knee—supporting Method   The patient sits upright on a stool. The operator stands by the patient's affected elbow, one hand fixing the affected upper arm, the other fixing the wrist, and one foot resting on the stool with the knee supporting the patient's cubital fossa, and, then, (1) flexes the patient's affected elbow at about 90 degrees and props forcibly the cubital fossa forward with the knee, (2) energetically performs traction with the hand fixing the wrist in the direction of the

longitudinal axis of the forearm, (3) gradually increases the degrees of flexion of the affected elbow (Fig. 100).

Immobilization

After reduction, the elbow joint should be immobilized at degrees less than a right angle and well bound with cubital 8–shape–bandaging. The forearm must be supported by a sling with a rectangular piece of cardboard (Fig. 101). The fixation is kept for 2—3 weeks. There is no restriction of movement except flexion and extension of the elbow joint. Once external immobilization is discarded, exercises for functional rehabilitation must be gradually initiated.

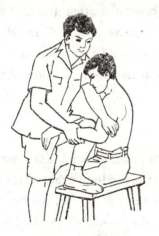

Fig.100　Pulling and knee–
supporting Method

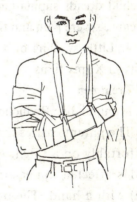

Fig.101　∞–shape bandaging
fixation for a dislocation of
the elbow joint

3. 4　Subluxations of the Capitulum Radii

Pathogenesis

Subluxations of the capitulum radii occur mostly in children younger than 4 years old. The mechanism of the lesion is sudden traction on the extending elbow joint, as in a fall or during dressing, that keeps the capitulum radii from restoring its normal position due to hinderance by the orbicular ligament after the traction.

Essentials for Diagnosis

1. A definite history of sudden passive traction of the affected limb.

2. Pain in the affected elbow or forearm. The child is reluctant to move the affected limb, not to mention to raise it up.

3. Definite tenderness at the lateral part of the elbow where the capitulum rests. The affected forearm is often pronated and the child dreads supinating it. Any passive flexion of the elbow will cause severe pain and thus meet the child's strong protest.

4. Little swelling or deformity at the elbow, nor any abnormality in X—ray films.

Treatment

Manipulative Reduction

The parent carries the child in arms, making him / her sit comfortably on a thigh. An assistant (or the parent) fixes the child's affected upper arm (suppose it is the left arm in the case) with a hand. The operator takes hold of the child's affected wrist with the right hand and presses the lateral aspect of the capitulum radii with the left thumb, and then, (1) slowly performs downward traction with the right hand while supinating the affected forearm, (2) forcibly presses the capitulum radii with the left hand (3) flexes the dislocated elbow joint. These maneuvers often produces a slight perceivable sound that reports completion of the reduction

(Fig. 102) and the child may soon feel relieved from the pain and able to flex the elbow joint or to raise the arm. If the first attempt fails, the maneuvers can be repeated. As a rule, there is no need for external immobilization though it is important to advise the parents to be cautious not to pull or tract the child's affected limb in a certain period of time in case reluxation occurs.

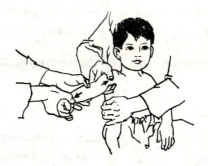

102–1   Traction with the thumb pressing the

dislocated capitulum radii

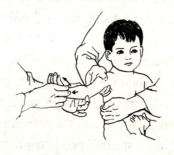

102–2   Traction plus supination of the forearm

with simultaneous thumb pressing

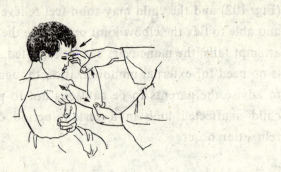

102-3　Flexion of the elbow plus thumb pressing

Fig. 102　Reduction of a subluxation of the capitulum radii

3.5　Dislocations of the Temporo-mandibular Joint

Pathogenesis

Dislocations of the mandibular articulation may be produced by opening the mouth too wide as in laughing, yawning or during a dental extraction or biting something hard. Clinically, anterior dislocations are the most common, which can further be classified as unilateral dislocations and bilateral dislocations. If the dislocation occurs repeatedly, habitual dislocation will generally be the result.

Essentials for Diagnosis

1. In the case of bilateral dislocations, there will be such signs as mandibular protrusion, a half-open mouth that can neither be closed nor opened wider at the patient's will, incapability of occlusion of the teeth, slurred speech, continual salivation, and dysphagia. In addition, a concavity can be felt in the areas in front of the tragus.

2. In the case of unilateral dislocations, there will be such

signs as obliquity of the lower jaw with deformity of the mouth especially angulus oris towards the unaffected side. Only in the area in front of the tragus of the affected side can a concavity be palpated.

Treatment

Manipulative Reduction

1. Intraoral Reduction   The patient sits on a low stool with the head resting against a wall. The operator stands in front of the patient, putting the thumbs (which have been protected with well fixed gauze in case they should be injured by the patient's teeth when the dislocation is reduced) into the patient's mouth on the occlusal surface of the lower molar teeth, with the other fingers supporting the mandibular body and angle of mandible of each side, then, (1) presses the lower molar teeth with both thumbs, exerting greater and greater force gradually, (2) fixes the mandibular body firmly with the other fingers and pushes it downward and backward. until the deformity and signs of the dislocation disappear, which means completion of the reduction (Fig. 103).

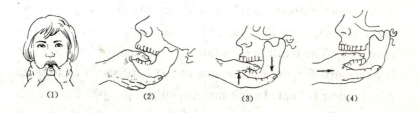

Fig. 103   Reduction of a dislocation of the temporo–mandibular joint (intraoral method)

Caution: During the operation, when a sound indicating completion of the reduction is heard, the thumbs must be moved immediately towards the lateral sides in case they are injured by the teeth.

This method can also be used for unilateral dislocations. In that case, the operator need not at all exert any strength on the teeth of the unaffected side.

2. Extraoral Reduction   The patient sits on a low stool with the head resting against a wall. The operator stands in front of the patient, putting thumbs on each upper part of the ramus mandible and fixing the mandibular body with the other fingers, and, then, (1) presses downward the ramus of mandible, exerting greater and greater strength, (2) slowly pushes it towards the posterior direction simultaneously.

These maneuvers will generally bring about good reduction.

Immobilization

4—tailed Strap Fixation   Use a wide bandage both ends of which have been cut into two in the median line. At the center of the bandage, a hole of 3—cm length should be made so as to support the mandible well. Apply the bandage to the head with the hole right under the chin and fix it by making knots with the four tails at the vertex and the occiput (Fig. 104). The fixation is usually maintained for 3—5 days. It is cautioned for the patient not to eat hard stuffs as long as the fixation is kept. It will not do, either, to open the mouth too wide. In the case of habitual dislocations, immobilization should last about two weeks and *Shiquan Dabu Wan* can be prescribed for oral intake.

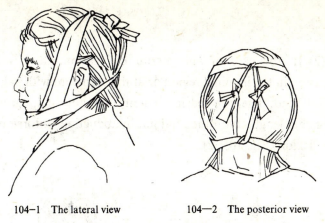

104-1   The lateral view   104-2   The posterior view

Fig. 104   4-tailed strap fixation

3. 6   Dislocations of the Hip Joint

Pathogenesis

The hip joint is the largest one of all the joints in human body. It is strong. Hence dislocation of this joint can only be produced by a very powerful force. Most victims are males in their youth under 40 years old. Clinically, there are posterior dislocations, anterior dislocations and central dislocations. Of all the three types, the first is the most common.

Essentials for Diagnosis

1. A definite history of injury by a violent force. The patient suffers from pains at the affected hip with loss of the function of this joint inspite of indistinct swelling.

2. Varying deformities

(1) In the case of a posterior dislocation, there will be protrusion of the clunis along with a shortened leg on the affected side. The hip joint is deformed with obvious flexion, adduction and intorsion. The injury may be complicated with a fracture of the acetabulum or with an injury of the sciatic nerve (Fig. 105-1).

(2) In the case of an anterior dislocation, there will be protrusion in the inguinal region or at the perineum with palpable femoral head. The affected lower limb may appear longer than the normal length, with the hip joint in abduction, extorsion and semi–flexion (Fig. 105–2).

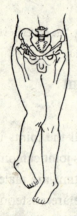 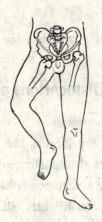

105–1　In a posterior dislocation　　105–2　In an anterior dislocation

Fig. 105　Forms of deformity in dislocations of the hip joint

(3) In the case of a central dislocation, the affected lower limb will become shorter. This injury is frequently associated with a fracture of the acetabulum; and X–ray films of the hip may help establish a correct diagnosis.

Treatment

Manipulative Reduction　　The operation can be performed under peridural anesthesia.

　1.　Posterior dislocations

　(1) Pulling and Lifting Flexed Hip　　The patient lies in dorsal position and the assistant fixes the patient's pelvis by pres-

sing the iliac parts on both sides with hands. Both the knee joint and the hip joint of the affectd limb are flexed in 90 degrees and the operator "rides" on the limb, facing the patient and, then, ① supports the popliteal fossa with the cubital fossa or grasps the popliteal fossa with both hands, ② gradually pulls the femoral segment of the limb so as to let the femoral head get close to the break of the joint sac, ③ simultaneously and slowly rotates the hip joint medially to make the femoral head slip into the acetabulum, ④ mildly rocks the limb until a click sound indicating completion of the reduction is heard, ⑤ slowly lets the affected limb extend straight (Fig. 106).

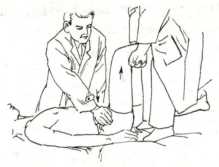

Fig. 106 Reduction of a dislocation of the hip joint by lifting—pulling method

(2) Rotation   The patient lies dorsally and the assistant fixes the patient's pelvis in the same way as in the above method. The operator stands on the patient's affected side, fixes the ankle of the affected limb with a hand while supporting and lifting the popliteal fossa with the cubital fossa of the other hand and, ① lets the affected thigh tightly press against the abdominal wall by adducting the thigh and flexing the hip joint to the utmost, then, ② makes the affected limb abduct, rotate outwardly and extend straight.

In the course of performing these maneuvers ceaselessly, a sound indicating completion of the reduction can be heard (Fig. 107).

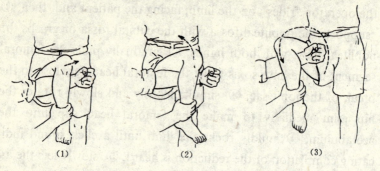

(1) Supporting upward from under the fossa with both the affected knee joint and the hip joint flexing

(2) Tracting, adducting and inwardly turning the limb

(3) Abducting and laterally turning the limb

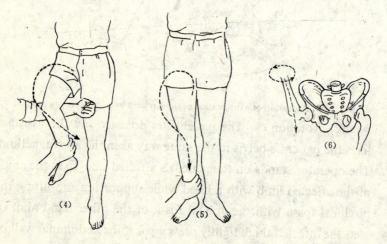

(4) (5) Extending the hip joint and the knee joint until the limb is stretched straight

(6) The track of movement of the femoral shaft during the reduction

Fig. 107 Steps in reduction of a dislocation of the hip joint by rotating method

2. Anterior Dislocations

(1) **Tracting and Pushing**   The patient lies dorsally. Two assistants respectively fix the patient's upper body and the ankle of the affected limb for countertraction. The operator stands on the patient's unaffected side, fixing the iliac bone with one hand and pushing the dislocated femoral head forward with the other hand. The reduction can be completed by harmonious collaboration of the three performers (Fig. 108).

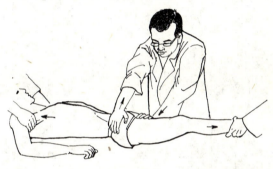

Fig. 108   Reduction of an anterior dislocation of the hip joint

(2) **Counter—rotation**   Preparations and manipulative performances of this method are very much similar to those for posterior dislocations except that the direction of rotation is just to the opposite (Fig. 109).

Immobilization

After the reduction, keep the patient lying dorsally, and skin traction or movement restriction with sand—sacks (as many as 4 —6 ones) should be applied. In the case of posterior dislocations, the hip portion should be maintained in a slightly abducent, neutral and extending position whereas in the case of anterior dislocations the affected limb in a slightly adducent, intorsion and extending position. The fixation should be kept for as long as 3—4 weeks.

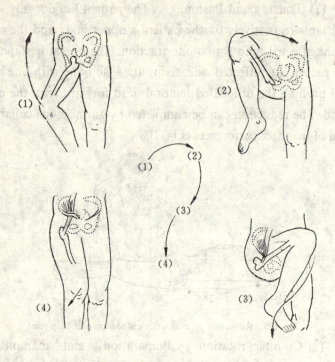

Fig. 109　Reduction of an anterior dislocation of

the hip joint by Counter-rotation

Continuous skeletal traction or skin traction for 6—8 weeks may be needed for central dislocations, which will produce not only an effect of reduction but also an effect of fixation. X-ray films at the initial period of the traction may help the surgeon master how the result of the reduction is. After the traction is discarded, exercises for functional rehabilitation can be practised, but weight-bearing should never be attempted too early. Besides, in certain cases, the doctor has to take into account the healing condition of associated fracture of the acetabulum.

4 Injuries of the Muscles,
Tendons and Ligaments

4.1 Manipulative Maneuvers

Uses of Maneuvers

Manipulatve maneuvers for injuries of the muscles, tendons and ligaments are widely applicable in practice to injuries such as fractures, dislocations, strains and sprains. Included in effects of these maneuvers are activating blood circulation and removing blood stasis, subduing swelling and alleviating pains, relieving rigidity of the muscles and tendons and dredging the channels and collaterals, expelling evil wind and clearing away cold, regulating *Qi* and blood, invigorating flexibility of the joints, releasing spasms of the muscles and tendons and promoting healing and repairment of the injured tissues.

Commonly Used Maneuvers and Their Indications

1. Pressing and Kneading

"Pressing" means to press energetically particular areas or parts of the victim's body with the palmar surface of the thumb, the middle part of the other fingers or the palm—base. The strength to be exerted is dependent upon the need of the condition and the endurance of the patient. "Kneading" means to press a certain area or acupoints with the thumb or other fingers or the palm and knead to and fro or rotatorily, without any release of the thumb, etc.,from the body surface of the patient. When kneading, the performer should practise the maneuver through the wrist movement. The above two maneuvers are frequently combined in clinical practice (Fig. 110).

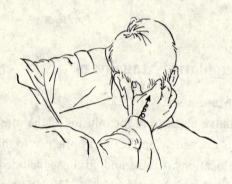

Fig. 110   Pressing—kneading maneuver: Pressing and kneading both
Fengchi (GB20) points with the thumb and the forefinger of a hand

2. Pushing and Rubbing

"Pushing" means to lay the palmar surface of the thumb or the palm—base on a part of the patient, with mild pressure, and to move the thumb or palm—base slowly and steadily to and fro horizontally or vertically along a straight line. "Rubbing" means to move the thumb or palm base with milder pressure and slightly higher speed than "Pushing". The two maneuvers are frequently combined in clinical application. As a rule, pushing upward is followed by rubbing downward, and pushing downward is followed by rubbing upward. If the part to be maneuvered is a small or narrow area, the manipulation is performed with the thumb, and if the part is wide enough, the manipulation is performed with the palm—base. It is significant to maneuver with most appropriate strength well matched by gentleness so as to produce an effect that the patient can feel a penetrative force from the rubbing though the manipulation is mildly done on the skin. Careless rubbing or wiping is in no case acceptable because it is harmful to the cutaneous tissue without a shade of curative effect(Fig. 111).

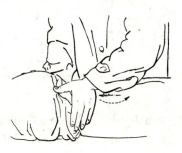

Fig. 111   Pushing—rubbing maneuver: Pushing and rubbing the
lumbodorsal portion with the thenar parts of the hands

This maneuver is a commonly—used treatment for injuries of the muscles and tendons, particularly applicable to old injuries and injuries caused by overstrain.

3. *Boluo* Maneuver

"*Boluo*" means to knead the related part with the thumb in a direction across the channels or collaterals, or to knead or pluck unidirectionally / reciprocatingly with the fingers but the thumb in a direction vertival to the muscle bundle(s) as if to play a plucked string instrument such as a guitar. The strength exerted and the frequency of plucking may vary greatly with different cases. This maneuver has an effect of relieving pains and spasms and releasing adhesion of tissues. It is applicable for cases with contracture and adhesion caused by acute or chronical injuries of muscles and tendons (Fig. 112).

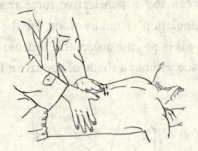

Fig. 112   Bolo maneuver: "Plucking" the back muscles with both thumbs.

(4) Pinching

"Pinching" means to nip muscles or ligaments tight and loose alternately with the thumb and the other fingers(Fig. 113). "Pinching" requires mild exertion of strength of the fingers, but the exertion must be made in a gradual and even way. There seems an intention to lift the muscle or ligament though actually not. During "pinching loose", the fingers should not be off the part being pinched. It is important to perform the maneuver along the muscular direction, in an order from the upper area to the lower portion. The maneuver has such effects as promoting

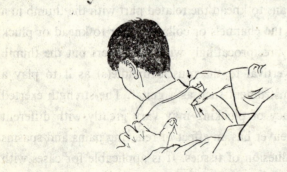

Fig. 113   Pinching maneuver: Pinching the shoulder muscles

flow of *Qi* and blood, removing blood stasis, alleviating pains, relieving spasms and releasing adhesion. It is frequently applied to old injuries, or injuries caused by overstrain, of the neck or limbs. In treatment of acute injuries of the muscles and tendons, this maneuver must be performed carefully in a mild and gentle way.

5. Flexing and Extending

This maneuver is applicable for cases with dysfunction of flexion and / or extension of joints as a means of passive movement. Performance of this maneuver requires the doctor (1) to hold the distal end of the limb to be treated with one hand and fix the joint area with the other hand and,(2) to flex and extend the limb slowly, evenly, continuously and forcibly. The mobility should be increased gradually, from small to as large as tolerable to the patient so as to restore the normal mobile range of the joint (Fig. 114).

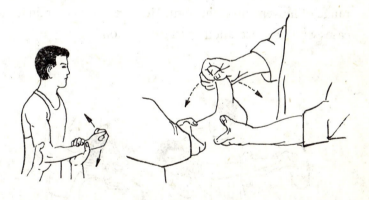

114—1   Flexing and extending   114—2   Flexing and extending
       the elbow joint   the ankle joint

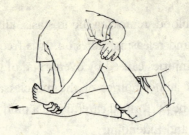

114-3 Flexing and extending the knee joint

Fig.114 Flexing—extending maneuver

6. Rotating and Rocking

This means to rotate, encircle or rock the limb to be treated. The doctor usually fixes the distal end of the limb (Fig. 115) to make it rotate, encircle or sway passively in one or more directions. The performance should be mild and gentle, and the range of movement is increased gradually. It is cautioned not to cause any severe pain to the patient. This maneuver can relax the tendons, relieve spasms, release adhesion and restore the normal range of movement of the joint. However, it is contraindicated to cases with new laceration or fragmentation.

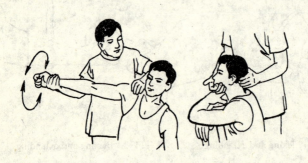

115-1   115-2

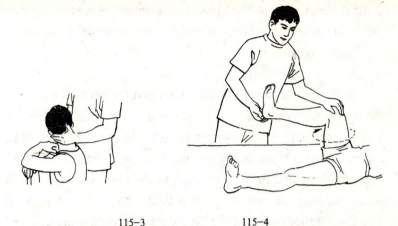

115-3   115-4

Fig. 115   Rotating—rocking maneuver

7. Rhythmic Tapping

This means to tap the part to be treated or the areas thereabout with the palm(s) or fist(s). The tapping must be rhythmic with moderate frequency, repeatedly from the left to the right or from the upper part to the lower. The exertion of strength should be mild and gentle, and a sensation of bounce should be felt by the performer immediately after each tapping (Fig. 116). This maneuver can promote the flow of *Qi* and blood, expel evil wind and cold, remove blood stasis due to injuries and make the

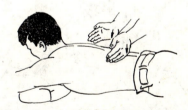

Fig. 116   Rhythmic tapping maneuver: Tapping the

lumbodorsal muscles with hypothenars

patient recover from tiredness. In treatment of new injuries or fresh strain, this maneuver is usually prescribed in combination with other maneuvers.

8. Oblique Pulling

This is a maneuver usually prescribed for patients with injuries of the neck or of lumbar region. For instance, in treatment of a lumbar injury, the patient is told to lie on the right side with a leg extending straight under the other that is in flexion. The operator stands behind the patient, pushing the posterior aspect of the anterosuperior iliac spine of the patient with one hand and pulling the anterior aspect of the shoulder for serveral times of simultaneous performance of pushes and pulls with the hands. The pushing—pulling distance can be gradually increased as the maneuver continues. It is important to advise the patient to try to get as relaxed as possible. When the distance is increased to where the possibly largest mobility is, an effort of steady pushing—pulling to the utmost position can be tried, which may sometimes be followed by a clear sound. If necessary, the patient can be told to lie on the opposite side and the operator changes the posture correspondingly and repeats what is described above (Fig. 117).

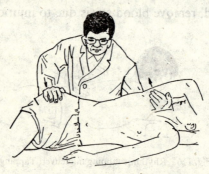

117—1

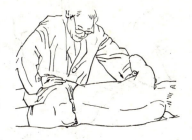

117-2

Fig. 117 Oblique pulling maneuver: Obliquely pulling the lumbar portion.

This maneuver is applicable for cases with injuries of the muscles and tendons, stiff–neck, lumbar sprain, luxation of the lumbar posterior joint, synovial incarceration and lumbar strain because it will produce such effects as releasing adhesion, relieving spasms and restoring functions of the joint.

9. Foulaging

This maneuver requires the operator to place the palms on either side of the affected part of the patient and knead, by relatively moving the palms to and fro, repeatedly from the upper portion to the lower for several times. The compressive strength by the hands should be in good equilibrium and the relative movement mild and harmonious (Fig. 118).

This maneuver is frequently used as the concluding relaxive method of a manipulative therapy. It can regulate the flow of *Qi* and blood in local tissues,relax muscles and tendons and activate the flow of *Qi* and blood in the channels and collaterals. The indications include injuries of muscles and tendons of the limbs, shoulders and knees.

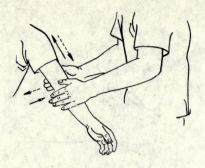

Fig. 118 Foulaging maneuver

10. Rolling

The commonly—used form is "palm—rolling", that is, to put the ulnar side of the dorsum of the hand on the patient's body, with the hand in arc—shape and the wrist flexed, and "roll" the hand to and fro from the upper part to the lower and from the left to the right along the distributive direction of the muscles (Fig. 119). This maneuver is applicable to old injuries and acute or chronical strain of the shoulder, back, the lumbar portion or the clunis region with such effects as promoting the flow of *Qi* and blood in the channels and collaterals, and relieving pains and spasms.

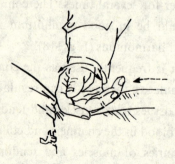

Fig. 119 Rolling maneuver: Rolling the hand on the lumbodorsal portion

11. Tracting and Shaking

The patient lies in dorsal or prone position. The operator fixes the distal end(s) of the limb(s) to be treated and performs downward traction along the axis. An assistant fixes the armpit(s) of the patient and pulls to the opposite direction for countertraction. The operator shakes the limb(s) up and down, or bilaterally, under the traction (Fig. 120).

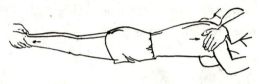

120-1 Tracting

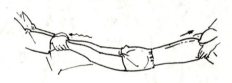

120-2 Shaking

Fig. 120 Tracting-shaking maneuver:Tracting and shaking the lumbar portion

This maneuver can also be used as the concluding maneuver in managing injuries of the muscles and tendons. It can produce such effects as relieving spasms, relaxing muscles and tendons, and releasing adhesion. The indications include acute or chronical injuries of the soft tissues, prolapse of lumbar intervertebral disc, disorder in flexion or extension of the limbs, etc.

12. Dorsal Extension of the Lumbodorsal Region

This method has two modes. (1) The patient and the operator stand back to back and arm in arm. The operator bends a little and bears the patient on his back, getting his / her feet off the ground to let them hang down naturally, and , then, begins to "jump" gently a few times so as to give the patient some shakes (Fig. 121). (2) The patient lies in prone position. The operator fixes the lumbar region of the patient with a hand and raises the affected leg with the other hand, and, then, swiftly lifts the affected leg higher to the posterosuperior direction so as to make the patient's lumbar region overextended (Fig. 122). This mode is also termed as "Raising Affected Leg".

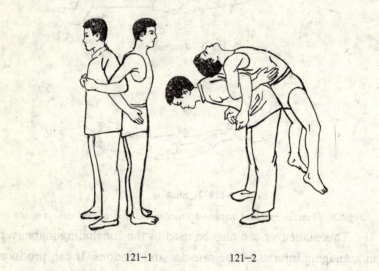

121—1   121—2

Fig. 121   Dorsal extension of the lumbar portion

Both modes of the maneuver are applicable to acute lumbar sprain, prolapse of the lumbar intervertebral disc, etc.

Cautions in Performance of the Maneuvers

1. First and foremost, the operator must have a good command of the condition of the patient and make a correct diagnosis so that the main problems may be ascertained in accordance with holism in TCM. On the basis of this, well—man-

aged maneuvers can be prescribed and performed.

2. The parts or points to be maneuvered must be precisely located and the posture of the patient must be most proper. In addition, it is essential to perform the maneuvers with best coordination of the assistant(s).

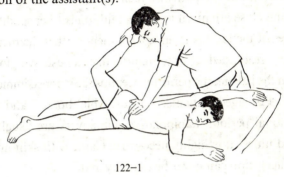

122—1

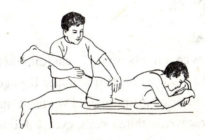

122—2

Fig. 122   Raising the leg dorsally

3. Skillful performance is very important. The maneuver must be penetrating when mildly performed, beneficial when persistent, not superficial when gentle, not detainable when mighty. The operator must perform the maneuvers with agility and nimbleness, consistence and harmoniousness, and well—exerted strength and best rhythm. When the patient has a sensation of soreness, numbness, senselessness, warmth and distention at the

site as the term *Deqi* in TCM implies, good clinical result can be expected.

4. During performance, it is also very significant to advise the patient to relax him— / her—self both mentally and physically. Inquiries about the patient's feelings must be made from time to time and close attention must be paid to his / her condition and the changes of the local part under treatment so that the therapy can be properly readjusted. If any premonitory faintish symptoms are noticed in the patient, the performance must be stopped immediately.

5. For aged patients, the less able—bodied and females in gestational period, manipulative maneuvers are usually not prescribed unless it is highly necessary. Cases with skin infections or local laceration can never be maneuvered.

4.2　Stiff Neck

Pathogenesis

Stiff neck is commonly found in clinical practice. Most of the victims are young people or people under the age of 50. The disease occurs more often in spring and winter. Usually, the patient will naturally recover within a week even without any treatment. However, recurrence is frequently to follow. Stiff neck should be timely and properly treated.

Individuals, especially those who are of weak constitution or who are very tired, may suffer from this disorder if they happen to sleep with their heads raised too high or rested too low as will cause overstrain of the neck muscles. Besides, exposure of the neck to cold wind is also an important pathogen of the disease.

Essentials for Diagnosis

1. Neck pain after sleeping or napping, which forces the patient to turn to a side.

2. Inability to turn the head freely. If a turning of the head is necessary, the patient usually turns the upper part of the body along with the head.

3. Spasms or tenderness of the neck muscles, which may present a cord shape.

Treatment

1. Maneuver Therapy   The patient sits upright on a stool. The operator stands behind the patient and (1) presses him / her on the points of Tianzhu (BL 10), Fengchi (GB20) with the thumb, forefinger and middle finger of a hand for 3—5 minutes, (2) performs Pushing maneuver downward along the muscle a few times, (3) practises Pinching maneuver on the spasmodic muscles for 2—3 minutes, (4) turns or rotates the patient's head clockwise and counterclockwise, or shakes it anteroposteriorly or leftward—rightwardly, (5) supports the patient's occiput with one hand and fixes the lower jaw with the other hand, (6) makes left and right turns of the patient's head until he / she can actively turn the head him— / her—self without difficulty, (7) suddenly turns the patient's head obliquely towards the affected side with careful and proper exertion of strength.

After these steps, a clear sound may occasionally be heard and the patient soon feels all right. To conclude the performance, the operator has to give further mild Pushing—rubbing to the patient's neck and shoulder as a means of regulatory relaxation (Fig. 123).

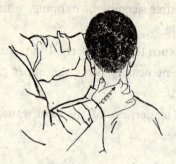

123-1　Pressing—kneading certain acupoints

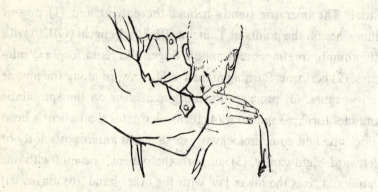

123-2　Pushing and rubbing muscles of the neck and the shoulder

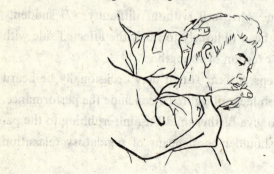

123-3　Abruptly pulling the patient's head to the unaffected side

Fig. 123　Maneuvers applicable to stiff neck

2. Acupuncture Therapy   The points Laozhen (EX26), Houxi(SI 3) can be used as the major points and Xuanzhong(GB39), Kunlun (BL60), Fengchi (GB20) as the adjunct points. Manipulation with strong stimulation is needed.

3. Medication   The drugs to be prescribed should be those of properties of expelling wind and clearing away cold and those of relaxing muscles and tendons and promoting blood circulation. For detailed information, please see relevant sections in General Introduction. *Refuling or Shangshi Zhitong Gao,* etc.can be prescribed for external application to the affected site.

4.3 Scapulohumeral Periarthritis

Pathogenesis

The disease is popularly termed in China as " senile shoulder", "Penetrating arthralgia of the shoulder","condensed arthralgia of the shoulder","frozen shoulder",etc. Most of the victims are people over the age of 50, especially the females. This disease may be produced by such causes as weak constitution of people over 50, overworking, invasion of evil wind, cold and dampness, overdue duration of fixation after a trauma. All of this will lead to chronical inflammation of the peripheral soft tissues around the shoulder, extensive adhesion, and restricted movement of the shoulder joint.

Essentials for Diagnosis

1. Pain of the affected shoulder, especially at night, with evident swelling and restricted movement of the shoulder joint, at the initial stage.

2. Severer restriction of shoulder movement, even unable to

do daily washing, combing and dressing at the advanced stage.

3. Lots of tender points in the area around the shoulder with restriction of both active and passive movement of the joint in adduction, abduction, backward extension, intorsion and upward elevation.

4. Long course of disease, ranging from a few months to 1—2 years, with possible natural cure in some cases in spite of such sequelae as muscular atrophy of the shoulder area and even stiff shoulder joint due to long—term illness.

Treatment

1. Maneuver Therapy   The patient sits on a stool. The operator stands on the affected side of the patient and (1) fixes the wrist of the affected limb with one hand, and performs such maneuvers as tracting, shaking, rocking and rotating, (2) places the thumb, forefinger and middle finger of the other hand on the patient's affcted shoulder, thumb on the anterior aspect and the other two fingers on the posterior, to perform pinching and pres- sing—kneading. The performance of each hand must be well coordinated with that of the other; the exertion of strength as well as the range of movement should be gradually increased until the patient's shoulder is fully invigorated. Then the affected upper

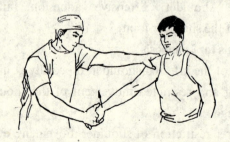

124—1   Pronating the affected limb under traction

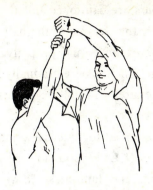

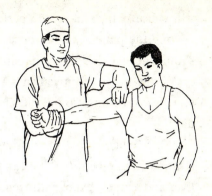

124–2 Raising the limb above the head

124–3 Abducting the limb with simultaneous extortion

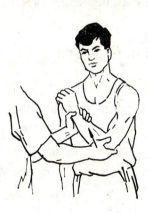

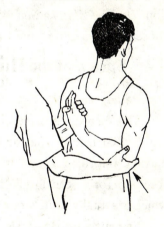

124–4 Adducting the limb to make it touch the other shoulder

124–5 Introsion of the limb with dorsal extension

Fig. 124 Maneuver applicable to scapulohumeral periarthritis

limb should be made to raise up, abduct, rotate laterally, adduct, extend backwardly and rotate medially (Fig. 124).

The maneuvers and the passive movements mentioned above

will cause pain, and so the performers are cautioned not to go beyong the patient's endurance. After the treatment, the patient should persist in doing rehabilitation exercises and properly increase the range of movement. As the functions are gradually restored, local pains around the shoulder area will subside day after day.

2. Medication   The drugs prescribed for internal administration should be those that can tonify *Qi* and blood, nourish the liver and kidney, expel pathogenic wind and dampness and warm the meridian channels. and collaterals, The frequently prescribed recipe is modified *Duhuo Jisheng Tang* (53). For external application, *Huoxue Zhitong San* (45), No 2 Washing Recipe (47) can be chosen for fumigation and washing.

4.4   Sprain of the Hip Joint in Children

Pathogenesis

This disorder is mostly found in children at the age of 7—10, more often in girls than in boys. The mechanism of the injury may be improper action in running, jumping or dancing. The common form seen in clinical practice is a sprain on one side, which is actually acute strain of the hip muscles and tendons.

Essentisla for Diagnosis

1. A history of moderate trauma or strain.

2. Severe pain at a hip one night after a trauma despite indistinct symptoms on the day of injury. The child walks like a cripple or simply refuses to walk.

3. The pain does not hurt when the patient is at rest, but if the child walks, it definitely does though it seems to begin sub-

siding when the hip joint is fairly invigorated. The child will suffer again if he / she tries to walk after a rest.

4. The affected lower limb may become longer than the unaffected, by 1.5—2cm in some cases. Strained muscles of the affected hip side can be observed, (in slight abduction and extorsion). Passive adduction and intorsion of the hip joint will cause pain with a sensation of elastic—like—fixation.

5. In contrast to 4, a few cases may have a shorted affected lower limb, which is in slight adduction and intorsion, than the unaffected, with restricted abduction and extorsion of the hip joint. Passive abduction will cause pain.

6. Flexion and extension of the affected limb is not restricted. There are no general symptoms, nor any abnormal findings in X—ray films.

Treatment

1. Maneuver Therapy   The child is told first to lie in prone position and the operator performs Pushing—rubbing maneuver with a palm on the area around the child's affected hip for 3—5 minutes so as to relax the muscles. Then the child lies dorsally and an assistant fixes his / her pelvis with both hands. The operator fixes the child's affected lower limb, one hand holding the knee and the other taking the ankle, and flexes the hip joint and the knee joint. If the patient happens to have a longer affected limb due to the injury, the operator should make adduction and intorsion of the hip joint and extend it afterwards. This process should be repeated 5—10 times, that is, until the lower limbs regain their equal lengths. The performance requires gradual increase of the range of movement and slow exertion of strength. In no case can the operator neglect the child's endur-

ance. If the child has got a shorter lower limb after the injury, the process should be changed to " flexion plus abduction—extorsion—extension" . The other requirements are similar (Fig. 125).

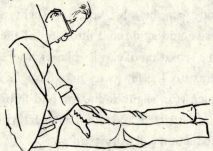

125-1　Pushing and rubbing the gluteal muscles

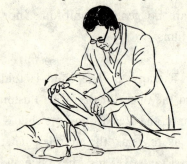

125-2　Flexing, adducting and medially turning the affected limb

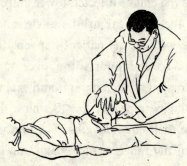

125-3　Flexing, abducting and laterally turning the affected limb

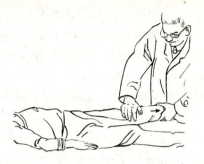

125—4 Medially turning and stretching straight the affected limb

Fig. 125 Maneavers applicable to sprains of the hip joint in children

The child should be prescribed a good rest for 1—3 days after the reduction. In addition, pressing—kneading and pushing—rubbing can be given to the affected hip, once a day.

2. Medication   *Huoxue Quyu Pian* (54), *Shujin Huoxue Pian* (55) , etc. are usually prescribed for oral intake. Besides, *Huoxue Zhitong San* (45) can be used for decoction hotcompress.

4.5 Acute Lumbar Sprain

Pathogenesis

This injury is frequently produced by improper exertion of strength in physical labour. For instance, if a person bends down with legs extending straight when carrying heavy objects, lumbar sprain will often be the result. The disease is clinically common, especially in youth and people at the age of 40—50.

Essentials for Diagnosis

1. A history of acute lumbar strain.

2. Local pain which becomes severer when coughing, sneezing or stooping down, but not worse when extending the lumbar

portion. The pain may be relieved when the patient is at rest. The patient is unable to stretch the spine straight and tends to support the lateral sides of the waist, an instinctive posture of standing akimbo to help bear the body weight. Movement of the lumbar portion is obviously restricted and normal walking has become a problem.

3. Tenderness at the points between or besides the spinous processes of the lumbar vertebrae, or at the sacrospinal muscle areas.

Treatment

1. Maneuver Therapy   The patient lies in prone position. The operator performs Pressing—kneading with thumbs on the patient's back along the spine from the shoulder height downward to the sacrococcygeal. When the thumbs pass across each of the following acupoints Shenshu (BL23), Zhishi (BL52), Dachangshu (BL25), Chengfu (BL36), Weizhong (BL40) and Chengshan (BL57), they should be kept there temporarily and press—knead each points three rounds. The above—described process should be repeated twice. Then, with a hand fixing the injury site of the patient and the other hand holding the distal segment of the affected thigh, the operator elevates the limb posterosuperiorly three times. For the 3rd time, the force exerted can be fairly greater, which is sometimes directly followed by a "click". To conclude the treatment, tapping a few times on either side of the spine is necessary. Posterior to the maneuver therapy, the lumbar portion of the patient must be refrained from any exertion or movement and bed rest on a board bed for 2 weeks should be prescribed for better recovery (Fig. 126).

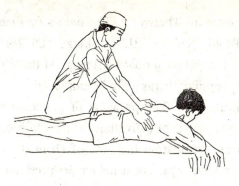

126-1　Kneading and pressing

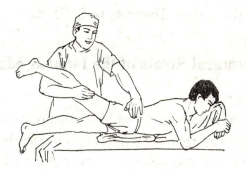

126-2　Raising the affected lower limb

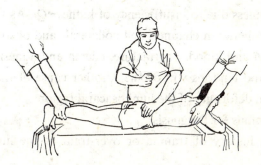

126-3　"Tapping" the lumbar soft tissues

Fig. 126　Manipulative maneuvers for soft tissue injuries of the lumbar portion

2. Acupuncture Therpy   The points frequently used are Weizhong (BL40), Kunlun (BL60), Shuigou(DU26) and Shenshu (BL23). The stimulation should be strong. At the site where there is tenderness, cupping therapy can be employed.

3. Medication   The principle of medication is to select drugs of the properties of activating the flow of blood to remove blood stasis and regulating the flow of *Qi* in the channels and collaterals to relieve pain. The usual recipes prescribed are *Fuyuan Huoxue Tang* (1), *Huoxue Quyu Tang* (3), *Dieda Wan* (56), etc. For external use, *Quyu Xiaozhong Gao* (57) can be applied to the injured site.

4.6   Chronical Strain of the Lumbar Muscles

Pathogenesis

This disease may be caused by constantly prolonged flexion of the lumbar portion or by prolonged weight-bearing in improper posture. It may also be the result of acute lumbar injury that has not yet been treated for too long a period. In any of the cases, the patient may become vulnerable to evils of wind, cold and dampness due to insufficiency of kidney—*Qi*. As the evils linger in the meridian channels and collaterals and obstruct normal flow of *Qi* and blood, contracture, edema and adhesion of local muscles and tendons will occur. Another cause of the disease is congenital deformity of the lumbosacaral region.

Essentials for Diagnosis

1. A history of trauma or overstrain of the lumbosacaral portion.

2. Frequent vague pain which attacks repeatedly and may

become severer now when tired and less severe then after a good rest. In some cases, there is also distending pain at the upper part of the clunis or of the thigh.

3. Tenderness at the spinous or transverse processes of the lumbar vertebrae, beside the spinous processes, or at the lumbosacaral joint, depending upon where the strain exists.

4. In some cases, X—ray films of the lumbosacaral portion may reveal hyperplasia of the vertebral body, osteoporosis and congenital deformity of the lumbosacaral portion.

Treatment

1. Maneuver Therapy   The treatment is similar to that used for acute lumbar sprain.Locate the site of tenderness and perform maneuvers in the same way as in treatment of acute lumbar sprain.It is also practical to employ Oblique—elevating,but the doctor must be cautious not to raise or pull the lower limbs in the case of aged patients or patients with invasion of evil wind,cold and dampness as these forcible maneuvers prove improper for them.The treatment can be practised once every other day and a course takes ten such treatments.

2. Acupuncture Therapy   The points frequently selected as main points are Shen—shu (BL23),Mingmen (DU4),Yaoyangguan (DU3),Weizhong (BL40) and Kunlun (BL60). The manipulation should be of reinforcement. In addition,puncturing with warmed needles heated by burning moxa, moxibustion and cupping therapy can be prescribed.

3. Medication   The principle is to warm the channels and collaterals to promote the flow of *Qi* and blood and to tonify the liver and kidney. The commonly prescribed recipe is modified *Duhuo Jisheng Tang* (53) or *Da Huoluo Dan*(58). For cases with

osteoporosis, *Guzhi Zhengsheng Wan* (59) can be added to the prescription. If the case is associated with invasion of pathogenic wind and cold, *Xiao Huoluo Dan* (60) can be given as a coordinative recipe, and *Zhengjiang Gao* (61) for external application.

The patient should be advised to take an active part in appropriate physical exercises, to take precaution against invasion of cold and dampness,to control sexual life and not to get exhausted.

4.7 Prolapse of Lumbar Intervertebral Disc

Pathogenesis

An intervertebral disc consists of a phaline cartilage disc,a fibrous ring and a pulpiform neucleus. The fibrous ring is a cartilage fibrous tissue,tough and tenacious. It is connected with the vertebral body and the upper and lower cartilage discs,effectively keeping the pulpiform neucleus from prolapsing in all directions. The pulpiform neucleus is elastic enough and is constrained between the cartilage disc and the fibrous ring. Once the pulpiform neucleus is under too great a pressure,whatever origin the pressure comes from,it may break through the fibrous ring and get out of place. The usual form is posterior prolapse,which will produce pressure symptoms of the nervous roots,the cauda equina nerve and the spinal cord.

Most victims of the disease are people at the age of 20—40,especially the males. The disease frequently follows an acute lumbar sprain or great tiredness. The injury mostly sits between L4 and L5 or between L5 and S1.

Essential for Diagnosis

1. Sudden pain in the lumbar region,with or without a history of trauma,which may radiate towards the posterior aspect of the thigh,the lateral aspect of the leg or foot. The pain hurts terribly in acute cases;in patients with chronical prolapse of the lumbar intervertebral disc,the pain may become worse or less from time to time.

2. Restricted movement of the lumbar portion. The physiological forward bending of the lumbar portion vanishes,but there is lateral flexion,mostly towards the affected side (Fig. 127).

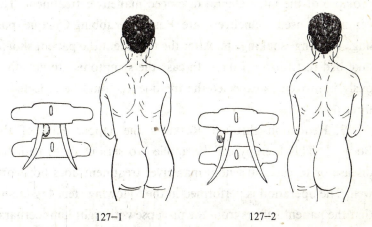

127-1   127-2

Fig. 127   Relation between nerve involvement and prolapse
of the lumbar interver tebral disc

3. Tenderness around the spinous process of the corresponding vertebral body,which may radiate downward.

4. Positive result in Laseque's test.The tensile force of the crural muscles and the strength of the extensor / flexor digitorum are weakened. Knee reflex and Achilles jerk are debilitated or incapacitated.

5. Narrowing of intervertebral space (or narrower in the an-

terior part and wider in the posterior part) between the corresponding vertebrae with possible labiate hyperplasia along the vertebral edge in X—ray films. It is possible to locate the injury site in iodized oil rentgenograph or in CT photograph.

Treatment

1. During acute attack,the patient should be kept in bed for two weeks and some cases with fresh mild prolapse will be relieved as the pulpiform neucleus has returned to its normal position in the fibrous ring.

2. Maneuver Therapy   Most of the patients with prolapse of the intervetebral disc need maneuver treatment. The commonly used maneuvers are Pushing—rubbing,Oblique—pulling. Tracting—shaking,etc. After the treatment,the patient should take bed rest for 5—7 days. In case the symptoms are not obviously improved as expected,the treatment should be repeated in three days.

3. Reduction through Rotating the Upper Part of the Body   This therapy can be applied to serious cases with the disease or to cases in whom maneuver treatment does not work well. The operation is performed in the following steps (assuming that the patient suffers from the prolapse with right lumbocruaral pain and a displaced spinous process toward the right side):

The patient sits on a stool and an assistant fixes his / her affected lower limb and the pelvis.

The operator stands on the patient's affected side and (1)fixes the posterior part of the patient's neck with the right hand (the arm under the patient's armpit),making the patient bow down the head slightly,(2)places the left thumb on the prolapsed spinous process,(3)forcibly presses the patient's neck to bring the upper part of his / her body down forwardly as much as possible (about bending down to 80—90 degrees),(4)pulls the upper part of the body of the patient with the right hand, making it turn towards the right side to the utmost while pushing the prolapsed spinous process to the left side with the right thumb.

This pulling—plus—pushing maneuver is often followed by a snap from the lumbar portion. If such a sound is not heard,it is necessary to repeat the maneuver. Once the sound comes, the patient will usually be relieved from the pain immediately.

It is important to advise the patient to lie on a board bed for 5—7 days after the operation (Fig. 128).

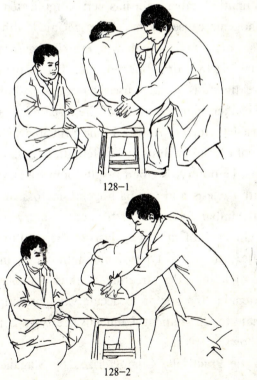

128—1

128—2

Fig. 128   Reduction of prolapse of the lumbar intervertebral disc by rotating maneuver

4. Sustained Traction Therapy　　This method needs a pelvic traction belt or a traction bed. Each lateral weight for traction may be 10—20 kg, and the traction can be applied 1—2 hours a time,once a day. If the therapy is combined with local Pressing—kneading,acupuncture treatment or local block technique,early better result can be expected.

4.8　Administration of Chinese Medicines in the Treatment of Traumatic Lumbar Pain

Traumatic lumbar pain has very complicated pathogenesis and pathogenic causes. It may be associated with pathological changes of the lumbar muscles,ligaments, bones, joints,intervertebral discs, nerves, etc. This explains why combined treatment is usually used clinically. Administration of Chinese medicines in treatment of the disease is one of the commonly used therapies. However, the principle of treatment on the basis of overall analysis and differentiation of symptoms and signs must be observed. Good results cannot be expected otherwise. Pathogenesis and the pathogenic factors of the acute or chronical lumbar pain due to traumatic injury must be made clear on the basis of careful analysis of the symptoms and signs. Then differentiation of types of the pain can be made ,and the principle guiding the treatment thus established,which,in turn,will enable the doctor to decide what prescription is most appropriate for the patient. Clinically,the types commonly seen are as follows:

1. Type Practically Characterized by Stagancy of *Qi* and Blood Stasis

Patients with this type of pain are characterized by a definite history of trauma. The pain is a twinge and just "stays" at a definite place where there is tenderness or tumefaction and ecchymosis. In a moderate case,the patient may just feel an endurable mild pain when bending the waist or looking up. In a severe case,the victim can not turn laterally at all,the patient's tongue looks dark—purplish and the pulse feels hesitant. This type may be found in patients with sprain or contusion of lumbar muscles and ligaments,acute lumbomuscular strain,acute prolapse of the lumbar intervertebral disc,and disorder of posterior lumbovertebral joint.

The principle of treatment is to activate the flow of blood to remove blood stasis and regulate the flow of *Qi* to relieve pain. The prescriptions may be modified *Fuyuan Huoxue Tang* (1), *Shengtong Zhuyu Tang*(62),or proprietary medicines such as *Huoxue Quyu Pian*(54), *Dieda Wan* (56) and *Yunnan Baiyao*(63),all for oral administration.

2. Type Practically Characterized by Blockage in the Channels and Collaterals

Patients with this type of pain are characterized by a long duration of illness with dull pain in the lumbar region,which sometimes involves the back,clunis and leg. The patient may also have a sensation of numbness and stickiness in these parts which becomes severer or milder now and then. Moderate movement may slightly relieve the pain,but a little more will worsen it. There may be a relatively broader area of tenderness due to prolonged stagnation of *Qi* and blood stasis that blocks free passage of the meridians. This type can be found in patients with chronical strain,lumbodorsal myofibrositis,congenital deformity of lumbodorsal structure,etc.

The principle of treatment for this type is to activate blood circulation and promote the flow of *Qi,* to relax the muscles and tendons and invigorate the meridian passage. The prescription to be used is modified *Tiaorong Huoluo Yin* (64). Radix Dipsaci, Squama Manitis and Radix Linderae can be added to the prescription according to practical need. The medication can also be composed of internal administration of *Shujin Huoxue Pian* (55) and external application of *Goupi Gao* (34) or *Zhengjiang Gao* (61).

3. Type Practically Characterized by Deficiency of *Yin* of the Liver and Kidney and Deficiency of *Yang* of the Kidney

Patients with this type of pain are characterized by a very long course of disease. The pain is primarily a sore with a feeling of weakness that seems to become less disturbing when the affected parts gets pressed and kneaded. The victim suffers from weakness of the lumbar portion and the knees,especially when tired. However,the pain subsides when the patient lies down . A case with deficiency of *Yang* may show asthenia and have a whitish face with a light—coloured tongue and a sinking,thready pulse. The limbs are not warm enough. A case with deficiency of *Yin* may have a dry mouth and throat with a reddish tongue and only a little tongur fur. The patient may suffer from insomnia and vexation and a feverish sensation in the palms and soles. The pulse is thready and rapid. This type can be found in patients of constant weak constitutions and feeble muscles,tendons and bones who happen to be injured or strained.

The principle of treatment is to tonify the kidney. Cases with *Yang*—deficiency should be treated with modified *Yougui*

Wan (65) that can warm and nourish kidney–*Yang* and cases with *Yin*–deficiency by modified *Zuogui Wan* (66) that can nourish kidney–*Yin*. If the lumbar pain is obstinate and if it is too difficult to distinguish between *Yin*–deficiency and *Yang*–deficiency, *Qinge Wan* (67),sometimes plus *Shujin Huoxue Pian* (55) and *Zhuangyao Jianshen Wan* (51) ,can be prescribed.

4. Type Practically Characterized by Invasion of Pathogenic Wind,Cold and Dampness

Patients with this type of pain are characterized by chronical lumbar pain. The pain is felt to be cold and sticky. There is no relief of the pain even when the patient lies still for a rest. Cloudy or rainy weather will make the pain severer,and application of warmth to the affected area can alleviate it. The patient has a whitish and greasy tongue fur and a sinking,slow and loose pulse. This type can be found in cases with chronical strain or with old injuries if they are further invaded by evil wind,cold and dampness.

The principle of treatment is to expel cold and clear away dampness,and to warm the channels and collaterals to promote the flow of *Qi*. The usual prescription is modified *Magui Wenjing Tang* (22) or *Xiao Huoluo Dan* (60) or *Shenjin Pian* (50). In addition, *Zhengjiang Gao Yao*(61) and *Kanli Sha* (48) can be given for external application.

5　Osteoarticular Infections

5.1　Suppurative Arthritis

Clinically, suppurative arthritis is mostly found in children,more often in boys than in girls. The joint involved is primarily either the hip joint or the knee joint,and secondarily the shoulder joint,or the elbow joint or the ankle joint. In any case,only one joint is diseased.

Pathogenesis

1. Invasion of Pathogenic Summer—heat and Dampness　During the period between mid—summer and mid—autumn, there is normally too much sun and dampness. A person may easily be exposed to them and is succeptible to their invasion.If the person then takes off his／her clothing to lie down in a cool environment to comfort him—／her—self,the normal cool may become pathogenic,hindering the body from dispersing the heat and dampness,and the two evils will thus reside between the *Ying* system and the *Wei* system. Hence the disease.

2. Residual Toxic Pathogens　Patients who were ill with sores or furuncles may once again be victims after recovery from the sores and furuncles because the toxic evils had invaded into the channels and collaterals and finally into the joint.

3. Blood Stasis　Patients with overwork or trauma may

have their limbs injured with stasis and stagnation of the stasis may turn into evil heat. Once the evil heat has invaded into any of the succeptible joints,the disease will occur.

In Western medicine,the pathogens of the disease are mostly staphylococus aureus,and sometimes diplococus pneumoniae or diplococus meningitidis. The route of infection may be through blood circulation or through pathogen—spreading from adjacent parts where there has been osteomyelitis. Open injury to the joint may also lead to the infection. The pathological manifestations include:(1) The synovium first gets conjested and distended,accompanied with leokocyte infiltration and increased exudate which presents a kind of serous fluid at the initial stage. As the articular cartilage remains uninvolved then,the patient can be completely cured by prompt proper treatment and the joint functions protected. On the other hand,in case the lesion continues,developed congestion,pachynsis or even necrosis of the synovium will be the result,causing impairment of the articular cartilage with suppurative exudate and there will be residual dysfunction of the joint.

Essentials for Diagnosis

1. Sudden onset with general symptoms such as malaise,anorexia,fever (body temperature being as high as $38.5\,°C — 40\,°C$),intolerance of cold,and sweating.

2. Congestion of the joint with pain and increased skin temperature. To relieve him— / her—self from the pain,the patient usually takes a particular posture to relax the joint,such as flexing the hip joint in an abducent and extorsion position or flexing the knee joint half way.

3. Dislocation or semi—luxation of the joint due to enlarged

sac (caused by accumulation of exudate) and muscular spasms.

4. Increased WBC, N and ESR in laboratary examination.

5. Broadened articular cavity and congested soft tissues in X—ray films at the initial stage. If there is impairment of the articular surface,the joint space will become narrower with adjacent osteoporosis and the joint will finally turn stiff with disappearance of the joint space.

6. To establish the diagnosis,it is very important to perform puncture for joint fluid examination and bacterial culture of the joint fluid. Subsequent drug sensitivity test of the bateria is also of great significance.

Treatment

1. At the Initial Stage   On the basis of the result in the bacterial culture and drug sensitivity test,sufficient quantities of effective anti biotic(s) should be used. In children and cases of severe condition,attention must be paid to cooling down the body temperature, fluid infusion,correction of metabolic imbalance of water and electrolytes, reinforcement of nutrient supplement and strengthening the body resistence.

As a measure of prophylaxis of deformity,proper local immobilization should be given,for it can prevent deformation of the joint due to body—weight pressure and relieve the pain as well as muscular spasms.

For a minor and superficial joint,puncture can be performed once a day. The dropsy must be thoroughly aspirated and the joint sac washed with normal saline and injected with effective antibiotic(s).

For a great joint such as the knee joint, if it is comfirmed after puncture that there exists dropsy or pus,two points must be selected for trocar puncture. After the trocars have been inserted into the joint sac,the needles are withdrawn,leaving the casings still in the sac. Two plastic or silica—lined pipes of 3—mm diameter are brought into the sac through the casings and left there. The pipes are then fixed on the skin with adhesive tapes,the one at the higher position as the inlet for daily dropping of antibiotic(s) and saline (2 000—3 000 ml), and the other at the lower position as the outlet for drainage of the dropsy or pus. A negative—pressure aspirating device is applied to the outlet. The above management will make it possible to remove the dropsy or pus and wash the sac successively until the inflammation is completely under control.

If it is necessary,open drainage can be performed by incision of the joint sac, and two pipes are respectively fixed at the upper end and the lower end of the opening for washing and drainage,once a day,after the incision is satured.

2. At the Advanced Stage   For cases with dislocation or semi—luxation of the joint,reduction through traction followed by splint / plaster fixation is necessary. Surgical treatment should be taken into consideration if there is dysfunction of the joint resulting from adhesion or deformity.

3. Administration of Chinese Medicines on the Basis of Overall Analysis and Differentiation of Symptoms and Signs   Administration of Chinese medicines should follow the principle of "elimination"(removing stagnant Qi and blood stasis), "reinforcement"(invigorating and nourishing vital Qi and blood to remove toxins of suppurative infections) and "tonification"(giving tonics).

At the acute stage,stress should be put on clearing away

heat and toxic materials and activating blood flow to remove obstruction in the channels. The proper prescription is modified *Wuwei Xiaodu Yin* (5).

When abscess has already begun to take shape,but not yet ulcerated,stress should be put on clearing away heat and toxic materials and on reinforcing the body vital *Qi* to promote pus—discharge. The usual prescription is modified *Tounong San* (68).

However,at the advanced stage when the abscess has begun to ulcerate with thin discharge and there is whitish granulation,a sign indicating retardation of wound healing,the course must have been very long and the patient must have been suffering from deficiency of both *Qi* and blood. The principle of treatment is therefore to invigorate *Qi* and enrich blood. The prescription to be used is *Bazheng Tang* (14).

External treatment with Chinese Medicine

At the initial stage, *Jinhuang Gao* (20), *Sihuang Gao* (28),etc. can be prescribed for external application. When the wound begins to heal, *Shengji Yuhong Gao* (30) will be beneficial.

Whether at the initial stage or after ulceration, *Jiedu Xiyao* (69) can be prescribed for external use,that is ,to wash the affected joint with the decoction of the drugs. Dressing change is routine for cases with ulceration after fumigation or washing.

5.2 Suppurative Osteomyelitis

Suppurative osteomyelitis is infection of the "bone" caused by suppurative bacteria. The "bone" here means such osseous tissues as bone marrow,substance of bone,periost,etc. Besides,even the soft tissues around the bone may be involved. In terms of TCM, this case is referred to as *Fuguju*.

Victims afflicted with this disease are mostly children younger than 10 years old. About 90% of the patients are youngsters under the age of 16, boys outnumbering girls. In most instances, the disease attacks the mytaphysis of the limbs, especially the mytaphysis of the tibia. Other vulnerable bones include the femur, the humerus and the radius. The pathogens most commonly found are staphylococus aureus (about 80% of all).

Pathogenesis

Acute hematogenous osteomyelitis is due to invasion of suppurative bacteria into the blood. Among the common essential foci are boil, carbuncle, follicolitis, tonsillitis and otitis media. Occasionally, a definite essential focus cannot be found. In any case, there must be pathogenic bacteria in the blood. However, the premise can not easily lead to the disease without an inducing factor such as weakened resistance due to prolonged illness, overwork, being ill with cold and local interruption of blood circulation in capillaries of the bone on account of capillary rapture, hemorrhage, stasis, which will provide a chance for the bacteria to settle down there to reproduce themselves. The severity of the symptoms is dependent upon the toxicity of the bacteria; the stronger the toxicity of the bacteria, the severer the symptoms.

Pathological Change and Development   Hemologenous osteomyelitis occurs mostly at the metaphysis of a long bone where the bone contains abundant spongiosa. In children, a wide—spread terminal capillary net—work exists at the metaphysis of a long bone and the blood flow there is slow. This provides a good shelter for the bacteria to reside and reproduce and finally to form emboli. Apart from this, local trauma may cause mild bleeding within osseous tissues and destruction of cells, both being favourable conditons for bacterial reproduction. A focus will then arise there that begins with concentration of neutrophil and serus exudation which will gradually become suppurative. The focus may.

1. be rapidly controlled and absorbed if the body resistance of the patient is powerful or the toxicity of the bacteria is mild and if proper treatment is promptly given.

2. not continue to develop but become chronical if the patient's body resistance is strong enough or the bacterial toxicity is weak. (The result is localized bone abscess.)

3. spread wider with inflammatory proliferation due to the fact that, as a rule, the toxicity of the bacteria is radical and the patient happens to be in poor health.

If the focus diffuses wider and perforates through the metaphysis bone substance, the abscess may amass under the periost, causing the periost to cleave from the bone to form subperiosteal abscess. The focus may further break through the periost to form subcutaneous abscess.

If the focus spreads within the marrow cavity, wide osteomyelitis may develop.

If the focus invades into the joint sac, it may lead to suppurative arthritis.

A bone layer may originate from the cleaved periost when subperiosteal abscess forms. This layer can gradually grow thicker and thicker and finally forms a cover outside the bone which cuts off blood supply for the diaphysis from the periost.

This plus embolism in the nourishing vessels for the bone will lead to wide osteonecrosis and the parts involved may become dead and completely isolated from the living bone (Fig. 129).

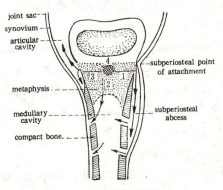

joint sac
synovium
articular cavity
subperiosteal point of attachment
metaphysis
medullary cavity
subperiosteal abcess
compact bone

1,2,3   The metastasic directions

4   The primary focus

Fig. 129   Metastasis of acute osteomyelitis

Essentials for Diagnosis

1. The Acute Stage

The disease has a sudden onset. The patient suffers from local pain, general malaise, tiredness, subsequent shiver and persistent high fever (39℃—40℃)in spite of perspiration. The appetite is poor and the tongue is reddish with yellowish greasy fur. The pulse proves slippery and rapid. Sometimes such toxic symptoms as nausea, vomiting, and enlarged liver and spleen can be observed.

These manifestations may be followed by intensified throbbing pain in the affected limb that will be completely restricted from any movement. The limb is circularly swollen, and the skin over the focus will have a burning sensation. There is evident tenderness at the metaphysis with muscular spasms in the near areas. The affected joint flexes and the child strongly rejects any examination.

Lab test shows increased hemogram (WBC as high as 30000 or more) and accelerated blood sedimentation rate. Blood culture proves positive.

At the initial stage, X—ray examination does not reveal any change in the bone substance but congestion of the soft tissues. Two weeks later, a same examination may present some periost response with bony destruction at the metaphysis. Dead bone can be found in 4 weeks.

2. The Chronical Stage

One or more sinuses usually appear that repeatedly discharge suppurative fluids and dead bone substances. The skin around the fistula grows thicker to form a kind of scar structure with pigmentation. If discharge of the suppurative fluids meets with difficulties, local swelling with intensified pain will occur in association with fever and general malaise.

If the disease is complicated with pathological fracture or dislocation, there will appear certain deformity. Cases with prolonged course may become pathologically thin with muscular atrophy of the affected limb. Other symptoms include a whitish face, listlessness, acratia, dizziness and night sweating.

In X—ray examinations, dead bone, cavity and shell—bone can be found, but the medullary cavity may occasionally be invisible.

Treatment

1. Acute Osteomyelitis

The treatment aims at early control of development of inflammation so as to prevent formation of any dead bone. At the initial stage, therefore, sufficient quantities of effective antibiotic(s) should be administered. This makes it possible to control further development of the disease or even to cure the disease completely. The treatment measures include.

(1) local drainage   After a definite diagnosis of the disease has been established, if administration of the chosen antibiotic(s) cannot control the symptoms, and puncture has affirmed that there is suppurative fluid under the periost or within the medullary cavity, local drainage should be performed so as to reduce the fluid pressure:① Make an incision, parallel to the bone, at the tenderest site of the metaphysis. ② Drill a series of holes with a bonedrill. If the pus in the medullary cavity should prove too much to be drained completely through the holes, an opening by a bone chisel may be necessary for two weeks 'drainage—washing.This requires to make an opening on the metaphysis and insert two pipes into the cavity for continual draining and rinsing with saline solution of effective antibiotic(s), 2 000 ml per day.

(2) Local Immobilization   The affected limb can be immobilized with plaster—supportor or skin traction so as to relieve muscular spasm and pain. It can also prevent subsequent fracture or dislocation.

(3) Support Therapy   Fluid infusion is necessary to maintain good balance between water and electrolytes. Blood transfusion (small quantities for many times) and large doses of Vitamin C are greatly helpful. The patient should also be given high—protein diet.

Administration of Chinese Medicines

Cases without pus at the initial stage should be treated

under the principle of clearing away heat and toxic materials, removing dampness and evacuating stagnated substances. A modified combined recipe of *Wuwei Xiaodu Yin* (5) and *Huanglian Jiedu Tang* (70) can be prescribed.

Cases with pus that has not yet ulcerated or with obstructed discharge of the pus should be treated under the principle of eliminating toxins from within the body to invigorate pus—drainage. The usually prescribed recipe is modified *Tuoli Xiaodu Yin* (71). The modification is dependent upon the condition of the patient. To the prescription, Gypsum Fibrosum, Folium Isatidis and Herba Patriniae are added for patients with fever, restlessness and thirst. Resina Boswelliae Carterii and Resina Commiphorae Myrrhae for patients with definite pain, Radix Ginseng and Radix Astragali seu Hedysari for patients with *Qi*—deficiency; Radix Rehmanniae, Radix Scrophulariae, Cortex Montan Radicis and Herba Dendrobii for patients with hyperactivity of fire due to *Yin*—deficiency; and *Angong Niuhuang Wan* (72) for patients with coma and delirium.

Besides, *Jinhuang Gao* (27), etc. can be prescribed for external application.

2. Chronical Osteomyelitis

Chronical osteomyelitis is usually the result of development of acute osteomyelitis that was not timely cured and so turned into a long—term condition. The patient is generally emaciated with deficiency of both *Qi* and blood and deficiency of both the spleen and kidney. There are also some remains of the pathogenic toxins. The principle of treatment of the condition is therefore to tonify blood and reinforce *Qi* and to warm the kidney and strengthen the spleen. The usual prescription is modified

Yanghe Tang:

Radix Astragali seu Hedysari	30 g
Radix Angelicae Sinensis	15 g
Radix Paeoniae Rubra	15 g
Radix Paeoniae Alba	15 g
Rhizoma Atractylodis Macrocephalae	9 g
Rhizoma Rehmanniae Praeparatae	30 g
Semen Sinapis Albae	6 g
Colla Cornus Cervi	9 g
(for temporary infusion)	
Poria	9 g
Fructus Psoraleae	9 g
Cortex Phellodendri	9 g
Radix Glycyrrhizae	3 g

Administration: Decoct these drugs with a proper amount of water and take the decoction.

For cases with poor appetite, *Xiangsha Liujunzi Tang* (73) can be prescribed. If the patient suffers from deficiency of both *Qi* and blood, the remedy is *Bazhen Tang* (14).

There are also some ointments, powders and pellets for external application. The frequently prescribed is *Dahuang Ruangao* (74) or *Shengji Yuhong Gao* (30). *Jiuyi Dan* (38) can be used along with the above—mentioned ointments to help extract out the pus and promote antiinflammatory effect, absorption of necrotic cells and tissue regeneration.

Surgery is necessary for cases with stubborn chronical sinus and dead bone in order to resect the sinus and remove the necrotic bone. This will help bring about early healing.

5.3   Osteoarticular Tuberculosis

Osteoarticular tuberculosis is known as "bone phthisis" or "*liutan*" in TCM terms. As a common contagious disease, it mostly attacks children or teenagers younger than 15, more boys than girls.

Pathogenesis

1. Direct Pathogenic Factors   The disease occurs as a result of invasion by bacilli tuberculae into the bone or joint. Actually, it is a secondary focus originating from the primary in the respiratory or digestive system.

2. Indirect Pathogenic Factors   If a person happens to be in a enfeebled constitution due to congenital defect or due to delivery of a baby, he / she will be vulnerable to this disease.

In some cases, the disease follows chronical strain due to long-term weight-bearing labour, or sometimes due to traumatic injuries that impair local osseous structure of the body. This impairment will greatly weaken the patient's resistance, thus providing a chance for the bacteria to invade in and cause the disease.

Besides, there are other factors that are responsible for the disease:

(1) The Muscle Fiber   Bone with abundant attached muscles like the iliac bone and the scapulae are hardly attacked by the bacteria. On the other hand, such bones as the vertebral body, the calcaneus and the short bones of the upper and lower limbs that have few or none muscles on them are easy to form a focus.

(2) The Terminal Arteroles   Osteoarticular tuberculosis

is seldom found in corticale bone structures because they have very good blood supply. Epiphysis and metaphysis are among the predilection sites of the disease as the tiny terminal arterioles in them can give but very poor blood supply.

(3) The Age   Children have relatively weak resistance to tubercle bacteria, for they have hardly been infected by these germs before. Once they are infected, they often become diseased and the microbes can easily spread to other parts from the focus. However, because children have very active metabolism and strong repairing ability, it is not at all difficult to cure this disease in them.

According to development of the disease, osteoarticular tuberculosis can be classified into 3 types:

Simple Bone Tuberculosis   This type may occur in a fast bone or in a spongy bone, In the former case, there will be hyperosteogeny and periosteal proliferation whereas in the latter case there will be destruction of the bone, resulting in dead bone or cavity in the bone without any new osteosis.

Simple Synovial Tuberculosis   In this type, the focus sits in most instances at the synovium of the hip joint or knee joint. The synovium generally becomes thicker with congestion, edema and a great amount of tuberculous exudate. Occasionally, synovial granulation tissue may spread inward along the cartilage edge, causing separation of the cartilage from the bone surface.

Tuberculosis of the Whole Joint   In case simple tuberculosis of the bone or synovium is not timely treated, the disease may keep developing and involve all the synovium, cartilage and the bone itself. The cartilage and the bone will then be impaired in various degrees which may lead to narrowing or complete loss of the joint space.

Essentials for Diagnosis

1. At the initial stage, the disease develops slowly with few evident symptoms. This may be followed by listlessness and asthenia, general lassitude with definite pain at night and dysfunction of the affected joint. The joint suffers severe pains when moving.

2. When the disease enters the intermediate stage, the involved joint will become swollen with exudate hydrops, but the skin over the joint is not red nor feverish. The patient may have muscular spasms around the joint and other symptoms such as hectic fever, night sweating, insomnia and loss of appetite .

3. At the advanced stage, there will be cold abscess near or at some distance from the focus that is easy to ulcerate with thin water—like or cheasy necrotic tissues. The opening of the sore forms a concavity and finally turns into a chronical sinus that remains unhealing for long duration. The patient gets thinner and thinner from day to day with listlessness and a dim complexion. Deficiency of both *Qi* and blood is the result in the end.

4. X—ray examination is diagnostically significant. Cases with tuberculosis of a spongy bone can be sorted into dead—bone type and disolved—bone type. In the dead—bone type, the dead bone occurs mostly at the center of the spongy bone where bone trabecula appears vaguely with increased density or visible dead bone. When the dead bone is absorbed completely, a cavity will be present. In the disolved bone type, the focus is usually located at the edge of the spongy bone with little or no dead bone, but, if it is tuberculosis of the bone shaft, the

manifestations will be hyperosteogeny, like the outcoating of a scallion stalk, if it is tuberculosis of the metaphysis, characteristics of tuberculosis of both spongy bone and bone shaft can be observed.

5. Lab Examination   Lab examination can reveal that ESR is increased whereas RBC and Hb decresed. Sometimes it is quite difficult to make an early diagnosis of the disease in certain cases, and , then, a bacterial culture or pathological examination of the puncture fluid will be necessary.

Treatment

1. Nourishment and Immobilization   Sufficient nourishment can improve the general condition, enhance the patient's resistance to the disease, and enable the patient to recover more quickly. Immobilization has the benefit of relieving the pain, preventing the focus from spreading to other parts of the body, and bettering selfrepairment of the tissues.

2. Use of Sufficient Quantities of Anti−phthisic Drugs

3. Administration of Chinese Medicines

At the initial stage, it is important to prescribe for the patient recipes that can warm and recuperate the kidney−*Yang*, disperse the pathogenic cold, remove obstruction and resolve phlegm. The usual prescription is augmented *Yanghe Tang*, that is, add to the original recipe:

Radix Angelicae Sinensis	15 g
Rhizoma Atractylodis Macrocephalae	15 g

And, for cases with abscess, add:

Spina Gleditsiae	9 g
Squama Manitis	9 g
Radix Astragali seu Hedysari	15 g

If the disease is already at the advanced stage, the principle should be to reinforce *Qi* and nourish blood. The usual prescription is *Renseng Yangrong Tang* (75). However, *Kangjiehe Tang* (76) and *Dabuyin Wan* (77)are more effective for cases with afternoon tidal fever, thirst without any desire for drinking, a reddish tongue with little fur, and a rapid thready pulse as the condition should be diagnosed as hyperactivity of fire due to *Yin*-deficiency and the remedial principle is thus to replenish the vital essence and to remove the heat. Administration: Take *Dabuyin Wan* (77) with the decoction of *Kangjiehe Tang* (76). If the patient has stubborn night sweating, add to *Kangjiehe Tang*:

Fructus Tritici Levis	9 g
Os Draconis Ustum	15 g

Proved Recipes   *Gulaodi* (78) is quite effective in treatment of osteoarticular tuberculosis. Other proved formulas with good efficacy include *Sichong Wan* (79) and *Jingong Wan* (80).

Preparations for External Use   When the abscess has not yet ulcerated, *Dingshe San* (81) can be applied to the joint. In case the abscess has ulcerated, vaseline gauze plus a small amount of *Wuwu Dan* (82) or *Zhuidu Dan* (83) can be used for sinus filling. If the patient has an ulcerous sore with only a little pus that remains unhealing for a long time, *Shengji Yuhong Gao* (30) can be chosen for dessing change.

Index of Recipes 方剂索引

Angong Niuhuang Wan(a proprietary)
   安宫牛黄丸 （成药）(72)   256,494
   Ingredients: omitted
   Administration: Take the proprietary boluses orally, 1 bolus once, once or twice a day.
   Efficacy: Being efficacious in clearing away the heart—fire, in removing toxic materials, in inducing recuscitation and in tranquilizing the mind.
   制用法: 每服一丸   日服 1～2 次。
   功能: 清心解毒, 开窍安神。

Bazhen Tang 八珍汤 (14)   33,250,257,355,491,494
   Ingredients:
   Radix Codonopsis Pilosulae   党参   10 g
   Rhizoma Atractylodis Macrocephalae   白术   10 g
   Poria   茯苓   10 g
   Radix Glycyrrhizae Praeparatae   炙甘草   6 g
   Rhizoma Ligustici Chuanxiong   川芎   6 g
   Radix Angelicae Sinensis   当归   10 g
   Remmanniae Praeparatae   熟地黄   10 g
   Radix Paeoniae Alba   白芍   10 g
   Administration: Add 2 dates and 3 slices of ginger to the prescription, boil the drugs in a proper amount of water to get about 500 ml of decoction and divide the decoction into 2—3 equal portions for oral intake, 1 portion a time, 2—3 times a

day.

Efficacy: Having an effect of reinforcing *Qi* and replenishing the blood.

制用法：水煎服。

功能：补益气血。

Bushen Huoxue Tang 补肾活血汤 (18)   34,355

Ingredients:

Rhizoma Rehmanniae Praeparatae	熟地	18 g
Fructus Corni	山萸肉	12 g
Fructus Lycii	枸杞子	12 g
Fructus Psoraleae	补骨脂	12 g
Semen Cuscutae	菟丝子	15 g
Herba Cistanchis	肉苁蓉	9 g
Commiphora Myrrha	没药	9 g
Flos Carthami	红花	9 g
Radix Angelicae Pubescentis	独活	9 g
Cortex Eucommiae	杜仲	9 g
Radix Angelicae Sinensis	当归	12 g

Administration: Boil these drugs in a proper amount of water to get about 500 ml of decoction and divide the decoction in to 2—3 equal portions for oral intake, 1 portion a time, 2—3 times a day.

Efficacy: Being efficacious in tonifying the liver and kidney, in strengthening the muscles, tendons and bones, in invigorating blood circulation and in allaying pains.

制用法：水煎服。

功能：补益肝肾，强壮筋骨，活血止痛。

Dabuyin Wan 大补阴丸 (77)   262,496

Inredients:

Rhizoma Rehmanniae Praeparatae	熟地黄	180	g
Plastrum Testudinis	龟板	180	g
Cortex Phellodendri	黄柏	120	g
Rhizoma Anemarrhenae	知母	120	g

Administration: Grind the drugs into a fine powder, mix the powder with some boiled swine spinal cord and well-heated honey, stir the mixture thoroughly and make boluses out of the mixture for oral intake, 9 grams once, twice a day.

Efficacy: Having such effects as nourishing *Yin* and clearing away pathogenic fire.

制用法: 上药共为细末，与煮熟之猪脊髓、已炼之蜂蜜，共捣为丸。每服9克，日服2次。

功能: 滋阴降火。

Dacheng Tang 大成汤 (7)　　　　　　　　32,147,152,354,428

Ingredients:

Radix Angelicae Sinensis　(fibrous root)	当归尾	12	g
Lignum Sappan	苏木	15	g
Flos Carthami	红花	9	g
Radix et Rhizoma Rhei	大黄	9	g
Mirabilitum	朴硝	9	g
Cortex Magnoliae Officinalis	厚朴	9	g
Pericarpium Citri Reticulatae	陈皮	9	g
Fructus Aurantii	枳壳	12	g
Caulis Akebiae	木通	6	g
Radix Glycyrrhizae	甘草	3	g

Administration: Boil these drugs in a proper amount of water to get about 500 ml of decoction and dinvide the decoction into 2—3 equal portions for oral intake, 1 portion a time, 2—3 times a day.

Efficacy: Being efficacious in eliminating extravasated blood and in regulating the flow of *Qi* so as to allay pains.

制用法: 水煎服。

功能: 攻下逐瘀, 理气止痛。

***Dahuang Ruangao* 大黄软膏(74)**   **257,494**

Ingredients:

Radix et Rhizoma Rhei   生大黄   100 g

Administration: Heat the drug in 300ml of water until it is boiled for 20 minutes, get the decoction by filtration , add to the boiled drug another 300 ml of water and reheat for 15 minutes before getting the second decoction by filtration. Mix the decoctions and condense the mixture to 100 ml to get a consensed decoction. To 100 grams of vaseline, add 30 ml of the condensed decoction and an ointment, *Dahuang Ruangao*, will be produced, Spread some of the ointment on a piece of gauze that is dependent upon the size of the wound and apply the gauze to the injured site, or *Dahuang*—vaseline gauze can be made for dressing change after it is sterilized through high—pressure process.

Efficacy: Having such effects as detoxifying poisons, eliminating dampness, promoting absorption of the necrotic tissues and dispelling pus.

制用法: 加水 300 毫升, 煎沸 20 分钟后过滤, 加水再煎沸 15 分钟过滤, 将两次大黄煎出液, 浓缩至 100 毫升, 即成 100% 的大黄煎出液。每 100 克凡士林加入 30 毫升大黄液, 即成 30% 大黄软膏。用时随伤口大小摊于纱布上外贴。或制大黄油纱布, 经高压灭菌, 以备换药。

功能: 解毒燥湿, 祛腐排脓。

***Dahuoluo Dan* (a proprietary)大活络丹(成药) (58)   237,483**

Ingredients: omitted

Administration: Take the proprietary boluses orally,   1 bolus once,   twice a day.

Efficacy: Being efficacious in promoting the flow of *Qi* in the channels and collaterals,   and in activating circulation of the blood so as to dredge the meridians.

制用法: 每服 1 丸，日服 2 次。

功能: 行气活血，通利经络。

Dieda Wan(a proprietary)跌打丸(成药)(56)   236,243,481,487

Ingredienmts:

Radix Angelicae Sinensis	当归	30 g
Eupolyphaga seu Steleophaga	土元	30 g
Rhizoma Ligustici Chuanxiong	川芎	30 g
Resina Draconis	血竭	30 g
Commiphora Myrrha	没药	30 g
Herba Ephedrae	麻黄	30 g
Pyritum	自然铜	60 g
Resina Boswelliae Carterii	乳香	60 g

Administration: Grind these drugs into a fine powder and make the powder into boluses with heated honey,   each weighing 3 grams,   for oral intake,   one bolus once,   twice a day.

Efficacy: Being efficacious in activating circulation of the blood so as to eliminate blood stasis,   in promoting reunion of the fractured bones and in benefiting self-repairment of the muscles and tendons.

制用法: 共为细末，炼蜜为丸，每丸重 3 克。每服 1 丸，日服 2 次。

功能: 活血破瘀，接骨续筋。

Dieda Wanhua You (a proprietary)跌打万花油(成药)(44)   37,356

Ingredients: omitted

Administration: Apply the remedy oil directly to the affected part or make gauze dressing with the oil for external application.

Efficacy: Being efficacious in subduing swelling, in alleviating pains, in eliminating toxic materials and in suppressing inflammation.

制用法: 可把药油直接涂擦患处，也可将纱布浸入药油贴敷患处。

功能: 消肿止痛，解毒消炎。

Dinggui San 丁桂散 (39)   37,356

Ingredients:

Flos Syzygii Aromatici	丁香	1 portion
Cortex Cinnamomi	肉桂	1 portion

Administration: Mix the drugs and grind the mixture into a fine powder. Dust some of the powder on a heated plaster and apply the plaster to the affected site.

Efficacy: Being efficacious in expelling pathogenic wind, dispersing stagnant cold and dredging the meridian passage by warming up the channels and collaterals.

制用法: 共为细末，加在膏药上，烘热后贴患处。

功能: 祛风散寒，温经通络。

Dingshe San 丁麝散 (81)   262,497

Ingredients:

Resina Garciniae	藤黄
Radix Aconiti Kusnezoffii	生草乌
Radix Aconiti	生川乌
Rhizoma Bletillae	生白芨
Radix Glycyrrhizae	生甘草
Rhizoma Atractylodis	苍术

Radix Ledebouriellae	防风
Radix Isaditis	板兰根
Moschus	麝香

Administration: Grind equal shares of the drugs into a fine powder and make a paste or ointment with the powder and water or some other liquids for external application.

Efficacy: Having such effects as activating circulation of the blood, neutralizing toxins, subduing swelling and alleviating pains.

制用法：共为细末，制成药膏外敷。

功能：活血解毒，消肿止痛。

Duhuo Jisheng Tang 独活寄生汤 (53)　　　　230,237,478,483

Ingredients:

Radix Angelicae Pubescentis	独活	12 g
Ramulus Loranthi	寄生	18 g
Radix Gentianae Macrophyllae	秦艽	9 g
Radix Ledebouriellae	防风	9 g
Rhizoma Ligustici Chuanxiong	川芎	9 g
Poria	茯苓	9 g
Ramulus Cinnamomi	桂枝	9 g
Radix Achyranthis Bidentatae	牛膝	9 g
Herba Asari	细辛	3 g
Cortex Eucommiae	杜仲	12 g
Radix Angelicae Sinensis	当归	12 g
Radix Rehmannia	生地	12 g
Radix Paeoniae Rubra	赤芍	12 g
Radix Ginseng	人参	4.5g
Radix Glycyrrhizae	生甘草	6 g

Administration: Boil these drugs in a proper amount of

water to get about 500 ml of decoction and divide the decoction into 2—3 equal portions for oral intake， 1 portion a time ， 2—3 times a day .

Efficacy: Being efficacious in activating circulation of the blood in relaxing the muscles and tendons ， in promoting the flow of *Qi* in the channels and collaterals,· in dispelling pathogenic wind and eliminating evil dampness.

制用法：水煎服。

功能：活血、舒筋，通络，散风祛湿。

Fuyuan Huoxue Tang   32,69,81,107,136,152,160,177,186,236,243,
复元活血汤 (1)   354,378,385,401,419,429,434,448,481,487

Ingredients:

Radix Angelicae Sinensis (fibrous root)	当归尾	15 g
Semen Persicae	桃仁	9 g
Flos Carthami	红花	9 g
Squama Manitis	山甲	9 g
Radix et Rhizoma Rhei	大黄	6 g
Radix Bupleuri	柴胡	12 g
Radix Trichosanthis	天花粉	12 g
Radix Glycyrrhizae	甘草	6 g

Administration: Boil these drugs in a proper amount of water to get about 500 ml of decoction and divide the decoction into 2—3 equal portions for oral intake， 1 portion a time ， 2—3 times a day.

Efficacy: Being efficacious in activating circulation of the blood， removing blood stasis and alleviating pains and swelling.

制用法：水煎服。

功能：活血化瘀，消肿止痛。

Goupi Gao (a proprietary)狗皮膏(成药)(34)   36,244,356,487

Ingredients: omitted

Administration: Heat the plaster to make it half—melt and apply it to the affected site.

Efficacy: Bening efficacious in clearing away pathogenic cold, alleviating pains, relaxing the muscles and tendons and activating the flow of Qi and the blood in the cheannels and collaterals.

制用法：烘热外贴患处。

功能：散寒止痛，舒筋活络。

Guipi Tang　归脾汤（17）   34,355

Ingredients:

Rhizoma Atractylodis Macrocephalae	白术	10 g
Radix Angelicae Sinensis	当归	3 g
Radix Codonopsis Pilosulae	党参	3 g
Radix Astragali seu Hedysari	黄芪	10 g
Semen Ziziphi Spinosae	酸枣仁	10 g
Poria	茯苓	10 g
Radix Aucklandiae	木香	3 g
Radix Poligalae	远志	3 g
Arillus Longan	龙眼肉	4.5 g
Radix Glycyrrhzae Praeparatae	炙甘草	4.5 g

Adiminstration: Boil these drugs in a proper amount of water to get about 500 ml of decoction and divide the decoction into 2—3 equal portions for oral intake, 1 portion a time, 2—3 times a day.

Efficacy: Having such effects as nourishing the heart, replenishing the spleen, invigorating Qi and tonifying the blood.

制用法：水煎服。

功能：养心健脾，补益气血。

Guishe San 桂麝散 （40）   37,356

Ingredients:

Herba Ephedrae	麻黄	15 g
Herba Asari	细辛	15 g
Cortex Cinnamomi	肉桂	30 g
Fructus Glidistsia Abmormalis	牙皂	10 g
Rhizoma Pinelliae	半夏	25 g
Flos Syzygii Aromatici	丁香	30 g
Rhizoma Arisaematis	生南星	25 g
Moschus	麝香	1.8 g
Borneolum Syntheticum	冰片	1.2 g

Administration: Grind the drugs into a fine powder and dust some of the powder on the surface of kind of medicinal adhesive plaster for external application to the affected site.

Efficacy: Having such effects as warming and resolving phlegm and dampness, alleviating pains and subduing swelling.

制用法: 上药共为细末，掺于膏药上，贴患处。

功能: 温化痰湿，消肿止痛。

Gulao Di 骨痨敌 （78）   262,497

Ingredients:

Rhizoma Drynariae	骨碎补	10 g
Radix Notoginseng	三七	10 g
Resina Draconis	乳香	10 g
Commiphora Myrrha	没药	10 g
Radix Astragali seu Hedysari	黄芪	10 g

Administration: Boil these drugs in a proper amount of water to get about 500 ml of decoction and divide the decoction into 2—3 equal portions for oral intake.

1 portion a time , 2—3 times a day.

Efficacy: Being efficacious in invigorating and tonifying *Qi* and blood and in strengthening the bones and tendons.

制用法: 水煎服。

功能: 补益气血, 强壮筋骨。

Guzhi Zhengsheng Wan 骨质增生丸 (59)   237,483

Ingredients

Rhizoma Rehmanniae Praeparatae 熟地	60 g
Caulis Millettiae Reliculatae	鸡血藤	45 g
Rhizoma Drynariae	骨碎补	45 g
Herba Cistanchis	肉苁蓉	30 g
Herba Pyrolae	鹿衔草	30 g
Herba Epimedii	淫羊藿	30 g
Semen Raphani	莱菔子	15 g

Administration: Grind these drugs into a fine powder, mix the powder with some heated honey and make boluses out of the mixture, eaching weighing 9 grams, for oral intake, 1 bolus once, twice a day.

Efficacy: Having such effects as nourishing the blood, relaxing the muscles and tendons and strenthening the bones.

制用法: 共为细末, 炼蜜为丸, 每丸 9 克。每服 1 丸, 日服 2 次。

功能: 养血, 舒筋, 壮骨。

Huajian Gao 化坚膏 (33)   36,356

Ingredients:

Semen Sinapis Albae	白芥子	60 g
Radix Euphorbiae Kansui	甘遂	60 g
Lumbricus	地龙	60 g
Cannobis Sativa	麻根	90 g
Radix Clematidis	灵仙	75 g

Semen Impatientis	急性子	105 g
Crinis Carbonisatus	血余	30 g
Fructus Mune	乌梅	120 g
Herba Speranskia Tuberculata	透骨草	75 g
Semen Crotonis Pulveratum	江子	30 g
Scorpio	全蝎	30 g
Radix Stephaniae Tetrandrae	防己	30 g
Radix Aconiti Kusnezoffii	生草乌	30 g
Herba Asari	细辛	9 g
Squama Manitis	生山甲	12 g
Sal-Ammoniac	紫碯砂	18 g
Oleum Sesami	麻油	2 500 g
Plumbumplumbi Oxydum	樟丹	1 250 g

Administration; Fry these drugs except Plumbumplumbi Oxydum and Sal-Ammoniac in a ceramic cauldron with the sesame oil until the drugs become dark brown, and now it is the time when Plumbumplumbi Oxydum can be added to them. Stir the mixture thoroughly to release the smoke completely and , then, put in sal-Ammoniac to get an ointment, Detoxify the ointment to make it ready for external use. Spread some of the ointment on a piece of cloth and apply it to the affected site.

Efficacy: Being efficacious in activating blood circulation, softening hard masses and alleviating pains.

制用法：取香油置锅内，除樟丹、碯砂外其它药炸枯去渣，炼油滴水成珠时下樟丹，将烟搅净后放紫碯砂，去毒，备用。取膏药适量摊于布上，外贴患处。

功能：活血，软坚，止痛。

Huanglian Jiedu Tang 黄连解毒汤 （70）   256,494

Ingredients:

Rhizoma Coptidis	黄连	
Radix Scutellariae	黄芩	
Cortex Phellodendri	黄柏	
Fructus Gardeniae	山栀	

Administration: Decide What quantities of the drugs are needed for a specific case, Boil the drugs in a proper amount of water to get the decoction for oral intake.

Efficacy: Being efficacious in purging pathogenic fire and neutralizing toxic substances.

制用法：按病情定药量。水煎服。

功能： 泻火解毒。

Huaruishi San 花蕊石散 （37）   36,356

Ingredients:

Ophicalcitum	花蕊石	1 portion
Sulphur	石硫磺	2 portions

Administration: Heat the drugs in a ceramic jar and, then, grind them into fine powder for external application: Dust some of the powder on the surface of the wound and dress the part with gauze.

Efficacy: Being efficacious in removing blood stasis and suppressing bleeding.

制用法：共入瓦罐煅研为细末。外掺伤面后包扎。

功能：化瘀止血。

Huoxue Jiu 活血酒 （41）   37,356

Ingredients:

Resina Boswelliae Carterii	乳香	15 g
Commiphora Myrrha	没药	15 g
Resina Draconis	血竭	15 g
Rhizoma seu Radix Notopterygii	羌活	15 g

Rhizoma Cyperi	香附	15 g
Squama Manitis	山甲珠	15 g
Pyritum Praeparatae	煅自然铜	15 g
Radix Angelicae Pubescentis	独活	15 g
Radix Dipsaci	川断	15 g
Os Tigris	虎骨	15 g
Rhizoma Ligustici Chuanxiong	川芎	15 g
Fructus Chaenomelis	木瓜	15 g
Bulbus Fritillariae Thunbergii	贝母	9 g
Cortex Magnoliae Officinalis	厚朴	9 g
Fructus Foeniculi Praeparata	炒小茴香	9 g
Cortex Cinnamomi	肉桂	9 g
Radix Aucklandiae	木香	6 g
Radix Aconiti Praeparatae	制川乌	3 g
Radix Aconiti Kusnezoffii Praeparatae	制草乌	3 g
Radix Angelicae Dahuricae	白芷	24 g
Cortex Cercis Chinensis	紫荆皮	24 g
Radix Angelicae Sinensis	当归	24 g
Moschus	麝香	1.5 g

Administration: Grind the drugs into a fine powder and soak the powder in white spirit, in a ratio of 15g of the powder to 500g of the liquor, for 7—10 days. Then the spiritous liquor can be administered for external application to the affected site or for oral intake.

Efficacy: Being efficacious in promoting the flow of *Qi* and blood in the channels, in activating circulation of the blood, in dispelling pathogenic wind and clearing away evil cold.

制用法：将药研为细末，每 15 克药散浸白酒 500 克，浸 7～10 天即成。外涂患处。也可内服。

功能: 通经活血, 祛风散寒。

Huoxue Quyu Pian 活血祛瘀片(54)   233,243,385,479,487

Ingredients:

Herba Siphonostegia	刘寄奴	45 g
Resina Draconis	血竭	15 g
Radix Angelicae Sinensis	当归	30 g
Radix Paeoniae Rubra	赤芍	30 g
Semen Persicae	桃仁	24 g
Flos Carthami	红花	24 g
Squama Manitis	山甲珠	24 g
Flos Syzygii Aromatici Masculina	公丁香	15 g
Radix et Rhizoma Rhei	大黄	15 g
Eupolyphaga seu Steleophaga	土元	24 g
Spina Gleditsiae	皂刺	24 g

Administration: Make tablets with these drugs in accordance with the manufacturing process, each tablet weighing 0.3 g, for oral intake, 8—10 tablets a time, 2—3 times a day.

Efficacy: Being efficacious in activating circulation of the blood, in promoting the flow of *Qi* and blood in the channels and collaterals, in removing blood stasis and in subduing swelling.

制用法: 依法制片, 每片重 0.3 克, 每次 8~10 片, 每日 2 ~3 次。

功能: 活血通络, 化瘀消肿。

Huoxue Quyu Tang 活血祛瘀汤 (3)   32,236,354,481

Ingredient:

Radix Angelicae Sinensis	当归	15 g
Eupolyphaga seu Steleophaga	土元	3 g
Pyritum	自然铜	9 g

Rhizoma Cibotii	狗脊	9 g
Semen Persicae	桃仁	9 g
Flos Carthami	红花	6 g
Resina Boswelliae Carterii	乳香	6 g
Commiphora Myrrha	没药	6 g
Rhizoma drynariae	骨碎补	15 g
Fructus Liquidambaris	路路通	6 g
Radix Notoginseng	三七	3 g

Administration: Boil these drugs in a proper amount of water to get about 500 ml of decoction, and divide the decoction into 2—3 portions for oral intake, 1 portion a time, 2—3 times a day.

Efficacy: Being efficacious in activating circulation of the blood so as to eleminate blood stasis, in removing obstruction in the channels and collaterals, in allaying swelling, in promoting repairment of the soft tissues and in helping fracture healing.

制用法: 水煎服。

功能: 活血化瘀，通络消肿，续筋接骨。

Huoxue Shujin Tang 活血舒筋汤 (21)   34,355

Ingredients:

Radix Angelicae Sinensis	当归	15 g
Caulis Millettiae Reticulatae	鸡血藤	18 g
Radix Salviae Miltiorrhizae	丹参	15 g
Flos Carthami	红花	9 g
Radix Gentianae Macrophyllae	秦艽	9 g
Radix Clematidis	灵仙	9 g
Rhizoma Curcumae Longae	姜黄	9 g
Rhizoma seu Radix Notopterygii	羌活	9 g
Radix Achyranthis Bidentatae	牛膝	9 g

Ramulus Mori   桑枝   12 g

Administration: Boil these drugs in a proper amount of water to get about 500 ml of decoction and divide the decoction into 2—3 equal portions for oral intake, 1 portion a time, 2—3 times a day.

Efficacy: Having such effects as invigorating and replenishing the blood, relaxing the muscles and tendons, and removing obstruction from the channels and collaterals.

制用法：水煎服。

功能：养血活血,舒筋通络。

Huoxue Zhitong San 活血止痛散(45)   38,186,230,233,357,448,478,479

Ingredients:

Radix Angelicae Sinensis （fibrous root)	当归尾	15 g
Flos Carthami	红花	15 g
Lignum Sappan	苏木	15 g
Radix Angelicae Dahuricae	白芷	15 g
Rhizoma Curcumae Longae	姜黄	15 g
Radix Clematidis	灵仙	15 g
Rhizoma seu Radix Notopterygii	羌活	15 g
Cortex Acanthopanacis Radicis	五加皮	15 g
Cortex Erythrinae	海桐皮	15 g
Radix Achyranthis Bidentatae	牛膝	15 g
Fructus Meliae Toosendan	川楝子	15 g
Rhizoma Smilacis Glabrae	土茯苓	15 g
Resina Boswelliae Carterii	乳香	6 g
Pericarpium Zanthoxyli	花椒	9 g
Herba Speranskia Tuberculata	透骨草	30 g

Administration: Boil these drugs in a proper amount of water and use the decoction to fumigate and ／ or rinse the affected part while it is hot; in the case of rinsing, it cannot be too hot though it should be warm enough.

Efficacy: Being efficacious in relaxing the muscles and tendons, in activating circulation of the blood , in invigorating the flow of *Qi* in the channels and collaterals and in alleviating pains.

制用法: 水煎熏洗患处。

功能: 舒筋活血, 通络止痛。

Huoxue Zhitong Tang 活血止痛汤 (2)   32,354

Ingredient:

Radix Angelicae Sinensis	当归	12 g
Rhizoma Ligustici Chuanxiong	川芎	6 g
Resina Boswelliae Carterii	乳香	6 g
Commiphora Myrrha	没药	6 g
Lignum sappan	苏木	6 g
Flos Carthami	红花	6 g
Herba Centallae	落得打	6 g
Eupolyphaga seu Steleophaga	土元	3 g
Radix Notoginseng	三七	3 g
Radix Paeoniae Rubra	赤芍	9 g
Lignum Cercis Cninensis	紫荆藤	9 g

Administration: Boil these drugs in a proper amount of water to ger about 500 ml of decoction and divide the decoction into 2—3 equal portions for oral intake, 1 portion a time, 2—3 times a day.

Efficacy: Being efficacious in activating circulation of the blood, in removing blood stasis and in alleviating pains and swelling.

制用法: 水煎服。

功能: 活血祛瘀, 消肿止痛。

Huoying Liqi Tang 和营理气汤 （10）   32,354

Ingredients:

Radix Angelicae Sinensis (fibrous root)	当归尾	12 g
Radix Paeoniae Rubra	赤芍	12 g
Lignum Sappan	苏木	12 g
Resina Boswelliae Carterii	乳香	9 g
Commiphora Myrrha	没药	9 g
Semen Persicae	桃仁	9 g
Rhizoma Ligustici Chuanxiong	川芎	9 g
Pericarpium Citri Reticulatae	陈皮	9 g
Radix Linderae	乌药	9 g
Radix Dipsaci	川断	15 g
Caulis Akebiae	木通	6 g
Radix Glycyrrhizae	甘草	6 g

Administration: Boil these drugs in a proper amount of water to get about 500 ml of decoction and divide the decoction into 2—3 equal portions for oral intake, 1 portion a time, 2—3 times a day.

Efficacy: Being efficacious in activating circulation of the blood so as to remove blood stasis and in promoting the flow of *Qi* in the channels so as to eliminate obstruction and thus to alleviate pains.

制用法：水煎服。

功能：活血化瘀，行气通络止痛。

Jianbu Huquan Wan 健步虎潜丸 （20）   34,250,355,491

Ingredients:

Colla Plastri Testudinis	龟板胶	2 portions
Colla Cornus Cervi	鹿角胶	2 portions
Os Tigris	虎骨	2 portions

Radix Polygoni Multiflori	何首乌	2 portions
Radix Achyranthis Bidentatae	牛膝	2 portions
Cortex Eucommiae	杜仲	2 portions
Herba Cynomorii	锁阳	2 portions
Radix Angelicae Sinensis	当归	2 portions
Rhizoma Rehmanniae Praeparatae	熟地	2 portions
Radix Clematidis	灵仙	2 portions
Cortex Phellodendri	黄柏	1 portion
Radix Ginseng	人参	1 portion
Rhizoma seu Radix Notopterygii	羌活	1 portion
Radix Paeoniae Alba	白芍	1 portion
Rhizoma Atractylodis Macrocephalae	白术	1 portion
Radix Aconiti Praeparata	附子	1.5 portions

Administration: Grind these drugs into a fine powder, mix the powder with a proper amount of honey, melt the mixture on a heater, and make small pills (in the size of mung beans) for oral administration. Take the pills with boiled dilute salty water before meals, 10 grams a time, 2—3 times a day.

Efficacy: Being efficacious in replenishing *Qi*, in nourishing the blood and in strengthening the muscles, tendons and bones.

制用法：上药共为细末，炼蜜为丸如绿豆大，每服 10 克，空腹淡盐水送下，每日 2～3 次。

功能：补气血，壮筋骨。

Jiangu Zhuangjin Gao 坚骨壮筋膏 (32)   36,356

Ingredients:

Constituent I: 第一组药：

Rhizoma Drynarriae	骨碎补	90 g
Radix Dipsaci	川断	90 g

Semen Strychni	马钱子	60 g
Borax	硼砂	60 g
Radix Aconiti Kusnezoffii	生草乌	60 g
Radix Aconiti	生川乌	60 g
Radix Achyranthis Bidentatae	牛膝	60 g
Lignum Sappan	苏木	60 g
Cortex Eucommiae	杜仲	60 g
Herba Lycopodii	伸筋草	60 g
Herba Speranskia Tuberculata	透骨草	60 g
Rhizoma seu Radix Notopterygii	羌活	30 g
Radix Angelicae Pubescentis	独活	30 g
Herba Ephedrae	麻黄	30 g
Cortex Acanthopanacis Radicis	五加皮	30 g
Semen Gleditsiae	皂角核	30 g
Flos Carthami	红花	30 g
Herba Lycopi	泽兰	30 g
Os Tigris	虎骨	24 g
Oleum Sesami	香油	5 000 g
Plumbumplumbi Oxydum	黄丹	2 500 g
Constituent II:	第二组药	
Resina Draconis	血竭	30 g
Flos Syzygii Aromatici	丁香	30 g
Radix Angelicae Dahuricae	白芷	30 g
Resina Boswelliae Carterii	乳香	30 g
Commiphora Myrrha	没药	30 g
Cortex Cinnamomi	肉桂	60 g
Rhizoma Nardostachyos	甘松	60 g
Herba Asari	细辛	60 g
Moschus	麝香	1.5 g

Administration: Make an ointment with the drugs in Constituent I, melt the ointment by supplying moderate heat and spreat some of it on a piece of gauze or cloth for external application.Grind the drugs in Constituent II into powder, Dust the ointment with the powder directly before application.

Efficacy: Having such effects as strenthening the bones and toughening the muscles and tendons.

制用法： 第一组药，熬成膏药后，温烊摊贴。第二组药，共为细末，临贴时撒于药面。

功能： 坚壮筋骨。

Jiedu Xiyao 解毒洗药 （69）   250,491

Ingredients:

Herba Taraxaci	蒲公英	30 g
Radix Sophorae Flavescentis	苦参	12 g
Cortex Phellodendri	黄柏	12 g
Fructus Forsythiae	连翘	12 g
Semen Momordiae	木鳖子	12 g
Flos Lonicerae	金银花	9 g
Radix Angelicae Dahuricae	白芷	9 g
Radix Paeoniae Rubra	赤芍	9 g
Cortex Moutan Radicis	丹皮	9 g
Radix Glycyrrhizae	甘草	9 g

Administration: Make decoction with these drugs and a proper amount of water and rinse the affected part with the decoction （or fumigate the part with the decoction steam） before dressing change.

Efficacy: Having such effects as clearing away pathogenic heat, removing toxic materials, activating circulation of the blood, subduing swelling, promoting absorption of the necrotic tissues and expelling pus.

制用法：上药煎汤，趁热熏洗患处。洗后换药。

功能：清热解毒，活血消肿，祛腐排脓。

Jiegu Dan 接骨丹 (11)   33,81,116,136,147,152,170,354,385,407,419,429,439

Ingredients:

Eupolyphaga seu Steleophaga	土元	60 g
Squama Manitis	穿山甲	60 g
Pyritum Praeparatae	制自然铜	90 g
Resina Draconis	血竭	30 g
Lumbricus	地龙	90 g
Radix Angelicae Sinensis (fibrous root)	当归尾	90 g
Herba Abri	鸡骨	150 g
Rhizoma Drynariae	骨碎补	120 g
Herba Ephedrae	麻黄	30 g
Semen Strychni Praeparatae	制马钱子	9 g
Pyrolusite Praeparatae	制无名异	120 g

Administration: Grind the above drugs into a fine powder and make tablets out of the powder (each tablet weighing about 0.3 g) for oral intake, 5—7 tablets once for adults, 3 times a day. The dosage should be reduced for children, depending on their body weight. The tablets are contraindicated for pregnant females.

Efficacy: Being Efficacious in activating circulation of the blood so as to remove blood stasis and in promoting fracture healing and repairment of the soft tissues.

制用法：以上各药共为细末，依法制片剂，每片重 0.3 克，成人每次 5~7 片，每日 3 次，口服。小儿酌减。孕妇忌服。

功能：活血化瘀，续筋接骨。

Jiegu Xujin Gao 接骨续筋膏 (25)   35,356

Ingredients:

Pyritum	自然铜	3 portions
Herba Schizonepetae	荆芥	3 portions
Radix Ledebouriellae	防风	3 portions
Cortex Acanthopanacis Radicis	五加皮	3 portions
Fructus Gleditsiae	皂角	3 portions
Radix Rabiae	茜草根	3 portions
Radix Dipsaci	续断	3 portions
Rhizoma seu Radix Notopterygii	羌活	3 portions
Resina Boswelliae Carterii	乳香	2 portions
Commiphora Myrrha	没药	2 portions
Rhizoma Drynariae	骨碎补	2 portions
Caulis et Folium Sambuci	接骨木	2 portions
Flos Carthami	红花	2 portions
Radix paeoniae Rubra	赤芍	2 portions
Eupolyphaga seu Steleophaga	土元	2 portions
Rhizoma Bletillae	白芨	4 portions
Resina Draconis	血竭	4 portions
Borax	硼砂	4 portions

Administration: Prepare 4 portions of crab powder, grind the above drugs into a fine powder, mix the two powders together with a proper amount of malt extract or honey, and heat the mixture in a pan to produce a paste for external application.

Efficacy: Having such effects as promoting reunion of the fractured bone and helping repairment of the muscles, tendons and ligaments.

制用法：共为细末，饴糖或蜂蜜调煮外敷。

功能：接骨续筋。

Jingong Wan　金蚣丸　(80)　　　　　　　　262,497

Ingredients:

Scolopendra	蜈蚣	30 g
Scorpio	全蝎	30 g
Bombyx Batryticatus	僵蚕	15 g
Squama Manitis	山甲珠	15 g
Radix et Rhizoma Rhei	川军	9 g
Realgar	雄黄	9 g
Cinnabaris	朱砂	6 g

Administration: Grind these drugs into a fine powder，mix the powder with some broomcorn millet gruel and make pills out of the mixture for oral intake，3 grams once，twice a day.

Efficacy: Being eficacious in softening hard masses，in dissolving lumps and in removing toxic sustances.

制用法：上药研细粉，与黄米饭共捣为丸。每服 3 克，日服 2 次。

功能：软坚、散结、消毒。

Jinhuang Gao 金黄膏 （27）   36,256,356,494

Ingredients:

Radix et Rhizoma Rhei	大黄	5 portions
Cortex Phellodendri	黄柏	5 portions
Rhizoma Curcumae Longae	姜黄	5 portions
Radix Angelicae Dahuricae	白芷	5 portions
Rhizoma Arisaematis Praeparata	胆南星	1 portion
Pericarpium Citri Reticulatae	陈皮	1 portion
Rhizoma Atractylodis	苍术	1 portion
Cortex Magnoliae Officinalis	厚朴	1 portion
Radix Glycyrrhizae	甘草	1 portion
Radix Trichosanthis	天花粉	10 portions

Administration: Grind these drugs into a fine powder,

mix the powder with a certain amount of vinegar / sesame oil / toilet water to produce a paste, or make an ointment with the powder and some vaseline in a ratio of 8 to 2, for external application.

Efficacy: Being efficacious in clearing away pathogenic heat and toxic materials dissipating blood stasis and promoting subsidence of swelling.

制用法：共为细末，可用醋、油、花露等调敷，或用凡士林 8／10，药散 2／10 的比例调制膏外敷。

功能：清热解毒，散瘀消肿。

Jiuyi Dan　九一丹 (38)　　　　　　　　　　36,257,356,495

Ingredients:

| Calcium Hydroxidum | 熟石灰 | 9 portions |
| Hydrargyri Oxydum Rubrum | 红升丹 | 1 portion |

Administration: Grind the drugs into a fine powder and dust the powder on the wound surface, or, make small rod—shaped pieces of the powder for insertion into the sore opening before covering the wound with sort of ointment or paste.Give dressing change every 1—2 days.

Efficacy: Having an effect in dispelling pus and promoting absorption of the necrotic tissues.

制用法：共为细末，掺于疮面，或制成条，插入疮内；再盖上软膏。每 1～2 日换药一次。

功能：提脓祛腐。

Kangjiehe Tang　抗结核汤 (76)　　　　　　　262,496

Ingredients:

Spica Prunellae	夏枯草	30 g
Radix Salviae Miltiorrhizae	丹参	15 g
Rhizoma Polygonati Odorati	玉竹	15 g

Concha Ostreae	生牡蛎	12 g
Radix Stellariae	银柴胡	12 g
Radix Stemonae	百部	12 g
Rhizoma Anemarrhenae	知母	12 g
Cortex Lycii Radicis	地骨皮	9 g
Carapax Trionycis	鳖甲	9 g
Cortex Moutan Radicis	丹皮	9 g

Administration: Boil these drugs in a proper amount of water to get about 500 ml of decoction and divide the decoction into 2—3 equal portions for oral intake, 1 portion a time, 2—3 times a day.

Efficacy: Being efficacious in nourishing *Yin* and in clearing away pathogenic heat.

制用法：水煎服。

功能：养阴清热。

Kanli Sha 坎离砂 (48)   38,245,357,488

Ingredients:

Herba Ephedrae	麻黄
Radix Angelicae Sinensis (fibrous root)	当归尾
Radix Aconiti Preparata	附子
Herba Speranskia Tuberculata	透骨草
Flos Carthami	红花
Rhizoma Zingiberis	干姜
Ramulus Cinnamomi	桂枝
Radix Achyranthis Bidentatae	牛膝
Radix Angelicae Dahuricae	白芷
Herba Schizonepetae	荆芥
Radix Ledebouriellae	防风
Fructus Chaenomelis	木瓜

Folium Artemisiae Argyi (in small pieces)　　生艾绒

Rhizoma seu Radix Notopterygii　　　　　羌活

Radix Angelicae Pubescentis　　　　　　　独活

Administration: Boil the drugs (all in equal shares) with a proper amount of vinegar—water (50% to 50%) mixture until a concentrated decoction is obtained, and , then, put in the decoction a proper amount of iron grains which have been heated red, stir the mixture; and this is just what *Kanli Sa* is .Make cloth bags (1—3 ones will be enough) and place *Kanli Sa* in them. Add to the bags of *Kanli Sa* some vinegar and they will naturally become warmer; then, apply the bags to the affected part.

Efficacy: Being efficacious in warming the channels so as to dispel pathogenic cold from them, in relaxing the muscles and tendons, in activating the flow of *Qi* and blood in the channels, in invigorating circulation of the blood and in alleviating pains.

制用法：以上诸药，用醋、水各半熬成浓汁，再将铁砂适量炒红拌入药汁即成。取坎离砂1～3袋，以食醋拌湿，装入布袋内，即自然发热，熨患处。

功能：温经散寒，活血通络，舒筋止痛。

Liqi Zhitong Tang 理气止痛汤 (9)　　　　　　　　　32,354

Ingredients:

Radix Salviae Miltiorrhizae	丹参	12 g
Pericarpium Citri Reticulatae Viride	青皮	9 g
Resina Boswelliae Carterii	乳香	9 g
Commiphora Myrrha	没药	9 g
Fructus Aurantii	枳壳	9 g
Rhizoma Cyperi Praeparatae	炙香附	9 g
Fructus Meliae Toosendan	川楝子	9 g
Radix Bupleuri	柴胡	9 g

Fructus Liquidambaris	路路通	9 g
Radix Aucklandriae	木香	6 g
Rhizoma Corydalis	延胡索	6 g

Administration: Boil these drugs in a proper amount of water to get about 500 ml of decoction and divide the decoction into 2—3 equal portions for oral intake, 1 portion a time, 2—3 times a day.

Efficacy: Being efficacious in activating blood flow so as to reinforce *Yingfeng* (the nutrition system), and in regulating the flow of *Qi* so as to alleviate pains.

制用法：水煎服。

功能：活血和营，理气止痛。

Magui Wenjing Tang 麻桂温经汤 (22)   34,245,355,488

Ingredients:

Herba Ephedrae	麻黄	6 g
Ramulus Cinnamomi	桂枝	9 g
Herba Asari	细辛	3 g
Radix Angelicae Dahuricae	白芷	9 g
Semen Persicae	桃仁	9 g
Flos Carthami	红花	9 g
Radix Paeoniae Rubra	赤芍	9 g
Radix Glycyrrhizae	甘草	6 g

Administration: Boil these drugs in a proper amount of water to get about 500 ml of decoction and divide the decoction into 2—3 equal portions for oral intake, 1 portion a time, 2—3 times a day.

Efficacy: Being efficacious in warming the channels, in clearing away cold, in invigorating blood circulation and in eliminating obstruction from the channels.

制用法：水煎服。

功能：温经散寒，活血通络。

No. 1 Washing Recipe　　**1号洗药（46）**　　　　**38,357**

Ingredients:

Herba Siphonostegiae	刘寄奴	15 g
Lignum Sappan	苏木	15 g
Flos Carthami	红花	9 g
Radix Salviae Miltiorrhizae	丹参	15 g
Radix Paeoniae Rubra	赤芍	15 g
Cortex Acanthopanacis Radicis	五加皮	15 g
Herba Leonuri	益母草	30 g
Radix Ledebouriellae	防风	9 g
Radix Angelicae Pubescentis	独活	9 g
Pericarpium Zanthoxyli	川椒	9 g
Rihzoma Curcumae Longae	羌黄	9 g
Herba Speranskia Tuberculata	透骨草	15 g

Administration: Boil these drugs in a proper amount of water and, then, fumigate the affected part with the decoction steam or rinse the affected part directly with the decoction while it is warm enough.

Efficacy: Being efficacious in activating circulation of the blood so as to remove blood stasis, in subduing swelling and in alleviating pains.

制用法：水煎熏洗患处。

功能：活血化瘀，消肿止痛。

No. 2 Washing Recipe　　**2号洗药（47）**　　**38,230,357,429,478**

Ingredients:

Radix Aconiti	川乌	9 g
Radix Aconiti Kusnezoffii	草乌	9 g

Pericarpium Zanthoxyli	花椒	9 g
Folium Artemisiae Aegyi	艾叶	9 g
Rhizoma Atractylodis	苍术	9 g
Radix Angelicae Pubescentis	独活	9 g
Ramulus Cinnamomi	桂枝	9 g
Radix Ledebouriellae	防风	9 g
Flos Carthami	红花	9 g
Herba Siphonostegiae	刘寄奴	9 g
Herba Speranskia Tuberculata	透骨草	9 g
Herba Lycopodii	伸筋草	9 g

Administration: Boil these drugs with a proper amount of water, and, then, fumigate the affected part with the decoction steam or rinse the affected part directly with the decoction while it is warm enough.

Efficacy: Being efficacious in warming up the channels and collaterals, in clearing away pathogenic cold, in relaxing the muscles and tendons, in dredginging the channels, in activating circulation of the blood and in alleviating pains.

制用法: 水煎熏洗患处。

功能: 温经散寒，舒筋通络，活血止痛。

Qing-e Wan 青娥丸 (67)   245,487

Ingredients:

Cortex Eucommiae	杜仲	480 g
Fructus Psoraleae	补骨脂	240 g
Juglandis Regiae	胡桃	50 g
Bulbus Allii	蒜	120 g

Administration: Gring the first two drugs into a powder, crush the later two into mash, mix them together and add to the mixture some rice-paste to produce pills (in the size of peas) for oral administration.Take the pills with boiled thin salty water or with warmed liquor, 10 grams a time, 1~3 times a day.

Efficacy: Being efficacious in tonifying the kidney and strengthening the bones.

制用法: 共为细末，米糊成丸如豆大。每服 10 克，淡盐汤或温酒送下，每服 1~3 次。

功能: 补肾壮骨。

Qingxin Yao 清心药 (4)　　　　　　　　　　　32,354

Ingredients:

Radix Angelicae Sinensis	当归	12 g
Radix Paeoniae Rubra	赤芍	12 g
Cortex Moutan Radicis	丹皮	12 g
Rhizoma Ligustici Chuanxiong	川芎	9 g
Semen Persicae	桃仁	9 g
Radix Scutellariae	黄芩	9 g
Fructus Gardeniae	栀子	9 g
Radix Rehmannia	生地	18 g
fructus Forsythiae	连翘	15 g
Rhizoma Coptidis	黄连	6 g
Radix Glycyrrhizae	甘草	6 g

Administration: Boil these drugs in a proper amount of waterto get about 500 ml of decoction and divide the decoction into 2—3 equal portions for oral intake, 1 portion a time, 2—3 times a day.

Efficacy: Having such effects as eliminating blood stasis, alleviating swelling and clearing away pathogenic heat and toxic materials.

制用法: 水煎服。

功能: 化瘀消肿，清热解毒。

Quyu Xiaozhong Gao　祛瘀消肿膏　(57)　　　236,481

Ingredients:

Resina Draconis	血竭	9 g
Acacia Catechu	儿茶	6 g
Commiphora Myrrha	没药	9 g
Resina Boswelliae Carterii	乳香	9 g
Rhizoma Corydalis	元胡	12 g
Pericarpium Zanthoxyli	川椒	6 g
Moschus	麝香	1.5 g
Borneolum Syntheticum	冰片	30 g
Semen Phaseoli	赤小豆	30 g
Lumbricus	地龙	30 g

Administration: Grind the drugs into a fine powder and mix the powder with a proper amount of honey or Saccharum Coranorum to get a paste for external application to the affected part.

Efficacy: Being efficacious in activating circulation of the blood to remove blood stasis, in subduing swelling and in alleviating pains.

制用法：上药共为细末，用蜜或饴糖调敷伤处。

功能：活血祛瘀，消肿止痛。

Renshen Yangrong Tang　人参养荣汤　(75)　　　262,496

Ingredients:

Radix Codonopsis Pilosulae	党参	10 g
Rhizoma Atractylodis Macrocephalae	白术	10 g
Radix Astragali seu Hedysari Praeparatae	炙黄芪	10 g
Radix Glycyrrhizae Praeparatae	炙甘草	10 g
Pericarpium Citri Reticulatae	陈皮	10 g
Radix Angelicae Sinensis	当归	10 g

Radix Paeoniae Alba	白芍	10 g
Medulla Cinnamomi	肉桂	1 g
Rhizoma Rehmanniae Praeparatae	熟地	7 g
Fructus Schisandrae	五味子	7 g
Poria	茯苓	7 g
Radix Polygalae	远志	5 g
Ziziphi Jujubae	大枣	10 g
Rhizoma Zingiberis Recens	生姜	10 g

Administration: Boil these drugs in a proper amount of water to get about 500 ml of decoction and divide the decoction into 2—3 equal portions for oral intake, 1 portion a time, 2—3 times a day.

Efficacy: Being efficacious in invigorating and tonifying *Qi* and blood and in tranquilizing the mind by nourishing the heart.

制用法: 水煎服。

功能: 补益气血, 养心宁神。

Shangyou gao 伤油膏 (43)   37,356

Ingredients:

Resina Draconis	血竭	60 g
Flos Carthami	红花	6 g
Resina Boswelliae Carterii	乳香	6 g
Commiphora Myrrha	没药	6 g
Acacia Catechu	儿茶	6 g
Succinum	琥珀	3 g
Borneolum Syntheticum	冰片	6 g

Administration: Grind the drugs except Borneolum Syntheticum into a powder, then put in Borneolum Syntheticum and grind the mixture. Resolve the new powder in 1 500 ml of heated sesame oil and condense the oil solution of the drugs with a proper amount of wax to produce an ointment for external application.

Efficacy: Having such effects as activating circulation of the blood and alleviating pains.

制用法: 除冰片、香油、黄蜡外，其它药为末，后入冰片再研，将末溶化于炼过的油内，再入黄蜡收膏。

功能: 活血止痛。

Shengji Xiangpi Gao　生肌象皮膏　(29)　　　　　　　　36,356

Ingredients:

Crinis Carbonisatus	血余	15 g
Plastrum Testudinis	生龟板	25 g
Radix Rehmannia	生地	25 g
Radix Angelicae Sinensis	当归	15 g
Gypsum Fibrosum	生石膏	30 g
Calamina	生炉甘石	50 g
Cera Flava	蜂蜡	90 g
Cutis Elephantus	象皮	20 g
Oleum Sesami	香油	500 g

Administration: Remove the residual cutaneous substances from Plastrum Cutaneous; cut Cutis Elephantus into small pieces and heat the pieces in a cauldron of sands until they become light brown and crisp, grind the heated pieces into a powder and sift the powder with a sieve （100 meshes per square centimeter）; cut Radix Rehmannia and Radix Angelicae Sinensis into slices; Grind Clamina and Gypsum Fibrosum into a powder and sift the powder with a sieve （100 meshes per square centimeter）; heat Oleum Sesami in a cauldron to about 250 degrees Centigrade until the oil drops will not break when the oil is let to fall in drops into a basin （ or the like）of water, put in Crinis

Carbonisatus, continue heating for about 10—15 minutes before getting it out; put in Plastrum Testudinis and fry it until it becomes dark brown (that is, for about 15 minutes), then , add in Radix Rehmannia and Radix Angelicae Sinensis and heat the three drugs together in the oil for 5 minutes; get the drugs out and filter the oil to remove residues before reheat it to 200 degrees centigrade; slowly put in the powder of Gypsum Fibrosum and Calamina and go on heating for 3—4 hours to get a dark brown mixture; melt Cera Flava and filter it before adding it to the dark brown mixture; stop heating 10 minutes later, stir the new mixture unceasingly while putting in the powder of Cutis Elephantus and a pastelike ointment will be obtained.Apply some of the ointment to the affected site.

Efficacy: Being efficacious in activating blood circulation and in promoting regeneration of the cells at the wounded surface.

用法: 生龟板除去残留皮质;象皮切成小块, 用砂子炒至脆黄, 研细过 100 目筛;生地、当归切片;生炉甘石、生石膏研细过 100 目筛。将香油置锅内, 加热至 250℃ 左右, 待熬至油可滴水成珠时, 投入血余, 10～15 分钟后捞出。再投入龟板, 炸至呈栗子皮色 (约 15 分钟), 再加入生地、当归, 5 分钟后将头三种药捞出。将锅中之油过滤去渣, 再加热至 200℃ 左右, 徐徐加入生石膏、生炉甘石, 熬 3～4 小时, 使其黑褐色。将蜂蜡熔化, 过滤后加入此油中, 10 分钟后去火, 不断搅拌, 并加入象皮粉, 搅至糊状即可。

功能: 活血生肌, 具有促进创面的组织细胞增生、分化, 增强血运的功效。

Shengji Yuhong Gao   36,37,250,257,262
生肌玉红膏 (30)   356,491,494,497

Ingredients:

Radix Angelicae Sinensis	当归	5 portions
Radix Angelicae Dahuricae	白芷	1.2 portions
Paraffinum	白蜡	5 portions
Calomeas	轻粉	1 portion
Radix Glycyrrhizae	甘草	3 portions
Radix Arnebiae seu Lithospermi	紫草	0.5 portions
Resina Draconis	血竭	1 portion
Oleum Sesami	麻油	40 portions

Administration: Soak the drugs Radix Angelicae Sinensis, Radix Angelicae Dahuricae, Radix Arnebiae seu Lithospermi and Radix Glycyrrhizae in the sesame oil for 3 days before heating them in a ceramic container on a moderate fire to make them slightly brown, remove the dry materials by filtration to leave in the container the oil only; heat the filtered oil again until it boils, put in Resina Draconis; when this drug dissolve thoroughly in the oil, add paraffinum and let the oil be boiling on a mild fire, then, pour the mixture of oil and paraffin into a mug that has been half-filled with water previously. A few minutes later, drop Calomeas into the mixture so as to produce an ointment. Spread some of the ointment on a piece of gauze and apply the gauze to the affected site.

Efficacy: Being efficacious in activating circulation of the blood, promoting absorption of the necrotic tissues, expelling toxic materials, alleviating pains, moistening the skin and helping tissue regeneration.

制服法：先将当归、白芷、紫草、甘草入油内浸三日，慢火熬微枯，滤清，再熬液，入血竭化尽，次入白蜡，微火化开，将膏倾入预放水的盅内，片刻，再把研细的轻粉末放入，搅拌成膏。将膏匀涂纱布上，贴患处。

功能：活血祛腐，解毒镇痛，润肤生肌。

Shenjin Gao　伸筋膏（31）　　　36,66,75,136,147,356,376,382,387

Ingredients:

Semen strychni	马钱子	9 g
Lumbricus	地龙	12 g
Herba Speranskia Tuberculata	透骨草	9 g
Huechys Sanguinea	红娘子	12 g
Squama Manitis	生山甲	9 g
Bombyx Batryticatus	僵蚕	12 g
Radix Stephaniae Tetrandrae	防己	9 g
Radix Clematidis	威灵仙	12 g
Radix Angelicae Sinensis (fibrous root)	当归尾	15 g
Radix et Rhizoma Rhei	生大黄	12 g
Folium Herba Lycopi	泽兰叶	12 g
Resina Boswelliae Carterii	乳香	9 g
Commiphora Myrrha	没药	9 g
Rhizoma Drynariae	申姜	9 g
Semen Vaccariae	王不留行	9 g
Herba Asari	细辛	9 g
Cortex Acanthopanacis Radicis	五加皮	9 g
Herba Siegesbeckiae	豨莶草	9 g
Folium Mahoniae	功劳叶	30 g
Scolopendra	蜈蚣	4 piece
Retinervus Luffae Fructus	丝瓜络	12 g
Herba Ephedrae	麻黄	12 g
Eupolyphaga seu Steleophaga	土元	12 g
Radix Angelicae Pubescentis	独活	9 g
Radix Aconiti Kusnezoffii	生草乌	9 g

Radix Euphorbiae Kansui	甘遂	30 g
Galla Chinensis	五倍子	9 g
Cortex Cinnamomi	肉桂	9 g
Radix Ledebouriellae	防风	12 g
Fructus Aurantii Immaturus	枳实	9 g
Fructus Arctii	牛蒡子	9 g
Crinis Carbonisatus	血余	9 g

Administration: Fry these drugs with 2 000 ml of sesame oil in a cauldron until they become dark brown, remove the dregs through filtration to get the oil; heat the oil again until the oil drops will not break when the oil is let to fall in drops into a basin (or the like) of water, add in 1 000 grams of Plumbumplumbi oxydum and stir thoroughly to produce an ointment.Spread some of the ointment on a piece of cloth and apply it to the affected site.

Efficacy: Being efficacious in removing stagnation from the channels, allev iating pains, relaxing muscles and tendons, activating blood flow, dispelling pathogenic wind and dredging the channels.

制用法: 取麻油 2 000 毫升置锅内, 将上药入锅内炸枯去渣, 炼油滴水成珠, 下樟丹 1 000 克, 搅匀即成。取药膏适量摊于布上, 贴患处。

功能: 散瘀止痛, 舒筋活血, 疏风通络。

Shenjin Pian 伸筋片(50)　　81,147,152,171,245,385,429,439,488

Ingredients: :

Semen Strychni Praeparata	制马钱子	21 g
Lumbricus	地龙	30 g
Resina Boswelliae Carterii	乳香	9 g
Coomiphora Myrrha	没药	9 g

Herba Ephedrae	麻黄	9 g
Cannabis Sativa	麻根炭	9 g
Cortex Acanthopanacis Radicis	五加皮	9 g
Radix Stephaniae Tetrandrae	防己	9 g
Resina Draconis	血竭	6 g
Rhizoma Drynariae	骨碎补	6 g

Administration: grind the drugs into a fine powder and make tablets of the powder, each weighing 0.3 g, for oral intake, 5 tablets a time, 3 times a day.

Efficacy: Being efficacious in activating circulation of the blood, in relaxing the muscles and tendons, in promoting the flow of *Qi* and blood in the channels and collaterals and in alleviating pains.

制用法: 上药共为细末, 依法制片, 每片重 0.3 克, 每服 5 片, 每日 3 次。

功能: 活血伸筋, 通络止痛。

Shenling Baizhu San 参苓白术散 (15)   34,355

Ingredients:

Semen Dolichoris Album	白扁豆	12 g
Radix Codonopsis Pilosulae	党参	12 g
Rhizoma Atractylodis Macrocephalae	白术	12 g
Poria	茯苓	12 g
Rhizoma Dioscoreae	山药	12 g
Semen Nelumbinis	莲子肉	10 g
Semen Coicis	薏苡仁	10 g
Radix Glycyrrhizae Praeparatae	炙甘草	6 g
Radix Platycodi	桔梗	6 g
Fructus Amomi	砂仁	

Adiminstration: Add 4 dates to the prescription, boil the

drugs in a proper amount of water to get about 500 ml of decoction and divide the decoction into 2—3 equal portions for oral intake, 1 portion a time, 2—3 times a day.

Efficacy: Having an effect in replenishing *Qi* in reinforcing the spleen and excreting dampness.

制服法: 水煎服。

功能: 补气、健脾、渗湿。

Shentong Zhuyu Tang 身痛逐瘀汤(62)   243,487

Ingredients:

Radix Gentianae Macrophyllae	秦艽	9 g
Rhizoma Ligustici Chuanxiong	川芎	9 g
Semen Persicae	桃仁	9 g
Flos Carthami	红花	9 g
Radix Angelicae Sinensis	当归	15 g
Rhizoma seu Radix Notopterygii	羌活	9 g
Commiphora Myrrha	没药	9 g
Faeces Trogopterorum	五灵脂	9 g
Rhizoma Cyperi	香附	9 g
Radix Achyranthis Bidentatae	牛膝	9 g
Lumbricus	地龙	9 g
Radix Glycyrrhizae	甘草	3 g

Administration: Boil these drug in a proper amount of water to get about 500 ml of decoction and divide the decoction into 2—3 equal portions for oral intake, 1 portion a time, 2—3 times a day.

Efficacy: Having such effects as activating circulation of the blood, promoting the flow of *Qi* in the channels and collaterals so as to dredge them, removing blood stasis, relieving stagnation—syndrome and alleviating pains.

制用法：水煎服。

功能：活血行气，祛瘀通络，通痹止痛。

Shuangbai San 双柏散 （24）   **35,356**

Ingredients:

Cacumen Biotae	侧柏叶	2 portions
Cortex Phellodendri	黄柏	1 portion
Radix et Rhizoma Rhei	大黄	2 portions
Herba Menthae	薄荷	1 portion
Herba Lycopi	泽兰	1 portion

Administration: Grind these drugs into a fine powder, mix the powder with some water and honey, and make a thick paste of the mixture on a heater for external application to the affected site.

Efficacy: Having such effects as clearing away heat and toxic materials from the blood and invigorating blood circulation.

制用法：上药共为细末，以水、蜜糖煮热调成厚糊状，外敷患处。

功能：清热解毒、凉血活血。

Shujin Huoxue Pian (a proprietary)舒筋活血片 （55）   **233,244,**
Ingrdients: **245,479,487**

Flos Carthami	红花
Cortex Periplocae Radicis	香加皮
Rhizoma Cyperi	香附
Folium Lycopi	泽兰叶
...	......

Administration: Take the tablets orally, 5 tablets a time, 3 times a day.

Efficacy: Being efficacious in relaxing the muscles and tendons, in promoting the flow of *Qi* and blood in the channels and collaterals, in activating circulation of the blood and in removing blood stasis.

制用法: 口服，每次 5 片，每日 3 次。

功能: 舒筋活络，活血散瘀。

Shujin Zhitong Shui　**舒筋止痛水** (42)　　　　　　　　**37,356**

Ingredients:

Radix Notoginseng (in powder)	三七粉	18 g
Rhizoma Sparganii	三棱	18 g
Flos Carthami	红花	30 g
Camphora	樟脑	30 g
Radix Aconiti Kusnezoffii	生草乌	12 g
Radix Aconiti	生川乌	12 g
Cortex Acanthopanacis Radicis	五加皮	12 g
Fructus Chaenomelis	木瓜	12 g
Radix Achyranthis Bidentatae	牛膝	12 g
Radix Angelicae Sinensis (fibrous root)	当归尾	18 g

Administration: Soak these drugs in 1 500 ml of alcohol (70% water solution) or in 1 000 ml of sorghum liquor for a month and the alcohol or liquor will become an alcoholic liniment for external application, Rub some of the liniment on the skin of the affected part, 2—3 times a day.

Efficacy: Being efficacious in relaxing the muscles and tendons, in activating circulation of the blood and in alleviating pains.

制用法: 密封浸泡一个月后备用，将药水涂擦患处，每日 2 ～3 次。

功能: 舒筋活血止痛。

Shunqi Huoxue Tang　**顺气活血汤** (6)　　　　　　**32,147,354**

Ingredients:

Radix Angelicae Sinensis (fibrous root)	当归尾	12 g
Radix Paeoniae Rubra	赤芍	9 g
Semen Persicae	桃仁	9 g
Fructus Aurantii	枳壳	9 g
Cortex Magnoliae Officinalis	厚朴	9 g
Rhizoma Cyperi	香附	9 g
Radix Aucklaudiae	木香	9 g
Fructus Amomi	砂仁	9 g
Flos Carthami	红花	6 g
Lignum Sappan	苏木	15 g
Caulis Perillae	苏梗	18 g

Administration: Boil these drugs in a proper amount of water to get about 500 ml of decoction and divide the decoction into 2—3 equal portions for oral intake, 1 portion a time, 2—3 times a day.

Efficacy: Being efficacious in activating blood circulation so as to eliminate blood stasis and in invigorating the flow of *Qi* so as to remove stagnation in the channels and collaterals.

制服法：水煎服。

功能：化瘀行气。

Sichong Wan 四虫丸 (79) 262,497

Ingredients:

Scorpio	全蝎
Scolopendra	蜈蚣
Eupolyphaga seu Steleophaga	土元
Lumbricus	地龙

Administration: Grind equal shares of the drugs into a fine powder and mix the powder with some water; make pills out of the mixture for oral intake, 3 grams once, twice a day.

Efficacy: Having such effects as promoting the flow of *Qi* and blood in the channels and collaterals, eliminating blood stasis and alleviating pains.

制用法：上药共为细末，水泛为丸。每服3克，日服2次。

功能：通络祛瘀止痛。

Sihuang Tang　四黄汤　(28)　　　　　　　　36,250,356,491

Ingredients:

Rhizoma Coptidis	黄连	1 portion
Cortex Phellodendri	黄柏	3 portions
Radix et Rhizoma Rhei	大黄	3 portions
Radix Scutellariae	黄芩	3 portions

Administration: Grind these drugs into a fine powder, mix the powder with a proper amount of water / honey to produce a paste, or make an ointment with the powder and some vaseline, for external application.

Efficacy: Being efficacious in clearing away pathogenic heat and toxic materials, subdueing swelling and alleviating pains.

制用法：共为细末，以水、蜜调服或用凡士林调制成膏外敷。

功能：清热解毒，消肿止痛。

Sijunzhi Tang　四君子汤　(12)　　　　　　　　33,355

Ingredients:

Radix Codonopsis Pilosulae	党参	10 g
Radix Glycyrrhizae Praeparatae	炙甘草	6 g
Rhizoma Atractylodis Macrocephalae	白术	12 g
Poria	茯苓	12 g

Administration: Boil these drugs in a proper amount of waterto get about 500 ml of decoction and divide the decoction into 2—3 equal portions for oral intake, 1 portion a time, 2—3 times a day.

Efficacy: Being efficacious in invigorating the spleen, in replenishing *Qi*, and in benefiting the functions of digestion and absorption.

制服法：水煎服。

功能：补益中气，调养脾胃。

Siwu Tang　四物汤（13）　　　　　　　　　　　　　33,355

Ingredients:

Rhizoma Ligustici Chuanxiong	川芎	6 g
Radix Angelicae Sinensis	当归	10 g
Radix Paeoniae Alba	白芍	12 g
Rehmanniae Praeparatae	熟地	12 g

Administration: Boil these drugs in a proper amount of water to get about 500 ml of decoction and divide the decoction into 2—3 equal portions for oral intake, 1 portion a time, 2—3 times a day.

Efficacy: Having an effect of nourishing and replenishing the blood.

制服法：水煎服。

功能：养血补血。

Suzhi Jiangqi Tang　苏子降气汤（52）　　　　　　　152,428

Ingredients:

Fructus Perillae	紫苏子	9 g
Rhizoma Pinelliae Praeparatae (water-soaked)	清半夏	9 g
Radix Peucedani	前胡	9 g
Pericarpium Citri Reticulatae	陈皮	6 g
Radix Angelicae Sinensis	当归	6 g
Cortex Magnoliae Officinalis	厚朴	3 g

Cortex Cinnamomi	肉桂	1.5 g
Radix Glycyrrhizae Praeparatae	炙甘草	3 g
Rhizoma Zingiberis Recens	生姜	3 slices

Administration: Boil these drugs in a proper amount of water to get about 500 ml of decoction and divide the decoction into 2—3 equal portions for oral intake, 1 portion a time, 2—3 times a day.

Efficacy: Being efficacious in checking the abnormal upward adverse flow of *Qi* in relieving cough and in removing phlegm.

制用法：水煎服。

功能：降气止逆，平冲定喘，镇咳化痰。

Taiyi Gao **太乙膏（35）**   36,356

Ingredients:

Radix Scrophulariae	玄参	100 g
Radix Angelicae Dahuricae	白芷	100 g
Radix Angelicae Sinensis	当归	100 g
Cortex Cinnamomi	肉桂	100 g
Radix Paeoniae Rubra	赤芍	100 g
Radix et Rhizoma Rhei	大黄	100 g
Radix Rehmanniae	生地	100 g
Semen Momordicae	土木鳖	100 g
Resina Ferulae	阿魏	15 g
Calomeas	轻粉	20 g
Ramulus Salix	柳枝	100 g
Crinis Carbonisatus	血余	50 g
Plumbumplumbi Oxydum	东丹	2 000 g
Resina Bowselliae Carterii	乳香	20 g
Commiphora Myrrha	没药	15 g

| Ramulus Sophorae | 槐枝 | 100 g |
| Oleum Sesami | 麻油 | 2 500 g |

Administration: Fry all the drugs except plumbumplumbi Oxydum with the sesame oil in a ceramic cauldron until they become dark brown, remove the dregs by filtration, then, put in Plumbumplumbi Oxydum and stir thoroughly to produce an ointment. Heat some of the ointment to melt it directly before use: Spread the melted ointment on a piece of cloth and apply it to the affected site.

Efficacy: Being efficacious in clearing away pathogenic heat, subduing swelling, removing toxic substances and promoting granulation.

制用法: 除东丹外，将余药入油煎，炸至药枯，去渣，再入东丹，搅拌匀成膏。用时取适量，烊化后摊于布上外贴患处。

功能: 清热消肿，解毒生肌。

Taohua San 桃花散 (36)   **36,356**

Ingredients:

| Calx | 白石灰 | 6 portions |
| Radix et Rhizoma Rhei | 大黄 | 1 portion |

Administration: Decoct Radix et Rhizoma Rhei with a proper amount of water and, then, pour the decoction onto the calx to make it into a powder; roast the powder subsequently until it becomes light brown, sieve the dried lime for external application; Dust some of the powder on the wound and dress the part with gauze.

Efficacy: Having a hemostatic effect.

制用法: 先将大黄煎汁，泼入白石灰内，为末再炒，以石灰变成红色为度，将石灰过筛备用。用时掺撒于患处，纱布包扎。

功能: 止血。

Taoren Chengqi Tang   桃仁承气汤 (8)   32,170,354,439

Ingredients:

Semen Persicae	桃仁	10 g
Radix et Rhizoma Rhei （to be put in one or two minutes before the decoction is ready)	大黄（后入）	12 g
Ramulus Cinnamomi	桂枝	6 g
Mirabilitum	芒硝	6 g
Radix Clycyrrhizae	甘草	6 g

Administration: Boil these drugs in a proper amount of water to get about 500 ml of decoction and divide the decoction into 2—3 equal portions for oral intake, 1 portion a time, 2—3 times a day.

Efficacy: Being efficacious in removing stagnation through purgation.

制用法：水煎服。

功能：泻下逐瘀。

Tiaorong Huoluo Yin   调荣活络饮 (64)   244,487

Ingredients:

Radix Angelicae Sinensis (fibrous root)	当归尾	12 g
Radix Paeoniae Rubra	赤芍	12 g
Semen Persicae	桃仁	9 g
Flos Carthami	红花	9 g
Radix et Rhizoma Rhei	大黄	6 g
Radix Angelicae Pubescentis	独活	9 g
Radix Gentianae Macrophyllae	秦艽	9 g
Radix Achyranthis Bidentatae	牛膝	9 g
Ramulus Cinnamomi	桂枝	6 g

Administration: Boil these drugs in a proper amount of water to get about 500 ml of decoction and divide the decoction into 2—3 equal portions for oral intake, 1 portion a time, 2—3 times a day.

Efficacy: Having such effects as activating circulation of the blood, relaxing the muscles and tendons and promoting the flow of *Qi* and blood in the channels and collaterals so as to ensure free passage in the meridain system.

制用法: 水煎服。

功能: 活血、舒筋、通络。

Tounong San 透脓散 (68)   250,491

Ingredients:

Radix Astrangoli seu Hedysari	生黄芪	15 g
Radix Angelicae Sinensis	当归	15 g
Squama Manitis	山甲珠	9 g
Spina Gledistsiae	皂刺	9 g
Rhizoma Ligustici Chuanxiong	川芎	9 g

Administration: Boil these drugs in a proper amount of water to get about 500 ml of decoction and divide the decoction into 2—3 equal portions for oral intake, 1 portion a time, 2—3 times a day.

Efficacy: Being efficacious in supplementing *Qi*, in expelling toxins, in dredging the channels and collaterals and in draining pus.

制用法: 水煎法。

功能: 益气托毒，通络透脓。

Tuoli Xiaodu Yin 托里消毒饮 (71)   256,494

Ingredients:

Radix Astrangali seu Hedysari	生黄芪	12 g

Flos Lonicerae	金银花	12 g
Radix Codonopsis Pilosulae	党参	12 g
Poria	茯苓	12 g
Spina Gledistsiae	皂角刺	10 g
Radix Platycodi	桔梗	10 g
Radix Angelicae Sinensis	当归	10 g
Rhizoma Atractylodis Macrocephalae	白术	10 g
Radix Paeoniae Alba	白芍	10 g
Radix Angelicae Dahuricae	白芷	6 g
Rhizoma ligustici Chuanxiong	川芎	6 g
Radix Glycyrrhizae	甘草	6 g

Administration: Boil these drugs in a proper amount of water to get about 500 ml of decoction and divide the decoction into 2—3 equal portions for oral intake, 1 portion a time, 2—3 times a day.

Efficacy: Having such effects as tonifying *Qi* and blood and dispelling toxic substances.

制用法：水煎服。

功能：补益气血，托里消毒。

Waiyong Jiegu Gao **外用接骨膏 (26)**   **35,356**

Ingredients:

Pyritum Praeparatae	制自然铜	30 g
Resina Boswelliae Carterii	乳香	30 g
Commiphora Myrrha	没药	30 g
Urina Humana	人中白	45 g
Resina Draconis	血竭	6 g
Galla Chinensis	五倍子	90 g

Administration: Gring the solid drugs in the recipe into a fine powder, mix the powder and the liquid Urina Humana with a certain amount of vinegar to make a thick paste, heat the mixture in a pan until it boils, and, then, spread some of the paste on a piece of cloth for external application to the affected site.

Efficacy: Having such effects as promoting reunion of the fractured bone and helping repairment of the affected muscles, tendons and ligaments.

制用法: 上药共为细末, 根据损伤的部位, 取药适量, 加醋调如稠粥状, 放火上熬沸取下, 摊于布上, 趁温敷伤处。

功能: 接骨续筋。

Wuwei Xiaodu Yin 五味消毒饮 (5)   32,69,170,250,256,
Ingredients: 354,378,439,491,494

Flos Lonicerae	金银花	30 g
Herba Taraxaci	蒲公英	30 g
Herba Violae	紫花地丁	30 g
Flos Chrysanthemi Indici	野菊花	15 g
Radix Semiaquilegiae	天葵子	9 g

Administration: Boil these drugs in a proper amount of water to get about 500 ml of decoction and divide the decoction into 2—3 equal portions for oral intake, 1 portion a time, 2—3 times a day.

Efficacy: Being efficacious in clearing away pathogenic heat and toxic material.

制服法: 水煎服。

功能: 清热解毒。

Wuwu Dan 五五丹 (82)   262,497

Ingredients:

Gypsum Fibrosum Praeparatae	熟石膏	15 g
Hydrargyri Oxydum Rubrum	红升丹	15 g

Administration: Grind the drugs into fine a powder for external application to the wound surface.

Efficacy: Having such effects as detoxifying poisons and promoting absorption of the necrotic tissues.

制用法：共研为极细末，撒于疮面。

功能：提毒祛腐。

Xiangsha Liujunzhi Tang　**香砂六君子汤** (73)　　　　**257,494**

Ingredients:

Radix Ginseng	人参	12 g
Rhizoma Atractylodis Macrocephalae	白术	9 g
Poria	茯苓	9 g
Pericarpium Citri Reticulatae	陈皮	9 g
Rhizoma Pinelliae	半夏	9 g
Radix Aucklandiae	木香	9 g
Fructus Amomi	砂仁	6 g
Radix Glycyrrhizae	甘草	3 g
Rhizoma Zingiberis Recens	生姜	3 slices
Fructus Ziziphi Jujubae	大枣	5

Administration: Boil these drugs in a proper amount of water to get about 500 ml of decoction and divide the decoction into 2—3 equal portions for oral intake, 1 portion a time, 2—3 times a day.

Efficacy: Having such effects as strengthening the middle—warmer and benefiting *Qi*, reinforcing the spleen and tonifying the stomach.

制用法：水煎服。

功能：益气补中，健脾养胃。

Xiao Huoluo Dan(a proprietary)**小活络丹(成药)(60)**　　**238,245,**

Ingredients:　　　　　　　　　　　　　　　　　**483,488**

Radix Aconiti	川乌	180 g

Radix Aconiti Kusnezoffii	草乌	180 g
Rhizoma Arisaematis	南星	180 g
Lumbricus	地龙	180 g
Commiphora Myrrha	没药	66 g
Resina Bosaelliae Carterii	乳香	66 g

Administration: Grind the drugs into a fine powder, mix the powder with some heated honey, and make boluses out of the mixture, each weighing 6 grams, for oral intake, 1 bolus once, twice a day.

Efficacy: Being efficacious in warming the channels and collaterals, in clearing away pathogenic cold, in activating circulation of the blood and in alleviating pains.

制用法：共为细末，炼蜜为丸，每丸重 6g，每服 1 丸，日服 2 次。

功能：温经散寒，活血止痛。

Xiaozhong Zhitong Gao 消肿止痛膏（23）   35,356

Ingredients:

Rhizoma Curcumae Longae	姜黄	1 portion
Rhizoma seu Radix Notopterygii	羌活	1 portion
Rhizoma Zingiberis	干姜	1 portion
Fructus Gardeniae	栀子	1 portion
Commiphora Myrrha	没药	1 portion
Resina Boswelliae Carterii	乳香	1 portion

Administration: Grind these drugs into a fine powder and mix the powder with a certain amount of vaseline, producing an ointment containing 60% of the powder for external application.

Efficacy: Having such effects as removing blood stasis, subduing swelling and alleviating pains.

制用法：共为细末，用凡士林调成 60% 软膏外敷患处。

功能: 祛瘀、消肿、止痛。

Yangpi Jingshi Tang **养脾进食汤** (16)   **34,355**

Ingredients:

Radix Codonopsis Pilosulae	党参	10 g
Rhizoma Atractylodis Macrocephalae	白术	10 g
Poria	茯苓	10 g
Pericarpium Citri Reticulatae	陈皮	10 g
Rhizoma Pinelliae	半夏	10 g
Cortex Magnoliae Officinalis	厚朴	10 g
Rhizoma Atractylodis	苍术	10 g
Fructus Amomi	砂仁	5 g
Radix Glycyrrhizae	甘草	5 g
Massa Fermentata Medicinalis	神粬	6 g
Fructus Hordei Germinatus Praeparatae	炒麦芽	6 g
Radix Aucklandiae	木香	3 g

Administration: Boil these drugs in a proper amount of water to get about 500 ml of decoction and divide the decoction into 2—3 equal portions for oral intake, 1 portion a time, 2—3 times a day.

Efficacy: Being efficacious in regulating the intestinal functions in improving appetite, in promoting digestion and in alleviating diarrhea.

制用法: 水煎服。

功能: 整肠健胃, 止泻增食。

Yougui Wan **右归丸** (65)   **245,487**

Ingredients:

Rhizoma Rehmanniae Praeparatae	熟地	240 g
Rhizoma Dioscoreae	山药	120 g
Fructus Corni	山萸肉	120 g

Fructus Lycii	枸杞	120 g
Semen Cuscutae	菟丝子	120 g
Cortex Eucommiae	杜仲	120 g
Colla Cornus Cervi	鹿角胶	120 g
Radix Angelicae Sinensis	当归	90 g
Radix Aconiti Praeparata	附子	60 g
Cortex Cinnamomi	肉桂	60 g

Administration: Grind these drugs into a fine powder, mix the powder with some heated honey and make boluses out of the mixture, each weighing 9 grams, for oral intake, 1 bolus a time, 3 times a day.

Efficacy: Having an effect in warming and tonifying the kidney and spleen.

制用法：共为细末，炼蜜为丸，每丸 9 克。每服 1 丸，日服 3 次。

功能：温补脾肾。

Yunnan Baiyao(a proprietary medicinal powder)云南白药(成药)(63) 243, 487

Ingredients: omitted

Administration: Administer the medicinal powder orally, 0.5 grams a time, 3—4 times a day.

Efficacy: Being efficacious in activating circulation of the blood, in supressing bleeding, in removing blood stasis and in alleviating pains.

制用法：口服，每次 0.5 克，每隔 4 小时服一次。

功能：活血止血，祛瘀定痛。

Zhenggu Tangyao   正骨汤药 (49)   39,357

Ingredients:

Radix Angelicae Sinensis	当归	12 g
Rhizoma seu Radix Notopterygii	羌活	12 g

Flos Carthami	红花	12 g
Radix Angelicae Dahuricae	白芷	12 g
Resina Boswelliae Carterii	乳香	12 g
Commiphora Myrrha	没药	12 g
Rhizoma Drynariae	骨碎补	12 g
Radix Ledebouriellae	防风	12 g
Fructus Chaenomelis	木瓜	12 g
Pericarpium Zanthoxyli	川椒	12 g
Herba Speranskia Tuberculata	透骨草	12 g
Radix Dipsaci	川断	12 g

Administration: Put all of the drugs in a cloth bag and steam the bag hot for external application to the affected part as drug fomentation.

Efficacy: Having such effects as activating circulation of the blood and relaxing the muscles and tendons.

制用法: 上药装入袋内, 放在锅内蒸热, 取出敷患处。

功能: 活血舒筋。

Zhenjiang Gaoyao (a proprietary plaster)镇江膏药(61)   238,244,
Ingredients: omitted   245,483,487,488

Administration: Heat the plaster and apply it to the affected part.

Efficacy: Having such effects as dispelling pathogenic wind from the body, alleviating pains, disolving masses in the organism, removing blood stasis and cheking adverse upward flow of stomach−*Qi*.

制用法: 烘热外敷患处。

功能: 祛风止痛, 化痞除瘀, 舒筋活血, 消散顺气。

Zhuangjin Yangxue Tang   壮筋养血汤 (19)   34,355
Ingredients:

Radix Angelicae Sinensis	当归	9 g
Radix Angelicae Dahuricae	白芷	9 g
Radix Achyranthis Bidentatae	牛膝	9 g
Cortex Moutan Radicis	牡丹皮	9 g
Rhizoma Ligustici Chuanxiong	川芎	6 g
Radix Dipsaci	续断	12 g
Radix Rehmannia	生地	12 g
Flos Carthami	红花	5 g
Cortex Eucommiae	杜仲	5 g

Adiminstration: Boil these drugs in a proper amount of water to get about 500 ml of decoction and divide the decoction into 2—3 equal portions for oral intake, 1 portion a time, 2—3 times a day.

Efficacy: Being efficacious in invigorating the flow of the blood and in strengthening the soft tissues.

制用法：水煎服。

功能：活血壮筋。

Zhuangyao Jianshen Tang 壮腰健肾汤(51) **147,170,245,425,439,487**

Ingredients:

Rhizoma Rehmanniae Praeparatae	熟地	15 g
Cortex Eucommiae	杜仲	9 g
Fructus Corni	山萸肉	9 g
Fructus Lycii	枸杞子	9 g
Fructus Psoraleae	补骨脂	9 g
Flos Carthami	红花	9 g
Rhizoma seu Radix Notopterygii	羌活	9 g
Radix Angelicae Pubescentis	独活	9 g
Herba Cistanchis	肉苁蓉	9 g
Semen Cuscutae	菟丝子	15 g

Radix Angelicae Sinensis   当归   15 g

Administration: Boil these drugs in a proper amount of water to get about 500 ml of decoction and divide the decoction into 2—3 equal portions for oral intake, 1 portion a time, 2—3 times a day.

Efficacy: Having such effects as regulating functions of the liver and kidney and strenthening the muscles, tendons and bones.

制用法：水煎服。

功能：调肝肾，壮筋骨。

Zhuidu Dan   **追毒丹** (83)   **262,497**

Ingredients:

Hydrargyri Oxydum Rubrum	红升丹	6 g
Radix et Rhizoma Rhei	大黄	6 g
Radix Angelicae Dahuricae	白芷	6 g
Borneolum Syntheticum	冰片	0.6 g

Administration: Grind the drugs into a fine powder for external application to the wound surface.

Efficacy: Having such effects as dispelling toxic substances and promoting absorption of the necrotic tissues.

制用法：共研细末，撒于疮面。

功能：提毒祛腐。

Zuogui Wan   **左归丸** (66)   **245,487**

Ingredients:

Rhizoma Rehmanniae Praeparata	熟地	240 g
Rhizoma Dioscoreae	山药	120 g
Fructus Lycii	枸杞子	120 g
Fructus corni	山萸肉	120 g
Radix Achyranthis Bidentatae	川牛膝	120 g

Semen Cuscutae	菟丝子	120 g
Colla Cornus Cervi	鹿角胶	60 g
Colla Plastrum Testudinis	龟板胶	60 g

Administration: Grind the drugs into a fine powder, mix the powder with some heated honey and make boluses out of the mixture for oral intake, 1 bolus a time, 3 times a day.

Efficacy: Having an effect in reinforcing both the essential liver—*Yin* and essential kidney—*Yin*.

制用法：共为细末，炼蜜为丸，每丸重 9 克。每服 1 丸，日服 3 次。

功能：填补肝肾真阴。

序

　　《英汉实用中医药大全》即将问世，吾为之高兴。

　　歧黄之道，历经沧桑，永盛不衰。吾中华民族之强盛，由之。世界医学之丰富和发展，亦由之。然而，世界民族之差异，国别之不同，语言之障碍，使中医中药的传播和交流受到了严重束缚。当前，世界各国人民学习、研究、运用中医药的热潮方兴未艾。为使吾中华民族优秀文化遗产之一的歧黄之道走向世界，光大其业，为世界人民造福，徐象才君集省内外精英于一堂，主持编译了《英汉实用中医药大全》。是书之问世将使海内外同道欢呼雀跃。

　　世界医学发展之日，当是歧黄之道光大之时。

　　吾欣然序之。

中华人民共和国卫生部副部长

兼国家中医药管理局局长

世界针灸学会联合会主席

中国科学技术协会委员

中华全国中医学会副会长

中国针灸学会会长

胡熙明

1989 年 12 月

序

  中华民族有同疾病长期作斗争的光辉历程，故而有自己的传统医学——中国医药学。中国医药学有一套完整的从理论到实践的独特科学体系。几千年来，它不但被完好地保存下来，而且得到了发扬光大。它具有疗效显著、副作用小等优点，是人们防病治病，强身健体的有效工具。

  任何一个国家在医学进步中所取得的成就，都是人类共同的财富，是没有国界的。医学成果的交流比任何其他科学成果的交流都应进行得更及时，更准确。我从事中医工作30多年来，一直盼望着有朝一日中国医药学能全面走向世界，为全人类解除病痛疾苦做出其应有的贡献。但由于用外语表达中医难度较大，中国医药学对外传播的速度一直不能令人满意。

  山东中医学院的徐象才老师发起并主持了大型系列丛书《英汉实用中医药大全》的编译工作。这个工作是一项巨大工程，是一种大型科研活动，是一个大胆的尝试，是一件新事物。对徐象才老师及与其合作的全体编译者夜以继日地长期工作所付出的艰苦劳动，克服重重困难所表现出的坚韧不拔的毅力，以及因此而取得的重大成绩，我甚为敬佩。作为一个中医界的领导者，对他们的工作给予全力支持是我应尽的责任。

  我相信《英汉实用中医药大全》无疑会在中国医学史和世界科学技术史上找到它应有的位置。

中华全国中医学会常务理事
山东省卫生厅副厅长

张奇文

1990年3月

出 版 前 言

　　中国医药学是我中华民族优秀文化遗产之一，建国以来由于党和国家对待中医药采取了正确的政策，使中医药理论宝库不断得到了发掘整理，取得了巨大的成绩。当前，世界各国人民对中国医药学的学习和研究热潮日益高涨，为促进这一热潮更加蓬勃的发展，为使中国医药学能更好地为全人类解除病痛服务，就必须促进中医中药在世界范围内的传播和交流，而要使这一传播和交流进行得更及时、更准确，就必须首先排除语言障碍。因此，编译一套英汉对照的中医药基本知识的书籍，供国内外学习、研究中医药时使用，已成为国内外医药学界和医药学教育界许多人士的迫切需要。

　　多年来，在卫生部门的号召下，在"中医英语表达研究"方面，已经作出了一些可喜的成绩。本书《英汉实用中医药大全》的编辑出版就是在调查上述研究工作的历史和现状的基础上，继续对中医药英语表达作较系统、较全面的研究，以适应中国医药学对外传播交流的需要。

　　这部"大全"的版本为英汉对照，共有 21 个分册，一个分册介绍论述中国医药学的一个分科。在编著上注意了中医药汉文稿的编写特色，在内容上注意了科学性、实用性、全面性和简明易读。汉文稿的执笔撰写者主要是有 20 年以上实践经验的教授、副教授、主任医师和副主任医师。各分册汉文稿撰写成后，均经各学科专家逐一审订。各分册英文主译、主审主要是国内既懂中医又懂英语的权威人士，还有许多中医院校的英语教师及医药卫生部门的专业翻译人员。英译稿脱稿后，经过了复审、终审，有些译稿还召开全国 22 所院校和单位人员参加的英译稿统稿定稿研讨会，对英译稿进行细致的研讨和推敲，对如何较全面、较系统、较准确地用英语表达中国医药学进行了探讨，从而推动整个译文达到较高水平，因此，这部"大全"可供中医院校高年级学生作为泛读教材使用。

这部"大全"的编纂得到了国家教育委员会、国家中医药管理局、山东省教育委员会、山东省卫生厅等各部门有关领导的支持。在国家教委高等教育司的指导下，成立了《英汉实用中医药大全》编译领导委员会。还得到了全国许多中医院校和中药生产厂家领导的支持。

希望这部"大全"的出版，对中医院校加强中医英语教学，对国内卫生界培养外向型中医药人才，以及在推动世界各国人民对中医药的学习和研究方面，都将产生良好的影响。

高等教育出版社

1990年3月

前　言

　　《英汉实用中医药大全》是一部以中医基本理论为基础，以中医临床为重点，较为全面系统、简明扼要、易读实用的中级英汉学术性著作。它的主要读者是：中医药院校高年级学生和中青年教师，中医院的中青年医生和中医药科研单位的科研人员，从事中医对外函授工作的人员和出国讲学或行医的中医人员，西学中人员，来华学习中医的外国留学生和各类进修人员。

　　由于中国医药学为我中华民族之独有，因此，英译便成了本《大全》编译工作的重点。为确保译文能准确表达中医的确切含义，我们邀集熟悉中医的英语人员、医学专业翻译人员、懂英语的中医药人员乃至医古文人员于一堂，共同翻译、共同对译文进行研讨推敲的集体翻译法，这样，就把众人之长融进了译文质量之中。然而，即使这样，也难确保译文都能尽如人意。汉文稿虽反映了中国医药学的精髓和概貌，但也难能十全十美。我衷心地盼望读者能提出批评和建议，以便《大全》再版时修改。

　　参加本《大全》编、译、审工作的人员达 200 余名，他们来自全国 28 个单位，其中有山东、北京、上海、天津、南京、浙江、安徽、河南、湖北、广西、贵阳、甘肃、成都、山西、长春等 15 所中医学院，还有中国中医研究院，山东省中医药研究所等中医药科研单位。

　　山东省教育委员会把本《大全》的编译列入了科研计划并拨发了科研经费，山东省卫生厅和一些中药生产厂家也给了很大支持，济南中药厂的资助为编译工作的开端提供了条件。

　　本《大全》的编译成功是全体编译审者集体劳动的结晶，是各有关单位主管领导支持的结果。在《大全》各分册即将陆续出版之际，我诚挚地感谢全体编译审者的真诚合作，感谢许多专家、教授、各级领导和生产厂家的热情支持。

愿本《大全》的出版能在培养通晓英语的中医人才和使中医早日全面走向世界方面起到我所期望的作用。

主编　徐象才

于山东中医学院

1990 年 3 月

目　录

说　明

　　本书是大型系列丛书《英汉实用中医药大全》中的第14分册。

　　中医骨伤科学有独特的诊断和治疗方法,可使患者骨折愈合快、肢体功能恢复满意。因此,在国内外越来越受到重视。

　　本分册共有总论、骨折、脱位、伤筋、骨关节感染等5章。书中有插图129幅,方剂索引83首,以方便读者查阅。其特点是:突出中医特色,着眼临床治疗,论述简明扼要,强调实用性。

　　本分册汉文稿承蒙长春中医学院骨伤科刘柏龄教授审阅。在《大全》英文稿泰安统稿会上,浙江中医学院的李磊同志参加审校了英文稿。

编　者

1 总论

1.1 正骨手法

正骨手法,在骨伤科占有重要地位,当骨折发生以后,如骨折端产生移位或成角畸形,必须通过手法整复,以恢复其骨折的解剖对位或功能对位,给骨折愈合和功能恢复打下有利的基础。骨折端对位越好,固定越稳定,病人才能及早地进行功能锻炼,骨折才能获得早期愈合。

骨折整复时间

只要周身情况允许,骨折整复时间越早越好。因骨折早期局部肿胀,疼痛较轻,肌肉未发生痉挛,最易获得 1 次复位成功。伤后 4～6 小时,由于局部瘀血未凝结变硬,也容易复位。时间越久,复位越困难。一般地说,伤后 7～10 天以内,均可应用手法复位。

病人如有休克、昏迷,内脏等损伤时,须在全身情况稳定之后才可进行整复。在此期间,应对伤肢妥善固定,以减轻病人的疼痛,避免局部继发损伤。如患肢有明显肿胀、水泡时,应在无菌操作下抽出泡液,临时夹板固定,抬高患肢,待肿胀消退后,再行复位。开放性骨折清创缝合后,争取 1 次整复对位。

整复前的准备

1. 麻醉的选择:根据病人的具体情况,选择有效的止痛和麻醉方式,伤后 6～8 小时,可于局部血肿内注射适量的 0.5～2%普鲁卡因,效果满意。时间久且骨折移位较重的,整复多有困难,病人痛苦较大,一般上肢可用臂丛神经阻滞麻醉,下肢选用股神经或坐骨神经阻滞麻醉或腰麻。

2. 人员准备:确定整复者和助手,并作好分工,参加整复者对伤员的全身情况、受伤的机理、骨折类型及移位情况等，应作全面的了解和复习，将 X 线所显示的骨折情况与病人实体联系起来，仔细分析，确定该骨折需要哪些整复手法，助手应如何配合等，做到认识一致，动作协调。将病员及伤肢置于恰当位置，并作好病人的思想工作，以取得病人的密切配合。

3. 物质准备：根据骨折的部位、类型及肢体大小，准备好所用的器材。如纸壳、夹板、棉垫、扎带、绷带、胶布、小压垫等，还应准备必要的抢救药品和设备，保证安全，防止在整复中发生意外。

正骨手法及其适应症

正骨手法是治疗骨折的主要手段之一，欲使移位的骨折复位，则必须施行一定的手法，手法操作的好坏，是骨折复位成功与否的关键。正骨手法甚多，概括有以下几种：

1. 触摸：为正骨复位的首用手法。即用拇指或拇、食、中 3 指，接触伤处体表，稍加按压，仔细触摸体察，结合 X 线照像，分析骨折端的移位情况，在术者脑子里构成骨折移位的立体形象，通过手摸达到心明的程度，给下一步手法提供依据。

2. 拔伸：即牵拉伸张之意。此手法主要是克服肌肉抗力，以矫正骨折断端的重迭移位，恢复肢体原来的长度，即所谓"欲合先离，离而复合"。此法对于成角、旋转移位的纠正也起辅助作用。操作时，要求术者与助手共同进行，一般，整复者两手握持骨折端，两助手握住伤肢的两端，徐徐用力，开始拔伸时，肢体保持在原来的位置，顺其伤骨的纵轴方向对抗牵引，将刺入软组织的骨折端，慢慢拔伸出来，而后再按整复步骤改变肢体的方向，用力牵引。拔伸力量的大小应视病人的肌肉强度为依据，小儿、老年人及女性患者，拔伸力不应太大；反之青壮年患者，肌肉发达，则应有足够大的拔伸力。在拔伸牵引的同时，应调正肢体的力线，以纠正畸形，提高复位的成功率。助手在拔伸时做到持续稳妥，切忌使用暴力（图1）。

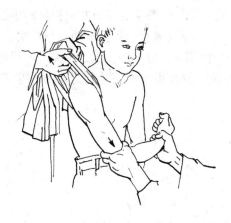

图1 拔伸手法示例

肱骨外科颈骨折（内收型）顺势牵引

3. 推按：即推送按压之意。术者用两手拇指或掌根部压于骨折端之高突处，用力按压，使突者复平，这是纠正骨折侧方移位的主要手法。此外，用拇、食、中3指捏住分离移位之骨块，推送至原位，按住勿使滑动（图2）。

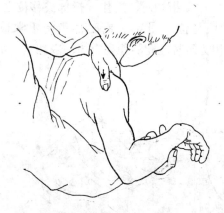

图2 推按手法示例

肱骨大结节骨折，用推按法整复

此手法一般与扳提手法配合应用。

4. 扳提：是与推按手法用力方向相反的手法。操作时术者用2~5指钩住陷下之骨折端用力扳动（与推按法协同），或用器具（如布带）作辅助，以手握住用力上提，或用指捏住下陷之骨折端用力提起。主要用于纠正骨折之侧方移位，使陷下者复起（图3）。

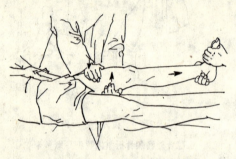

图 3 扳提手法示例

股骨干骨折整复法，一手推按，一手扳提

5. 揑挤：常用整复细小部位的骨折，如指（趾）骨折，术者用拇指与食、中2指相对，揑住骨折部或移位之骨块用力挤，使移位之小骨块复位（图 4）。有时，用两手掌根部按于骨折部，余指相扣用力对挤，此法稳妥有力，以纠正骨折移位，如跟骨骨折。

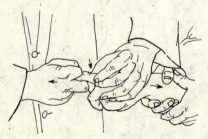

图 4 用指捏法整复指骨骨折

6. 分骨：凡是两骨并列部位发生骨折，如尺桡骨、胫腓骨、掌骨和蹠骨，骨折段因骨间肌或骨间膜的收缩而互相靠拢，复位时，应以两手拇指与其它4指相对，由骨折部的掌背侧夹挤骨间隙，使靠拢的骨折断端分开，恢复正常的骨间隙，骨折端则自然对位，相应稳定（图5）。

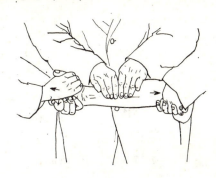

图5　分骨手法示例

尺桡骨干骨折，用分骨法整复

7. 折顶：此法用于两种情况，一是骨折端对位良好，而仅有明显成角畸形者，可在拔伸的基础上，1手按于骨折成角突出处，1手握伤肢远端，用反折力将成角扳回，恢复骨的正常轴线；一是用于肌肉发达，骨折端移位较大，而且一般拔伸力量不易拉开其重迭者。如股骨干骨折、前臂双骨折等，即在加大骨折端成角畸形的基础上，用力拔伸，同时以指顶压远侧骨折端，使之向远侧移动，至两断端骨皮质相对、顶住时，骤然将远端反折拉直，恢复骨干之正常轴线，骨折即可复位。此法操作时，术者与助手要做到动作协调，稳妥，敏捷。骨折端有伤及血管、神经或刺伤皮肤之可能，应注意防止（图6）。

8. 回转：回乃回绕之意，转即旋转。当骨折发生螺旋形骨折，或由外力作用造成骨折面背对背移位，整复时将远侧断端由移位之原路绕回，使骨折面互相对合。某些部位骨折由于肌肉牵拉，使骨折断端发生旋转，整复时，必须在拔伸的基础上，由助手将远侧断端绕其纵轴旋转，以远端凑近端，术者配合使用推

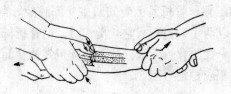

6-1　加大成角

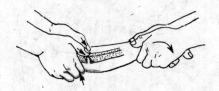

6-2　顶按折端，扳回成角

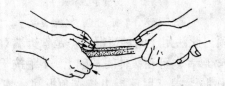

6-3　折端对位

尺桡骨双骨折用折顶法纠正其重迭移位

图 6　折顶手法示例

按、扳提手法使骨折复位（图7）。施用回转手法时，必须对骨

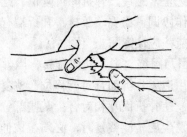

7-1　折端背对背移位回转法

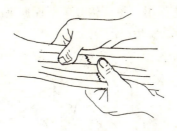

7-2 已复位

图7 回转手法示例

桡骨斜形骨折，折端背对背移位，用回转法整复

折移位机理有清楚的了解，方能行之有效。

9. 屈伸：此手法常用于整复关节部位骨折，在拔伸牵引的基础上，配合推按手法，根据骨折的类型，使关节或伸直或屈曲，或者屈伸活动数次，将移位之骨折复位。如肘、腕、踝部骨折常用此法（图8）。

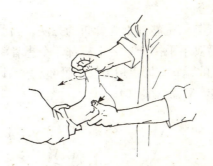

图8 屈伸手法示例

屈伸法整复踝骨骨折

10. 摇晃：经过以上手法一般骨折即可复位，但横断或锯齿型骨折，骨折断端间可能有一定间隙，为使骨折面紧紧接触，术者可用两手固定骨折部，助手在维持牵引的情况下，同时轻轻摇动伤肢的远端，使骨擦音逐渐变小或消失，骨折端即紧密地吻

合，增加其稳定性；如果属关节内骨折，也可通过摇晃手法，可对关节面产生模造作用，尽量恢复关节面原来的形态和光滑度，以防创伤性关节炎的发生（图9）。

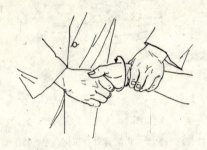

图9 摇晃手法示例

桡骨远端粉碎骨折，用摇晃法使骨折复位，并"模造"关节面

11. 叩击：某些稳定型骨折，如干骺端骨折，经手法整复对位满意，以夹板固定后，术者双手固定伤处，助手以手掌轻轻叩击骨折远段之远端，使骨折端紧密嵌插，骨折端更加稳定，有利于骨折愈合。

12. 气鼓：是整复肋骨骨折的方法。当肋骨骨折有前后移位时，助手双手平按于患者上腹部，令患者深呼吸而后用力咳嗽，在咳嗽的瞬间，助手用力按上腹部，术者以拇指下压高突的骨折端，多能复位（图10）。

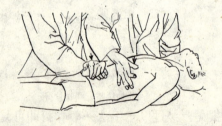

图10 气鼓整复手法示例

用气鼓整复法，整复肋骨骨折

13. 摩捋：此法常为整复骨折的最后步骤，术者用拇指或

与食指按于伤处，稍用力下按，并顺伤肢的筋肉走行方向或骨干纵轴往反捋摩，达到顺筋捋骨，散瘀止痛的作用。也可借此手法检查骨折整复的效果。如正骨满意，即可夹缚固定。

正骨复位的要求

1. 解剖对位：骨折之畸形和移位完全纠正，恢复骨的解剖学形态。解剖对位可使骨折端稳定，骨折愈合快，功能恢复好。对每一个骨折都应争取解剖对位。

2. 功能对位：所谓功能对位，即骨折在整复后，无重迭移位，旋转、成角畸形得到纠正，肢体力线正常，长短相等。骨折愈合后，肢体的功能可以恢复到满意程度，不影响病人生活和一般生产劳动。究竟对位到什么程度才合乎功能对位的要求，在不同部位骨折，不同年龄、职业等，各有不同的要求，如老年人虽骨折对位较差，而骨折愈合后，对其生活并无多大影响。然而对于舞蹈演员、体育运动员，其骨折对位要求较高，如对位不良多影响功能。关节内骨折对位要求也高。长骨干骨折，在上肢主要要求灵活，虽然有轻度成角和侧方移位，对肢体功能影响不大。儿童骨折不能遗留下旋转和成角畸形，轻度的重迭及侧方移位，在发育过程中可自行矫正。

正骨复位时注意事项

1. 树立满腔热情、全心全意为伤病员服务的思想，做好病人的思想工作，树立战胜疾病的信心，取得病人的密切合作。

2. 切忌使用暴力。拔伸牵引应徐徐用力，恰到好处，勿太过或不及。不得施用猛力，整复时着力点部位要准确，用力的大小、方向都应根据病情而定。不得用手指在伤处摩擦，避免增加软组织损伤。

3. 手法操作过程中，注意力要集中，仔细体会手下的感觉，观察伤处外形变化，注意病人反应，以判断手法的效果，并防止意外事故发生。

4. 整复骨折最好 1 次达到成功。多次复位增加软组织损伤，肿胀更加严重，再复位难以成功，而且有造成骨折迟延愈合或关节僵硬之可能。

5. 对于身体虚弱、孕妇，或者有其它严重并发症、多处复杂骨折等，整复时应特别慎重，如感复位有困难时，不得勉强行事，宁可暂缓复位或大体上改善骨折移位状况，待采取一定的积极治疗措施，条件允许后再设法弥补。不能只顾局部而忽视全身。

1.2 夹缚固定

为了维持骨折整复后的良好位置，保证骨折正常的愈合过程，在整复后必须采取适当的固定措施。固定是治疗骨折的一项重要措施。较好的固定应有以下作用：

保持伤肢于一定恰当的位置，使骨折处于相对稳定状态，给骨折愈合创造条件。

保持整复后的效果，避免骨折部位承受有害的伤力，防止骨折再移位。

为早期功能活动创造有利条件。

能够逐步纠正整复后的残留畸形或移位。

保护伤处，减少疼痛，避免增加新的损伤。

局部外固定形式

1. 小夹板局部外固定：适用于一般骨干骨折，如肱骨、桡尺骨、胫腓骨骨折等。

2. 超关节夹板固定：适用于关节面完整的关节内骨折或接近关节的干骺端骨折。如肱骨外科颈骨折、肱骨髁上骨折、踝部骨折等。

3. 小夹板局部外固定或超关节夹板固定合并骨牵引：小夹板局部外固定合并骨牵引，适用于骨折部软组织多，肌肉力量大的股骨干骨折、不稳定性胫腓骨骨折。超关节夹板固定合并骨牵引，适用于关节面已遭到破坏的关节内骨折。如肱骨髁间骨折等。

4. 竹帘、纸壳或木板分骨垫固定：适用于掌、跖骨骨折。

5. 小竹片和上纸壳：适用于指（趾）、跖骨骨折。

6. 绷带与胶布固定：适用于肋骨骨折、锁骨折。

夹板固定的作用

1. 扎带、夹板、压垫的外部作用力：捆缚扎带有一定的作用力，这种作用力通过夹板、压垫和软组织传导到骨折段或骨折端，以对抗骨折发生再移位。如3垫固定的挤压，杠杆力可防止骨折再发生成角移位；2垫固定的挤压剪切力可防止骨折再发生侧方移位。总之，扎带、夹板、压垫能有效地防止骨折侧方移位或成角移位，持续牵引可防止骨折的重选移位。

2. 肌肉收缩的内在动力：骨折经整复后，夹板只固定骨折局部，一般不超过上、下关节，在一定范围内可进行关节屈伸和功能活动，又不妨碍肌肉的纵向收缩活动，肌肉在骨干的纵向收缩力，可使两骨折端产生纵向挤压力，从而使上、下骨折端紧密吻合，增强其稳定性。另一方面，由于肌肉收缩时体积膨大，肢体的周径也随之增大，可对压垫、夹板产生一定的挤压作用力。同时，骨折端亦承受了由夹板、压垫产生的同样大小的反作用力，从而加强了骨折端的稳定性，起到了矫正骨折端残余移位的作用。肌肉舒展放松时，肢体周径恢复原状，夹板也恢复了原来的松紧度。根据以上原理，可按照骨折不同类型和移位情况，在相应的位置放置压垫，并保持夹板的适当松紧度，即可把肌肉收缩的不利因素，转化为对骨折愈合的有利因素。肌肉收缩活动，必须在医护人员正确指导下进行，并非盲目的、无限制的活动，否则可引起骨折再移位。为此，必须根据骨折类型、部位、病情的不同阶段及患者不同年龄等，进行不同方式的练功活动。

3. 伤肢处于与移位倾向相反的位置：肢体骨折后的移位可由暴力作用的方向、肌肉牵拉和远侧端肢体的重力等因素引起。因此，骨折复位后，应防止肢体重力引起骨折再移位的倾向，将伤肢处于与移位倾向相反的位置。并配合一定的活动，就可成为维持骨折对位、对线或矫正残余成角移位的有利因素。如肱骨髁上伸直型骨折，应将肘关节固定在屈曲位。

夹板材料和制作要求

夹板材料要求

可塑性：选材要根据肢体各部体形，弯曲成各种形状。

韧性：能有足够的支持力而不变形、不断折或不裂折。

弹性：能适应肌肉收缩和舒张时所产生的肢体内部的压力变化，不因肢体变形而失去夹板的支持固定作用。

夹板必须有一定程度的吸附性和通透性，以利肢体表面散热，不致发生皮炎等。

质量轻：过重则增加肢体的重量，增加骨折端的剪力，影响肢体练功活动。

能被 X 线穿透，以利放射线检查。

来源广，价低廉。

临床常用的夹板材料有：柳木板、竹板、杉树皮、硬纸壳、胶合板、铝板、塑料板等。

夹板的制作

夹板大小、厚薄要合适，所选用的小夹板，必须根据欲固定部位的体形，精心地加以制做、塑形。如选用竹板时，必须刨光，其厚度一般为 1.5～2.5mm，长度及宽度应视损伤部位之不同情况而异。如固定前臂时，掌背侧板宽约 3～5cm，内外侧板宽约 2cm，长约 12～18cm。板之边角要削光滑，放在温水中浸泡数小时后，取出，用酒精灯烘烤至软，再用屈板器制成所需要的弯曲形状（图 11）。

不超关节固定适用于骨干骨折，其夹板的长度，以等于或接近骨折段肢体的长度，但不妨碍上、下关节活动为度；超关节固定，其夹板长度应超出关节外 2～3 厘米，能以捆缚扎带为度。

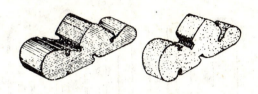

图 11　木制曲板器

夹板的总宽度相当于所要固定的肢体周径的$\frac{4}{5}$或$\frac{5}{6}$左右，每块夹板间要有一定的空隙。在夹板接近皮肤的一面，需贴上衬垫或外套，衬垫和外套必须是质地柔软，有一定的吸水性、可散热，对皮肤无刺激。其厚度为 0.2 厘米，表面平整。

　　制做夹板应制备大、中、小 3 种型号，根据肢体的部位应配套，以便用之方便（图 12）。

压垫的应用

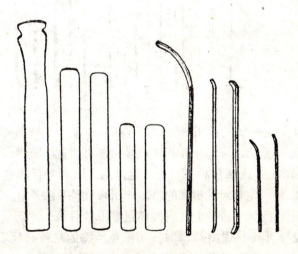

12-1　肱骨外科颈骨折固定板（连肩板）

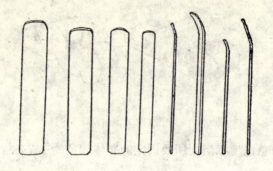

12—2　桡骨远端骨折固定板

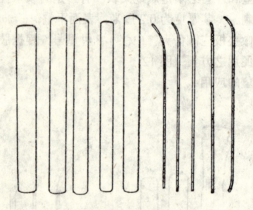

12—3　胫腓骨干骨折固定板

1. 小压垫的作用：一定形式的小压垫，可增加夹板对局部的有效固定力，以防止骨折块或骨折端再移位，或借以纠正骨折端残余畸形，或加强对关节的固定作用，以利骨折的愈合。但不可以依赖固定垫对骨折端的挤压作用来代替手法整复，否则将引起压迫性溃疡，或缺血性肌肉坏死等不良后果。

2. 小压垫取材与制做：小压垫所需的材料必须质地柔软，有一定的韧性和弹性，并能维持一定的形态，有一定的支持力，能吸水，可散热，对皮肤无刺激。常用的材料有：毛头纸、棉花、棉毡、绷带、纱布等。小压垫的形状、厚薄、大小应根据骨折的部位、类型、骨折移位情况而定，其形状原则上应与体形相符合，以保持压力的平衡。其大小、厚度、硬度应适宜。常用压垫有以下几种形态：

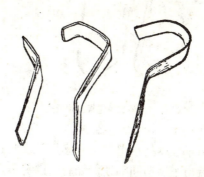

12-4　掌骨骨折固定板

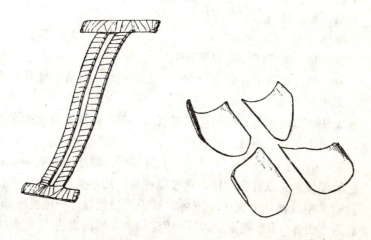

12-5　腰椎骨折固定板("工"字板用　　12-6　肘部固定板（硬纸壳）
　　厚竹板做成,外包棉花、绷带)

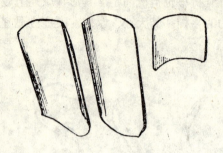

12-7 踝部固定板（硬纸壳）

图 12 塑形配套备用的小夹板示例

平垫：适用于肢体的平坦部位，多用于四肢长管骨骨折。

塔形垫：适用于关节凹陷处，如肘、踝关节。

梯形垫：适用于肢体斜坡处，如肘后部、足踝部。

高低垫：适用于锁骨或复位后固定不稳的尺桡骨骨折。

抱骨垫：呈半月状，用于鹰嘴及髌骨骨折，可用绒毡制成。

葫芦垫：适用于桡骨小头。

横垫：用于桡骨下端。

合骨垫：用于下尺桡关节分离。

分骨垫：适用于并列之骨骨折。如尺桡骨、掌骨及跖骨骨折等（图 13）。

大头垫：用棉花和绷带包扎夹板的一头，做成蘑菇状的固定垫，适用于肱骨外科颈骨折。

3. 小压垫的放置：一般于正骨复位后，将小压垫放于体表一定的部位，并以胶布贴住，再包以棉垫，用小夹板固定。要根据骨折类型、移位情况，小压垫安放于适当位置，一定要准确。安放的方法有：1 垫固定法，2 垫固定法和 3 垫固定法。

1 垫固定法：主要直接压迫骨折部，多用于肱骨内上髁或肱骨外髁骨折。

2 垫固定法：用于有侧方移位的横形骨折。骨折复位后，将两垫分别置于两骨端原有移位的一侧，以骨折线为界，两垫不要超过骨折线，以防骨折再发移位。

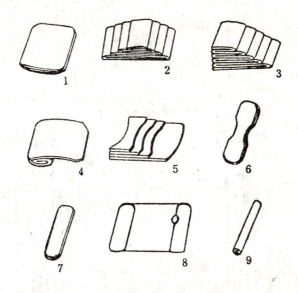

图 13　纸压垫

1. 平垫；2. 塔形垫；3. 梯形垫；4. 高低垫；5. 抱骨垫；

6. 葫芦垫；7. 横垫；8. 合骨垫；9. 分骨垫。

3 垫固定法：用于有成角畸形之骨折，1 垫置于骨折成角移位的角尖处，另两垫尽量置于靠近骨干两端的对侧，3 垫形成杠杆力，防止骨折再发生成角移位（图 14）。

4. 应用压垫时注意事项：压垫大小、厚薄，压卷之粗细、长短应根据受伤的部位而选用。压垫过薄，垫卷过细则压力过小，起不到固定作用；相反，则压力过大，有压伤皮肤的危险。若固定后局部皮色暗红，是压力过大之表现，应及时纠正。

小夹板固定方法

各个部位及不同类型的骨折，均有不同的固定方法。现以长骨干为例说明小夹板固定方法：将用的固定器材准备齐全，骨折

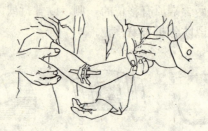

14-1　一点加压法示例
肱骨外髁骨折小压垫放置

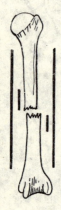

14-2　二点加压法示例

肱骨干骨折二点加压法，纠正折端
侧方移位

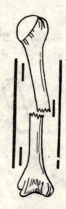

14-3　三点加压法示例

肱骨干骨折三点加压法，纠正折端
成角移位

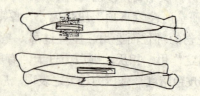

14-4　分骨卷放置法示例
尺桡骨干双折分骨卷放置部位
图14　小压垫放置法

整复成功后，需加压垫者应将压垫安放适当位置，将棉垫包缠于伤处，将夹板分别置于棉垫之外，均匀排列，板之间距为 1～1.5 cm 为宜，板之两端勿超过棉垫，骨折线最好位于夹板之中部，由助手扶住夹板。术者以扎带捆缚，先扎中间 1 道，缠绕两周后抽紧打结，再扎两端 2 道，一般 3 道即可。两端者应距板端1.5 cm 为宜，但不能滑脱。扎带的松紧度应适宜，肌肉丰满者可紧一些，一般要求横拉扎带能上下移动 1 cm 为适合。如需外附长板者，可在小夹板外层以绷带包扎。如需牵引者，可按牵引处理。小夹板固定后 3～5 天，由于肢体肿胀扎带有渐紧的趋势，而后由于肢体消肿，扎带逐渐变松，应及时调整扎带松紧度。

小夹板固定后注意事项

1. 适当抬高患肢，以利肢体肿胀消退。

2. 密切观察伤肢的血液循环情况，如发现有循环障碍，必须及时放松扎带，否则可发生严重后果。

3. 若在骨突处有严重疼痛，应及时检查，以防发生压迫性溃疡。

4. 注意经常调整扎带的松紧度。

5. 应将固定后的作用及可能出现的问题，告诉病人及家属，发现问题及时就诊。

6. 及时指导病人进行练功活动。

1.3　辨证用药

运用中药治疗骨折，是骨科的一大特点。临床实践证明，凡用中药治疗骨折均能达到：消肿止痛快、骨痂生长早、骨折愈合好、功能恢复满意。

我们认为：人体是一个完整的有机体，五脏六腑、四肢百骸、气血经络、皮肉筋骨都有密切关系。骨骼是由脏腑而化生，赖气血以濡养，经脉所贯通。肢体某处受伤，则往往影响全身，常出现脏腑、经络、气、血功能失调。为此，中医治疗骨伤，是在整体观念指导下，以辨证施治为基础，调整机体生理机能，消除因骨折后所产生的病理反应，以达到治愈骨折之目的。人体一旦遭受损伤，则经络受损，气机凝滞，营卫离经，瘀滞于筋肉之间，不通则痛，通则不痛。为此，中医治疗骨伤时，重点在调理气血，内治之法必须以活血化瘀为先，血不和则瘀不能去，瘀不能去则骨不能接。根据骨伤的发展过程，一般分为初、中、后3期，但这3期各有不同的特点和具体情况，所以在临床中必须辨证施治、处方用药。

初期（1~2周）

用药法则有以下几种：

1. 行气活血，消肿祛瘀法：临床上骨伤病人，凡是有气滞血瘀，肿胀疼痛均可应用，本法所用药物大都为活血祛瘀药为主，再配以行气通络药物。常选用复元活血汤（1），活血止痛汤（2），活血祛瘀汤（3）等。

2. 活血消肿，清热解毒：骨折初期，局部瘀血肿痛，皮肤色红灼热，周身发热，体温升高可用本法。常选用清心药（4）和五味消毒饮（5）加减。

3. 行气导滞、攻下逐瘀法：由于外伤后常合并内脏功能失调。如胃肠胀满，不思饮食，呕吐等，采用活血行气导滞，可用顺气活血汤（6）。如腹胀疼痛，呕吐，大便不通，舌红苔黄，应以攻下逐瘀，可选用大成汤（7），桃仁承气汤（8）。

4. 和营理气法：外伤后常可引起胸闷，咳嗽，胁肋刺痛，呼吸加重，咳嗽不畅或咳血诸症，多是肋骨骨折致肝气不舒和肺气不宣，可用理气止痛汤（9）和营理气汤（10）。

中期

一般骨折经过3~6周后，骨折局部肿痛消退，骨折端也基本稳定，全身症状消除。除保持骨折断端稳定之外，在用药时应以补骨生新、续筋接骨为主，一般可服接骨丹（11）。

后期

一般在骨折 7 周后,骨折端已有骨痂形成, 即可认为临床愈合,此期用药主要有以下几种方法:

1. 补益气血法: 凡是外伤筋骨、内伤气血或因长期卧床出现气血亏损、筋骨萎缩等症均可应用本法。常用方剂有四君子汤 (12)、四物汤 (13)、八珍汤 (14) 等。

2. 补养脾胃法: 损伤已久, 耗伤正气: 气血、脏腑亏损导致脾胃虚弱、运化失职。出现饮食不消、四肢疲乏无力, 形体消瘦, 肌肉萎缩, 脉搏虚弱无力, 治疗宜补养脾胃, 以促进气血生化, 使筋骨、肌肉加速恢复。临床常选用参苓白术散 (15)、养脾进食汤 (16)、归脾汤 (17)。

3. 补养肝肾法: 本法又称强壮筋骨法。中医认为, 肝主筋, 肾主骨, 主腰脚。故损伤后期, 老年虚弱, 骨折愈合迟缓, 骨质稀疏, 肢体无力, 此为肝肾不足之表现, 治疗应以补肝肾为主, 可用补肾活血汤 (18)、壮筋养血汤 (19)、健步虎潜丸 (20) 等。

4. 温经通络法: 本法是用温热性的祛风散寒药物, 配以调和气血的药物, 以达驱除体内宿留之风寒湿邪, 使气血通畅, 关节滑利。常选用活血舒筋汤 (21)、麻桂温经汤 (22) 等。

1.4 外用药

贴敷药

是将药物制剂直接贴敷在损伤局部, 使药力发挥作用。常用有以下几种:

1. 药膏: 将药制成细末, 然后选加饴糖, 蜜、油、水、酒、醋或凡士林等, 调匀如糊状, 涂敷伤处。对闭合损伤者药膏多以饴糖配制, 饴糖与药物之比为 3∶1。也可用饴糖八成、米醋二成调拌。对有伤口者, 却用药物与油类熬炼或拌匀后制成油膏, 因其柔软有滋润作用。常用有以下种类:

消瘀退肿止痛类：适用骨折、伤筋初期肿胀疼痛者，可用消肿止痛药膏（23）、双柏散（24）等。

接骨续筋类：适用于骨折对位良好，肿痛消退的中期患者，可用于骨折迟缓愈合或骨不连。常用的有接骨续筋药膏（25）、外用接骨膏（26）。

消热解毒类：适用于伤后感染，局部红、肿、热、痛者。可选用金黄膏（27）、四黄膏（28）。

生肌拔毒长肉类：适用于局部红肿已消，但伤口未愈。可选用生肌象皮膏（29）、生肌玉红膏（30）等。

2. 膏药：膏药是将药物制成细末，配合香油、黄丹或蜂蜡等基质炼制而成。如骨折中、后期，筋脉不舒疼痛者，可用伸筋膏（31），坚骨壮筋膏（32）。若关节粘连活动受限者，可外贴化坚膏（33）。适用于风湿者可用狗皮膏（34）。创面溃疡者可用太乙膏（35）。

3. 药散：是将药物制成极细的粉末，用时可直接掺于伤口，或加在其它膏药上。

止血收口类：适用于一般伤口出血，如桃花散（36），花蕊石散（37）。

祛腐拔毒类：适用于创面腐肉未去或肉芽组织过长的伤口，常用的有九一丹（38）。

生肌长肉类：适用于脓水稀少，新肉难长的创面，可选用生肌玉红膏（30）。

温经散寒类：适用于局部寒湿停聚，气血凝滞、疼痛，损伤后期患者。如丁桂散（39），桂麝散（40）等。

4. 搽擦药

酒剂：指外用药酒和伤药水。如活血酒（41）和舒筋止痛水（42）等。具有活血止痛，舒筋活络，追风祛寒的作用。

油膏与油剂：用香油把药物熬煎去渣后，制成油剂，也可加黄蜡制膏。具有温经散寒，消散瘀血作用。常用的有伤油膏

(43)，跌打万花油（44）等。

5. 熏洗药

熏洗疗法在伤科比较重要，常用在骨伤后期。本法是将药物置于锅或盆中加水煮沸后，先用热气熏蒸患处，稍冷后，以药水浸洗患处，每日2次，每次30～40分钟。具有舒筋活血，松解关节的作用。适用于关节强直拘挛，酸痛麻木或兼夹风寒者，多用四肢关节损伤。常选用活血止痛散（45），1号洗药（46），2号洗药（47）。

6. 热熨药

是一种热疗方法，多选用温经散寒、行气活血止痛的药物，加热后用布裹，热熨患处。

坎离砂（48）：是铁砂加热后与醋水煎成的药液搅拌后制成。使用时加醋少许拌匀装布袋中，数分钟后会自然发热，热熨伤处，多用于陈伤兼有风寒症。

熨药：将药装入袋中，放在锅中蒸热后，趁热敷患处。适用于各种风寒湿、肿痛症。常用正骨烫药（49）。

其它：如粗盐、黄砂等，炒热后装入袋中，趁热敷患处。

1.5　练功与导引

功能活动的作用

练功活动对治疗骨关节及软组织损伤，提高疗效，减少后遗症有着重要意义。练功活动是治疗骨折的重要手段，在治疗骨折及其它损伤过程中，在各个不同阶段，根据具体情况，循序渐进地进行筋肉、关节及全身各部的功能活动，能促进全身气血运行，增强体质，恢复各关节的固有功能，能比较好地解决局部与全身、固定与活动的相互关系。合理的功能活动具有以下作用：

1. 改善和消除全身和局部的损伤症状：在医生指导下进行合理的练功活动，使伤员看到骨折后，虽经固定，但是能够活动，从而使伤员增强信心，保持乐观，解除精神上的压力，改善全身症状。由于伤肢的局部活动，能够促进血液循环，使肿胀、疼痛迅速消退。相反，若不进行功能锻炼，由于广泛石膏固定，则肿胀疼痛消退明显延缓。

2. 促进骨折愈合：伤肢关节功能活动与全身锻炼，能促进血液流通，因而代谢旺盛，营养充足，为骨折的修复提供了物质基础，加速骨折愈合，保证骨折愈合与功能恢复同时并进，缩短疗程。

3. 防止肌肉萎缩和关节僵直：人身各器官不用就会退化，肌肉长期不运动，也会产生萎缩，软弱无力。积极合理地进行练功活动，肌肉则不会产生明显萎缩。关节长期被固定，久之则产生僵硬。如果经常进行练功活动，关节囊和周围的韧带则不会发生粘连；关节内的滑液不断分泌和循环，关节软骨则不会产生退变。一旦骨折愈合解除固定后，即可获得功能满意的结果。

4. 预防骨质疏松：骨质疏松也是由于长期不活动的结果。临床研究证明，一个用石膏固定躯干和四肢的患者，即使在最理想的饮食和充足的维生素调养下，5～6周内也要失去骨钙总量的 1%，若按体重 70 公斤骨钙总量 1200 克计算，失去的钙要达到 12～24 克。这种废用性骨质疏松，骨钙丢失在局部超关节石膏固定时表现更为突出，所以静止和缺乏功能活动是造成骨质稀疏的一个重要因素。为此，广泛的固定对骨折病人是极其不利的，只有进行合理的功能活动，才可以避免骨质疏松的发生。

5. 积极地练功活动，可以预防其它并发症，如坠积性肺炎，泌尿系结石等。

练功时注意事项

1. 练功的方式应以肌肉和关节的主动活动为主，不应予以被动的扳动和牵拉。

2. 练功应有利于骨折愈合，不得因练功而产生疼痛，或对骨折产生不利的伤害。如旋转，剪力或重复受伤机理。

3. 练功时必须在医生的正确指导下进行，活动内容视病情而定，严格掌握循序渐进的原则，练功的次数由少到多，幅度由小到大，时间由短到长。患者在练功时思想必须集中。动作要缓慢，局部与整体的练功相结合。

练功的步骤和具体方法

在上肢练功主要目的是恢复上肢诸关节功能，特别是手部掌指和指间关节的功能。下肢主要是恢复负重和行走的功能，要保持各关节的稳定性。在各组肌肉中，尤其要加强臀大肌、股四头肌和小腿三头肌的力量。才能保持正常的步态。

1. 各阶段练功的形式和步骤

(1) 初期：此期局部疼痛、肿胀，骨折不稳定，软组织损伤需要修复。练功的目的是促进软组织肿胀消退，防止肌肉萎缩，预防关节粘连。练功的形式主要是肌肉收缩锻炼。在不妨碍局部固定的前提下，可以活动某些关节，但不能太用力，如前臂稳定性骨折，可练习握拳动作，并可轻微地活动肩，肘关节。但前臂的旋转活动应严加避免。下肢，股骨干和胫腓骨骨折，应加强踝关节、趾关节的活动，同时注重股四头肌的舒缩锻炼，但应禁止抬高和扭转活动。全身的活动则根据病情而定，一般不需绝对卧床；上肢骨折经复位固定后，应立即下床活动；下肢骨折除伤肢外,不应限制其它肢体的自由活动。

(2) 中期：此期局部疼痛消失，肿胀消退，软组织损伤修复，骨折端亦趋向稳定，骨痂开始出现。除继续有利地进行肌肉舒缩锻炼外，只要病人的肌肉有力，骨折部不痛，上肢病人可作一些自主性关节活动，幅度比初期加大，同时还可进行几个关节活动。下肢病人可开始逐渐抬高患肢，如不痛不抖时，先练习一个关节活动，而后逐步作几个关节的协同活动。未牵引的病人可开始扶拐下床练习行走；牵引病人可通过全身活动带动患肢关节活动。

(3) 后期：局部软组织已恢复正常，肌肉坚强有力，骨折已达临床愈合。此期练功活动极为重要，主要应加大诸关节的活动范围和肢体负重能力，仍以主动练功为主，可配合按摩。下肢可扶双拐下床行走，逐步进行膝、踝关节活动，由不负重转为轻微负重。上肢则应采取各种方法活动诸关节，以尽快恢复其固有的功能。

2. 身体各部位练功方法

(1) 头颈部练功法　颈部练功法可采取站位或坐位，站立时两足分开与肩同宽，两手叉腰进行锻炼。

前屈后伸法：在练习前先进行深呼吸，在呼气时使颈部尽量前屈，使下颌接近胸骨柄上缘，然后在吸气时使颈部后伸至最大限度。反复 7~8 次（图 15-1）。

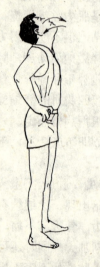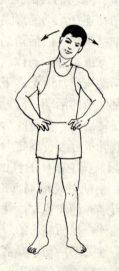

15-1　颈部前屈后伸法　　　　15-2　颈部侧屈法

颈部侧屈法：亦在深呼吸下进行，吸气时使头向左偏，呼气时头部还原；然后吸气时头向右偏，呼气时头部还原。反复 7~8 次（图 15-2）。

颈部伸展法：在深吸气时，使头颈尽量伸向左前方，在呼气时使头颈还原；然后在深吸气时使头颈伸向右前方，呼气时还原。反复 7～8 次（图 15-3）。

颈部旋转法：头部先向左侧旋转，继而向右侧旋转，反复 2 ～3 次。最后使头颈部作回旋动作，先向左侧，再向右侧（图 15-4）。

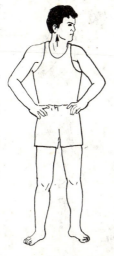 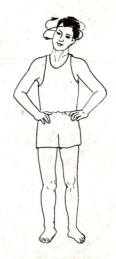

15-3 颈部伸展法   15-4 颈部旋转法

图 15 颈部练功法

通过以上练功，可增强颈部肌肉力量，灵活颈部诸关节，调和气血，以达到内在平衡。可治疗颈部扭挫伤、失枕、颈椎病等。

（2）腰部练功法

腰部前屈后伸法：两足分开站立，两手叉腰，作前屈后伸动作。活动时尽量放松肌肉（图 16-1）。此法能活动腰骶关节，使腰部肌肉一松一紧，缓解肌肉的痉挛，起到舒筋活血、消肿止痛的作用。

腰部两侧弯屈法：两足分开站立，两手叉腰，左右弯腰活动至最大限度为止（图 16-2）。其作用与上法同。

腰部回旋法：站立两足分开与肩同宽，两手叉腰，依靠腰部和下肢力量，先使腰部由左向右顺时针转动，而后再逆时针转动。动作要求柔和协调，有节奏（图16-3）。其作用，促使腰骶关节和骶髂关节活动自如，疏通经络气血。

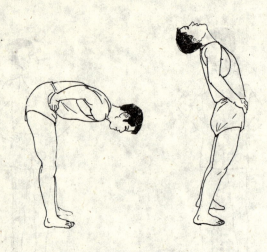

16—1　腰部前屈后伸法

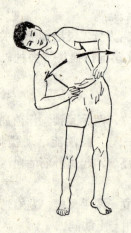

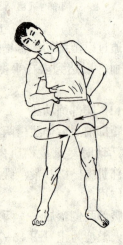

16-2　腰部两侧弯屈法　　　16-3　腰部回旋法

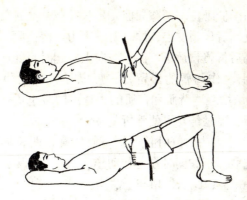

16-4 撑弓导引

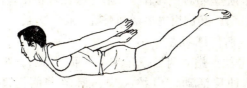

16-5 飞燕点水导引

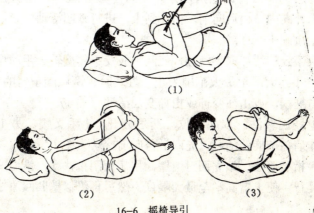

(1)

(2)   (3)

16-6 摇椅导引
图16 腰部练功法

撑弓导引：仰卧位，两膝屈曲，足膝并拢，两肘关节附于床面，以两足及两肘作为支点，同时向下用力，腹、腰、臀部逐渐向上挺起，而后再慢慢放下。注意在向上挺起时不能屏气，每次挺起在原位上，作短暂的停留，一般以呼吸 3 次为起落（图16-4）。其作用增强腰背肌和臀肌的力量。同时也适合于单纯腰椎压缩性骨折，通过练功可使骨折复位。

飞燕点水导引法：俯卧位，两下肢伸直，两臂伸直放于体侧，使头、上肢、下肢同时作背伸动作，使其背肌紧张，作到尽量背伸（图16-5）。此法作用与上法同。

摇椅导引法：仰卧位，两侧髋、膝关节屈曲，两臂环抱双腿，先练髋伸屈活动，伸的限度以臂伸直范围为标准，屈的限度以双大腿前侧完全贴胸壁为宜。最后，抱住双腿使背部作摇椅式活动（图16-6）。其作用主要增加臀肌、腹肌力量。

（3）肩、肘部练功法

前屈后伸法：站立两足分开，手下垂，将肩、肘向前伸直，然后作前后伸展活动，以扩大肩、肘关节的活动范围（图17-1）。

弯腰划圈法：站立两足分开，向前弯腰 90°，患臂自然下垂，由外向内，由后向前，由小到大，进行划圈活动，至最大限度为止（图17-2）。

双手云旋法：取半蹲位，使两上肢及手作旋转云手动作。其范围由小到大，至最大范围为止。旋转时，两膝随前臂的旋动，作左右摇摆，或由屈变伸或由伸变屈活动（图17-3）。

上肢旋转法：取站立位，两足分开，1 手叉腰，另 1 手握拳，作肩关节旋转活动，先向后再向前旋转（图17-4）。

手指爬墙法：站立面对墙壁，用病侧四指扶墙，沿墙缝徐徐向上爬行。使上臂高举至最大限度。然后再沿墙壁归回原处（图17-5）。

高举摸顶法：患侧肘关节屈曲，先摸同侧头顶,再摸对侧头顶（图 17-6）。

后伸摸背法：使前臂放于旋前后伸位，练习后伸摸背，加大肩关节后伸、内旋活动（图 17-7）。

滑车操练法：患者立于滑车之下，以绳穿过滑车，双手各持绳之两端，用健侧向上提拉患肢。防止用力过大（图 17-8）。

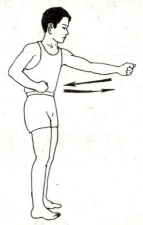

17-1　前后伸展法

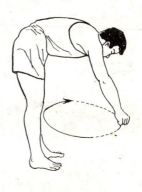

17-2　弯腰划圈法

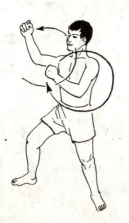

17-3　双手云旋法

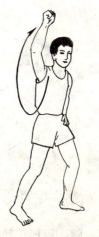

17-4　上肢旋转法

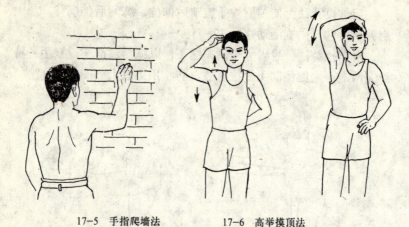

17-5 手指爬墙法   17-6 高举摸顶法

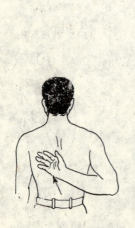
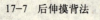

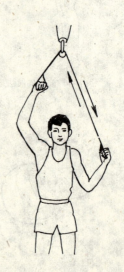

17-7 后伸摸背法   17-8 滑车举肩法

图17 肩、肘部练功法

(4) 腕、手部练功法

腕及手部诸关节功能极为重要，不但要保持其功能位，而且要旋转自如，动作灵活。适用于腕及手部骨折的后期。

抓空练习法：将五指用力张开，再用力抓紧握拳。

旋前旋后法：将前臂贴于胸侧，手握棒，使前臂作旋前旋后活动（图18-1）。

背伸掌屈法：各指用力握拳，作腕关节背伸掌屈活动（图18-2）。

手运球法：手握两枚核桃或健身球，在手中运转活动（图18-3）。

(5) 髋、膝、踝练功法：髋、膝、踝是人体负重的三个重要关节，损伤后关节功能恢复的满意与否，对人体的站立、负重、走路、步态及劳动能力关系甚大。尤以膝、踝关节损伤后遗症较多，必须抓紧功能锻炼。

肌肉收缩法：股骨干骨折及膝部损伤，最易引起股四头肌萎缩，不管在损伤的早期或晚期，都应抓紧锻炼股四头肌收缩活动。

直腿抬高法：仰卧位，膝关节伸直，徐徐将伸直的下肢抬高，然后再逐渐放回原处。以恢复肌肉力量，逐渐增加次数恢复

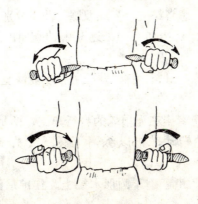

18-1　旋前旋后法

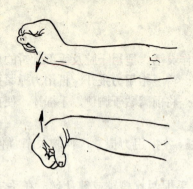

18-2　背伸掌屈法

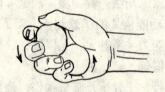

18-3　手运球法

图18　腕、手部练功法

耐力。如抬举轻松时，可在足底加重量练习。

蹬空操练法：取仰卧位，两腿伸直，先作踝关节屈伸活动，然后强屈髋、膝关节向外上方作蹬空动作（图19-1）。

旋转摇膝法；患者站立，半屈双膝，两手分别放于膝上，作膝关节旋转活动，可由屈到伸，逐渐由伸到屈，反复活动（图19-2）。

上下台阶锻炼：对髋、膝、踝三关节功能恢复甚为有利（图19-3）。

蹬车活动：患者坐在无前轮的自行车上，两足放于足蹬上，以健侧带动后轮转动，借以练习下肢三大关节的功能（图19-4）。

足蹬滚木法：患者蹬于圆形木棍上，作前后滚动练习（图19-5）。

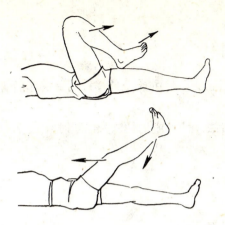

19—1 蹬空练习法

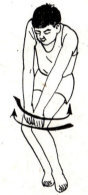

19—2 旋转摇膝法

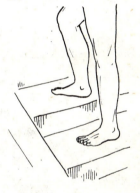

19—3 上下台阶法

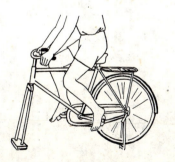

19—4 蹬车活动法

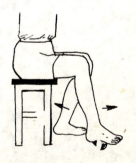

19—5 足蹬滚木法

图 19 髋、膝、踝练功法

足背伸跖屈法：仰卧或坐位，练习踝关节背伸和跖屈活动，至最大限度。

足踝旋转法：仰卧或坐位，先作顺时针旋转，再作逆时针旋转。

2 骨折

2.1 锁骨骨折

发病

锁骨骨折多数由间接暴力所致，因跌倒时肩部，肘部或手掌撑地时引起。骨折以中外$\frac{1}{3}$部位最多见。骨折近端因胸锁乳突肌的牵拉而向后上移位（图20），骨折远端或碎骨片可刺伤臂丛神经和锁骨下血管。远端骨折较少见。

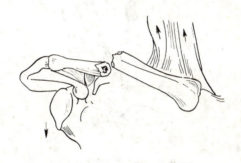

图 20　锁骨中 1／3 骨折移位情况

诊断要点

1. 有外伤史，尤其摔伤史。

2. 锁骨部肿胀，疼痛，肩下垂，手臂主动抬高因疼痛而受限。

3. 局部压痛，易触及移位的骨折近端和骨擦音。　·

4. 注意检查患肢血运、感觉及活动情况，以排除臂丛神经和血管损伤。

5. 锁骨部正位 X 线片可明确诊断。小儿多为青枝骨折，成人多为斜形或粉碎性骨折。

治疗

复位

患者坐在较低的方凳上，双手插腰，用1%普鲁卡因注入局部血肿内。助手站在患者背后，一足踏于方凳腿边，屈膝抵住患者两肩胛区之间，双手握住两上臂，徐徐用力向后外上方牵拉，令患者挺胸抬肩，头偏向患侧。术者站在患者前面，以两手拇、食、中指摸住骨折远近断端，按压骨折近端，提拉骨折远端，使骨折复位（图21）。

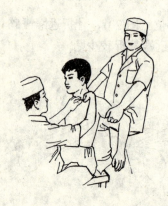

图21 锁骨骨折手法复位

固定

1. 后"8"字形绷带固定法：在腋窝部垫棉垫，自患侧开始，经腋下达对侧肩部，再经对侧腋下返回患侧肩上，如此往复，拉紧固定。然后在骨折部位放置"夹形垫"，在骨折近端放置"方平垫"，再用带衬垫之硬纸壳盖在上面，绷带通过前胸绷带环拉紧结扎（图22）。

2. 绷带环固定法：在腋窝部垫棉垫，用绷带做成两个绷带环，套在肩部，用两条绷带在肩后方分别扎紧。

3. 肩部胶布固定法：用宽6 cm的胶布，肘部正对胶布中点，分别由肘前后方经肩前后方拉紧后，粘贴于胸前和背后。本法适用于锁骨远端骨折（图23）。

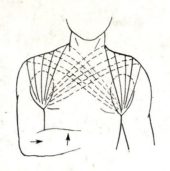

图22 锁骨骨折"∞"形绷带固定

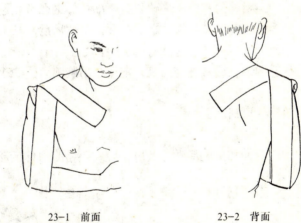

23-1 前面　　　　　　　　　23-2 背面

图23 锁骨外端压垫胶布固定法

4. 腋卷纸壳压垫固定法：在局麻下，患者坐位，术者以前臂挎住患侧上臂，手部尺侧缘按住患侧肩胛骨外缘，使肩部后伸，纠正骨折重叠移位。另手拇、食指按压后上翘之骨折近端，使之复位（图24）。术毕，术者维持对位，助手将腋卷放于患侧腋下（棉絮包裹硬纸壳圆筒，外缠绕绷带，长12cm，粗8cm，绷带从圆筒中心贯穿，作捆扎用）。将方垫放在骨折近端，棉垫

衬里，硬纸壳覆盖，拉紧腋卷之绷带两端在硬纸壳上打结，再互

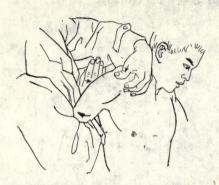

图 24　锁骨外端骨折整复法

相从健侧腋下绕到胸前打结，一端从胸腰部扎好之绷带绕过后自行打结，另端与肩前绷带打结。之后，绷带绕过肩后，与上述绷带系住，再通过腰部绷带，扦回，向上拉紧，系于上带上。然后，患臂贴近胸侧，绷带缠绕固定，前臂悬吊胸前（图 25）。

药物

按 3 期用药原则。

练功

早期作肩后伸和挺胸活动，及肘、腕、手指的屈伸活动；中

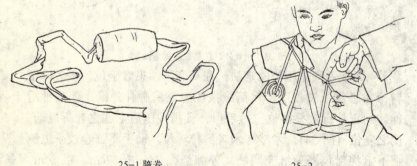

25—1 腋卷　　　　　　　　　25—2

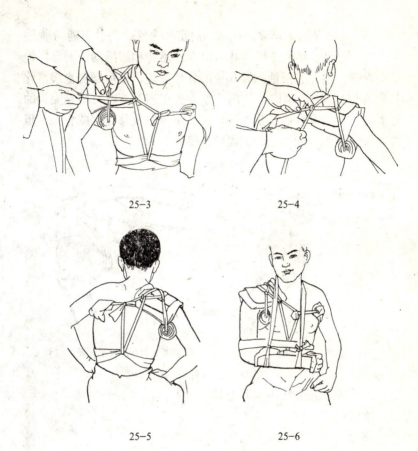

25-3 25-4

25-5 25-6

图 25 腋卷纸壳压垫固定法

期逐步加大活动量；后期骨折愈合解除固定后，作肩关节各方向活动。

2.2 肱骨外科颈骨折

发病

肱骨外科颈骨折多为间接暴力引起，跌倒时，肘部或手掌撑地，暴力向上传导至肩部所致，多见于成年人。

诊断要点

1. 肩部肿胀，疼痛，压痛，肘部冲击痛，伤肢不能抬举。

2. 无明显移位骨折，其畸形，骨擦音和假活动不明显；外展型骨折，虽在腋下能触及移位的骨性突起，但肩部仍饱满，此与肩脱位相鉴别（图26）；内收型骨折在肩外下方可摸到突起的骨折端；伴肩脱位者，呈方肩，在腋下可触及移位之肱骨头，但搭肩实验阴性，此与单纯肩脱位相鉴别。

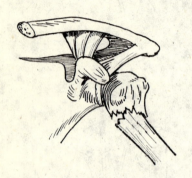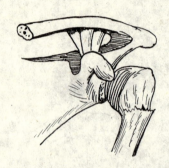

肱骨外科颈外展型骨折　　　　　肱骨外科颈内收型骨折

图 26　肱骨外科颈骨折

3. 肩部正轴位 X 线片有助于诊断。

治疗

整复

1. 无移位骨折：肩部外敷伸筋膏（31），用连肩夹板固定。前臂悬吊胸前 3—4 周。

2. 外展型骨折：患者端坐或仰卧位。局麻后，下助手握前臂及肘部，使肘屈 90°；上助手用宽布带绕过腋下，其间垫以棉垫。两助手顺骨折远端纵轴方向牵引约 10 分钟后，术者双手握住骨折断端，使拇指向内向后按压骨折近端，其余手指向外向前提拉骨折远端，同时下助手在拨伸下逐渐内收上臂，使肘部移向胸前，以纠正骨折端向前向内成角及移位（图27）。

3. 内收型骨折：下助手先将伤肢外展 70°，前屈 30°位

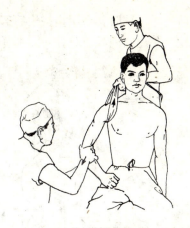

27-1 外展型骨折外展牵引

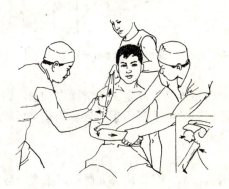

27-2 外展型骨折复位法

图 27

作对抗牵引 10 分钟后，术者双手握住骨折部位，使拇指向内向后按压骨折远端，其余手指向外向前提拉骨折近端，下助手逐渐加大伤肢外展 90°以上，以纠正骨折端向前向外成角及移位（图 28）。

　　4. 伴肩脱位型骨折，在全麻下，助手保持肩关节外展 90—150°位，使骨折远断端对准骨折近断端，同时便于使破裂的关节囊张开，使肱骨头还纳复位，术者双拇指从腋下向上向后向外推顶肱骨头的前下缘，同时其余手指按住肩部以作支点，助手轻轻顺势移动患肢，并逐渐内收，肱骨头即可复位，骨折按内收型整复。

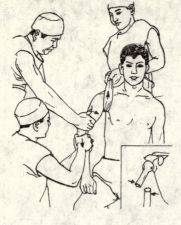

图 28　内收型骨折复位法

固定

外展型骨折用连肩板固定，前臂固定胸前，内收型骨折用外展架固定，伴肩脱位型骨折用带连肩板的小夹板固定，前臂悬吊胸前。

药物

按 3 期用药原则。早期肩部如肿胀严重者，应加大活血化瘀药剂量，佐以清热解毒药。可用复元活血汤（1）和五味消毒饮（5）加减。

练功

由于肩部挫伤，如果较长时间固定，肩关节容易粘连，因此要注意肩关节的功能锻炼。早期作手指和腕部的屈伸活动；中期骨折稳定后，作前臂和肘部的屈伸旋转活动，并开始进行肩关节的各方向活动；后期骨折愈合，加大肩关节各方向的运动范围，预防肩关节粘连。

2.3 肱骨干骨折

发病

肱骨干骨折可发生于任何年龄，以成人多见。多为直接暴力所伤，如产伤、机器卷压伤等。投掷、跌倒等间接暴力亦可致伤。以横形和螺旋形骨折多见，桡神经损伤可发生在肱骨中 $\frac{1}{3}$ 骨折。

诊断要点

1. 上臂肿胀、疼痛、侧突畸形，不能高举。
2. 有挤压痛、假活动，骨擦音和肘部冲击痛。
3. 正侧位 X 线片，可明确骨折部位，类型及移位程度。
4. 如有腕下垂，手不能伸直，虎口背侧感觉丧失，应考虑到桡神经损伤。

治疗

肱骨干骨折，不强求完全复位，轻度的重叠移位和成角畸形，不影响上肢功能。

整复

臂丛麻醉或局麻后，患者坐位，肘屈 90°位，两助手分别握住伤臂上端及肘部，轻力拔伸。术者双手握住骨折部位进行复位。如为肱骨上段骨折（三角肌止点之上）。下助手将伤臂下垂贴近胸壁，术者两拇指向内按压骨折远端，其余手指向外端提骨折近端，使骨折复位。如为肱骨中段骨折（三角肌止点之下），下助手宜将伤臂外展 40—50°位，术者两拇指向内按压骨折近端，其余手指向外端提骨折远端，使骨折复位（图 29）。复位时，如骨折断端明显滑动，且无骨擦音，为软组织嵌入，可用摇摆法或回旋法，使软组织脱出骨折断端，如为肱骨中下 $\frac{1}{3}$ 骨折，宜用拔伸法和推按法，勿用折顶法或回旋法，以免损伤桡神经。

骨折断端无重叠或有分离移位，宜用合骨法，以使骨折断端接触。桡神经损伤者，如系轻度损伤，一般能够自行恢复，整复时，注意手法轻柔，勿加重其损伤。

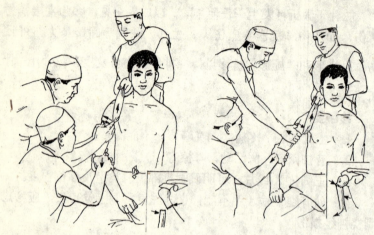

29-1　肱骨干上1／3骨折复位法　　29-2　肱骨干中1／3骨折复位法

图29

固定

1. 肱骨上段骨折：用带连肩板之小夹板三点加压固定，伤臂贴胸侧，绷带绕胸壁固定，前臂悬吊胸前，肱骨中段骨折，用不包括肩肘关节的小夹板固定，胸壁间放置棉垫，使伤臂保持外展30°位，肱骨中下$\frac{1}{3}$骨折，宜用超肘关节小夹板固定，前臂悬吊胸前。

2. 悬吊皮肤牵引加小夹板固定法：适宜上臂严重肿胀、重叠移位者。患者仰卧位，肩关节前屈90°，肘关节屈曲90°，前臂旋前，顺前臂长轴作皮肤牵引，同时在前臂用宽布带向上悬吊牵引，4块小夹板，用3根连筋带捆扎固定。

3. 肩肘胶布加小夹板固定方法：适宜骨折断端有分离的骨折。术者固定骨折端，一助手向上推挤骨折远端，另一助手在肘尖部放 1 棉垫，取宽 4～6 cm 胶布 1 条，自肩锁部向后上，绕过肩部，沿上臂向下，绕过肘尖部，沿上臂前方向上，绕过臂部向后，止于肩胛冈处，贴紧后再捆扎小夹板。

药物

按 3 期用药原则。

练功

早期作腕关节的屈伸和手的握拳活动；中期开始行肘关节和肩关节各方向活动；后期加大肩肘关节活动范围。应特别注意防止肩凝症的发生。骨折稳定后，就要循序渐进地行肩关节的活动锻炼。

2.4 肱骨髁上骨折

发病

肱骨髁上骨折临床常见，多为 4～8 岁的儿童。由于受伤暴力不同，临床分为伸直型，屈曲型。伸直型骨折严重移位时，近侧骨折端对肱动、静脉直接压迫或刺激，造成前臂缺血，后果严重。同时近侧骨折端能损伤正中神经、桡神经和尺神经，检查时应予注意。

诊断要点

1. 肘部肿胀，疼痛，髁上挤压痛。

2. 肘三角关系正常，骨擦音明显，肘关节功能丧失。

3. 伴血管损伤者，尺、桡动脉搏动减弱或消失，末梢循环差，肌肤温度降低。

4. 伴神经损伤时，出现相应的正中神经、桡神经和尺神经损伤体征。

5. 肘部正、侧位 X 线片有助于诊断。应与肘关节脱位、肱骨小头骨骺分离相鉴别。

治疗

整复

1. 无移位或青枝骨折：不需整复，外敷伸筋膏（31），用三角巾悬吊胸前2周。较重的青枝骨折，应纠正之。注意正常肱骨下端有25°前倾角。如是伸直型，整复时，术者一手握前臂，使肘屈90°，1手拇指推按肘尖部，其余4指扳提肘窝上部，使肘关节小于90°，然后用"∞"字形绷带固定，或用瓦形硬纸壳绷带固定2～3周。

2. 有移位骨折：局麻或臂丛麻醉后,患者坐位或仰卧位，一助手握患侧上臂，另助手握患侧腕及前臂，患肘微屈位，持续对抗牵引，纠正重叠移位。若骨折远端有旋前畸形，应在助手牵引下，使前臂旋后，反之亦然。然后，术者双手分别置于上臂远端的前后方，虎口朝向伤肢远端。其2—5指固定骨折远端之外侧，双拇指置于骨折远段之内侧，并用力向外推挤，纠正骨折向内侧移位，然后纠正前后移位。伸直型骨折，术者用双拇指按压肘尖，虎口朝向远端方向，其余手指扳提肘窝上部，助手在牵引下徐徐屈曲肘关节。但要注意，推拉力勿过大，肘屈曲勿过小，以免将骨折远段推向前移位，而影响骨折的稳定性（图30）。屈曲型骨折，术者双拇指按压肘窝部，虎口朝向远端，其余手指扳提肘后上方，令助手在牵引下徐徐伸直肘关节。尺偏型骨折，允许矫枉稍有过正。骨折复位后，术者双手固定肘上骨折处，由助手握住前臂略伸直肘关节，并将前臂向桡侧伸展，使骨折断端桡侧骨皮质嵌插，以防止肘内翻发生。

固定

1. 瓦形硬纸壳固定法；外展型骨折，复位后，用胶布剪成近似三角形纸板共4块。先在肘尖部及内侧垫以压垫并外裹棉垫，用4块硬纸壳分别扣于肘部内、外、上、下侧，纸壳尖端互相重迭后，以4根连筋带扎缚，肘内、外侧各用1根连筋带将中间两根带扎紧，以加强固定效力，再用"8"字形绷带包缠，固定肘关节屈曲90°位。前臂悬吊胸前（图31）。屈曲型骨折，则固定肘关节伸直位（图32）。

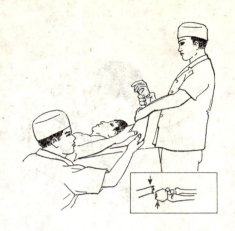

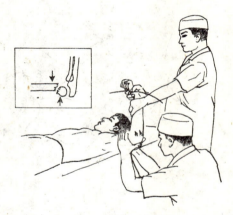

图 30　伸直型肱骨髁上骨折复位法

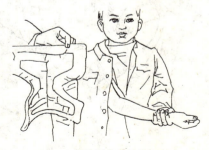

31-1　固定用的薄棉垫

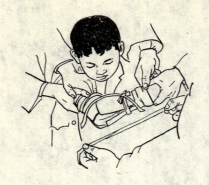

31—2

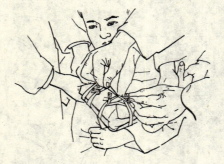

31—3

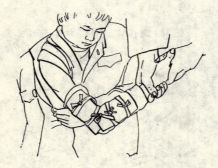

31—4

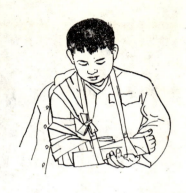

31—5

图 31　伸直型肱骨髁上骨折固定法

2. 鼎式小夹板固定法

木板 4 块，宽度均为上臂最

大周径的 $\frac{1}{5}$ 左右，前侧板上自肱

骨大结节，下至肘窝部，后侧板
上自腋窝，下至鹰嘴下，两板之
下端，均烤成向前弯曲弧形。内
侧板自腋下至鹰嘴下 3 cm，外
侧板自肩峰至鹰嘴下 3 cm。伸
直尺偏型骨折，梯型垫两块，1
块放在尺骨鹰嘴部，推挤骨折远
端向前，1 块放在内髁部推挤骨

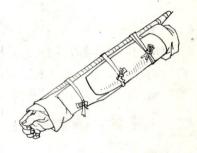

图 32　屈曲型肱骨髁上骨折固定法

折远端向外，塔形垫 1 块放在外髁上方，推挤骨折近端向内。肘
上部包以棉垫。3 条连筋带捆扎，前臂悬吊胸前（图 33）。

药物

早期内服活血祛瘀片（54），肿胀重者内服复元活血汤（1）
加川芎、姜黄；中期服接骨丹（11）；后期内服伸筋片（50），外
用 2 号洗药熏洗。

练功

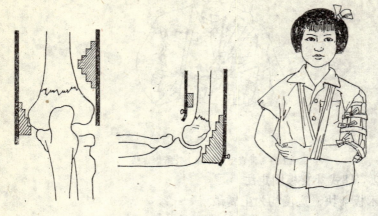

33-1　固定示意图　　　　　　33-2　固定外观

图 33　伸直型肱骨髁上骨折固定法

早期进行手指及腕的伸屈活动；中期逐渐练习肩关节的各方向活动；后期约 4 周左右，骨折临床愈合，去除外固定后，逐渐进行前臂的旋转和肘关节的屈伸活动。

2.5　肱骨外髁骨折

发病

临床较多见，多发生于 5～10 岁的儿童，多为间接暴力引起。由于受伤时暴力的大小，肘关节内外翻位置及前臂旋转方向不同，骨折块有不同程度的移位。临床可分：无移位骨折、有移位骨折和旋转移位骨折 3 种类型。

诊断要点

1. 有外伤史，尤其跌倒伤。

2. 肘关节外侧肿胀，疼痛。肘关节功能丧失，常处于 130°半屈曲位。

3. 局部压痛，有时有骨擦音。

4. 肘关节正侧位 X 线片可明确骨折移位情况，但要注意骨折块大部分为软骨，不显影，比 X 线片显示实际为大。

治疗

整复

1. 无移位骨折：外敷伸筋膏（31），肘用"8"字绷带固定，肘屈 90°位，前臂悬吊胸前 3 周。

2. 单纯移位骨折：患者取仰卧位，助手握住患侧上臂，术者一手握住患肢前臂，使之旋后，肘半屈曲，腕背伸位，以放松伸肌群的牵引，另手握住肘部，使拇指按压骨折块。余 4 指扳住肘内侧，使患肘内翻，以加大肘关节外侧间隙。同时拇指用力按压骨折块，使之复位，然后使肘在 135°位作屈伸活动，使骨折块复位稳定（图 34）。

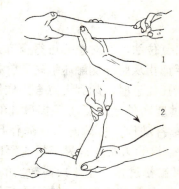

1. 伸直挤捏　　2. 屈曲挤捏

图 34　肱骨外髁骨折复位法

3. 翻转移位骨折

（1）右侧为例，臂丛麻醉后，取仰卧位。两助手分别握住患侧上臂和前臂，轻轻拔伸，术者先用右手拇指向肱骨远端外后方空隙处推移骨折块，再用左拇指向内下方按压骨折块的滑车端，使之插入骨折面内，右手拇、食指由外下方向外上方推压骨折块外髁端，此肘翻转移位纠正，再按单纯移位整复之。

(2) 助手及体位准备同上。术者用左食指按压住骨折块的滑车端，拇指扣住肱骨外上髁端，将骨折块向后方稍推移，滑车端推向后内下方，肱骨外上髁端由外下方推向外上方。再用右拇指将骨折块向内挤压，推至肱骨外髁上脊平整，表示骨折块复位良好（图35）。

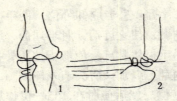

桡骨纵轴线正常通过肱骨小头骨骺中心

1. 正位　　2. 侧位

图 35

(3) 摇晃牵抖复位法，在对患儿进行全麻或臂丛麻醉下，患肢外展。术者1手拇指从肘外侧触压翻转的骨折片，使移向关节间隙内，其余4指托住患肘，起到支点合力作用，也可保护在摇晃时，防止肘部过度内外翻。另1手握患儿的腕掌部作伸肘屈肘，左右摇晃与牵抖动作，协调配合。先作尺侧摇晃（即肘内翻），在摇晃中有牵抖的力量。摇晃牵抖的幅度，从小到大，动作细柔均匀，不可粗暴过猛。压1次或数次的手法动作过程中，当听到清脆响声时，且骨擦音消失，表示骨折块已翻转复位。如未复位，可加用屈肘旋前或旋后，迅速伸直的牵抖，同时内翻肘关节，即可复位。

固定

1. 四方形压垫置于外髁部，肘部包裹棉垫，4块瓦形硬纸壳用连筋带捆扎固定。肘半屈135°位，悬吊胸前。

2. 肘伸直前臂旋后位，外髁部放置四方形压垫，4块夹板从上臂中段至前臂中下段，连筋带捆扎，2周后改肘屈90°位。

3 至 4 周去掉外固定。

药物

按 3 期用药原则

练功

早期作手指的屈伸活动；半月后作腕关节的屈伸及肩关节的各方向活动；骨折愈合去掉外固定后，积极练习肘关节屈伸、旋转功能。

2.6　肱骨内上髁骨折

发病

肱骨内上髁骨折在青少年中多有发生。一般是在跌倒时，肘外翻力与前臂屈肌收缩牵拉所致。由于暴力大小不同，骨折按移位情况分为 4 型：无移位型、移位型、嵌入关节型、嵌入关节并移位型（肘关节脱位型）。

诊断要点

1.　有明显外伤史。

2.　肘内侧肿胀，疼痛，有压痛和骨擦音，肘三角关系发生改变。

3.　有时因骨折块嵌入关节腔内，触及不到骨折块。

4.　肘部正侧位 X 线片可观察骨折块移位程度.

5.　注意检查尺神经损伤症状与体征。

治疗

整复

无移位型：肘后硬纸壳绷带"∞"字固定，肘屈 90°，前臂旋前，手腕屈曲位，悬吊胸前。

移位型：右侧为例，在局麻下，患肘屈曲 90°，助手握住前臂及腕部，前臂旋前，手腕屈曲位，使前臂屈肌群松弛。术者左手握住肘部，右拇、食指推按骨折块向后上方，使之复位。

嵌入关节型：

1. 助手握持同上，术者左手握住前臂上端外侧，右手拇、食指向远端按推前臂屈肌群，同时助手快速使前臂旋后，肘关节伸直并外翻，手腕关节背伸，可连续作几次，骨折块一般能脱出关节腔，再按Ⅱ型骨折处理。

2. 患肢屈肘 40°，肩外展 90°，助手握住前臂及手部，使前臂极度旋前外展，使肘内侧间隙开大。术者 1 手握住肘上部外侧，1 手握住肘下部内侧，将尺骨近端向外推挤，造成肘关节外侧半脱位，以解除尺骨半月切迹对骨折块的钳夹。这时，术者可在肘内下侧，摸到骨折块的边缘，令助手数次极度背伸手腕关节，骨折块可脱出关节腔。否则，再将前臂极度旋后，使骨折块被牵拉排挤出尺骨半月切迹，术者 1 手向外推挤肱骨下端，1 手向内推挤尺、桡骨上端。助手用力背伸手腕关节，随着肘关节复位，骨折块可被牵拉和推挤出关节腔，再按Ⅱ型骨折复位（图36）。

固定

1. 硬纸壳固定法：四方形棉布垫 1 块，放置在内上髁部，外包棉垫，用四块瓦形硬纸壳固定。屈肘 90°，前臂旋前，手腕屈曲位悬吊胸前。

2. 小夹板固定法

内上髁下部用梯形压垫，外髁上方用塔形压垫，外包棉垫，小夹板 4 块，分别放置在上臂下端前后及内外侧，3 根连筋带捆扎固定，肘屈 90°，前臂旋前，手腕屈曲位悬吊胸前。

药物

按 3 期用药原则。

练功

早期不限制肩关节活动，但避免握拳和腕关节活动；中期行手指、腕关节屈伸和前臂的旋转活动；后期行肘关节屈伸活动。

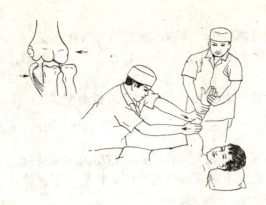

36-1　由第四型转为第三型者复位法之一,先使肘外展,内侧关节间隙张开,造成
　　　肘关节向后、外侧脱位,骨折块逸出尺骨半月切迹的内侧缘

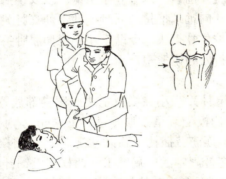

36-2　利用尺骨半月切迹的内缘将骨折块挤出肘关节

图36　肘关节脱位型肱骨内上髁骨折复位法

2.7　尺骨鹰嘴骨折

发病

尺骨鹰嘴骨折临床较少见，多发生于成人。多数由间接暴力所致，偶见直接暴力。前者为横形骨折，后者为粉碎性骨折。儿童可为骨裂。

诊断要点

1. 有外伤史，多见跌倒损伤，偶见于打击伤。

2. 肘后部肿胀，疼痛，肘三角关系有改变。

3. 肘关节伸直受限，肘后压痛，有时有骨擦音或可触及骨折端间隙。

4. 肘部正侧位 X 线片可明确骨折类型。

治疗

整复

尺骨鹰嘴骨折属关节内骨折，应尽力解剖复位。

1. 骨裂或无明显移位的粉碎性骨折：不需整复，硬纸壳固定肘关节微屈位 3—4 周。

2. 有移位的骨折：在局麻下，患者仰卧位，肘微屈位。助手握住患者手腕及前臂。术者立于患侧，以双手拇指按压尺骨鹰嘴上端内外侧，向远端推挤。同时令助手伸直肘关节，使两骨折面接触。术者按住骨折块，令助手小幅度伸屈肘关节数次，以利肱骨滑车对骨折处的模造塑形。

固定

1. 前臂超肘关节小夹板固定法：鹰嘴部放置梯形压垫。4 块小夹板，后侧板上端呈弧形超过肘上 7 cm，内、外、前侧板齐肘关节，3 根连筋带捆扎，绷带包缠，固定屈肘 20—30°位。

2. 闭合穿针固定法：局麻下，两枚克氏钢针，在骨折上下端，平行骨折线由内侧向外侧穿出。插针时，避开尺神经。然后，用带孔的木块或钢丝，使钢针两端靠拢，以加压固定骨折块。此法适用于移位较大的横形骨折。

药物

按 3 期用药原则。

练功

早期练习手腕伸屈及肩关节各方向活动；解除固定后，逐渐练习肘关节伸屈活动和前臂的旋转活动。

2.8 桡骨头骨折

发病

桡骨头骨折比较常见，多为间接暴力引起。在儿童则为桡骨头骨骺分离。根据骨折部位和移位情况，可分为青枝型、裂纹型、劈裂型、嵌插型、倾斜型、翻转型和粉碎型。

诊断要点

1. 有明显外伤史，多为跌倒伤。
2. 肘部外下方肿胀，疼痛，瘀斑
3. 局部压痛。倾斜型和翻转型可触及移位的桡骨头。
4. 前臂旋转及屈曲受限。
5. X 线拍片可了解骨折类型。

治疗

整复：一般对青枝型、裂纹型、劈裂型、嵌插型骨折不需整复。

1. 倾斜型：患者坐位或仰卧位，局麻或臂丛麻醉下，前臂旋后、肘微屈位。一助手握住上臂，一助手握住前臂，对抗拔伸牵引。术者两拇指在桡骨头的外后侧抵住骨折块的下缘，向上、向前、向内侧推按。同时助手旋转前臂及屈伸肘关节。骨折块复位满意后，保持肘屈 90°,前臂中立位 (图 37)。

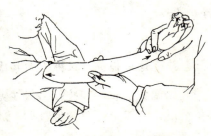

图 37　桡骨头骨折的整复方法

2. 翻转型：准备同上，术者 1 手拇指抵住骨折块之上缘，向内侧和前侧推按，另手拇指抵住骨折块下缘，向上向前方推按，使骨折块变成倾斜型，再按倾斜型整复。如整复失败者，可用针拨复位法：消毒铺巾，克氏针避开桡神经，自骨折块的外后方刺入，针尖抵住骨折块，向前上方及内侧推顶，以拨正骨折块（图38）。

固定

前臂超肘关节固定法：长方形压垫1块，放置在桡骨小头后外侧，小夹板4块，前侧夹板近端呈凹形，后侧夹板过肘上，夹板放好后，连筋带捆扎，使肘屈90°，前臂中立位，悬吊胸前。

药物

按3期用药原则。（参见1.3节）

练功

早期作手腕屈伸活动和肩关节各方向活动；中期逐渐作前臂旋转功能锻炼；后期逐渐作肘关节屈伸锻炼和加大前臂旋转活动范围。

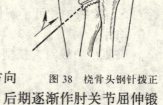

图38 桡骨头钢针拨正

2.9 尺骨上$\frac{1}{3}$骨折合并桡骨头脱位

(Monteggia 骨折)

发病

尺骨上$\frac{1}{3}$骨折合并桡骨头脱位，又称孟他其氏骨折，多见于儿童和青年。常为间接暴力引起，直接暴力较少见。根据暴力作用方向和骨折移位情况，临床上可分为伸直型、屈曲型和内收型（图39），而以伸直型为多见。

诊断要点

1. 有明显外伤史，尤其跌伤史。
2. 前臂上段及肘关节外侧肿胀疼痛，有瘀斑，压痛。

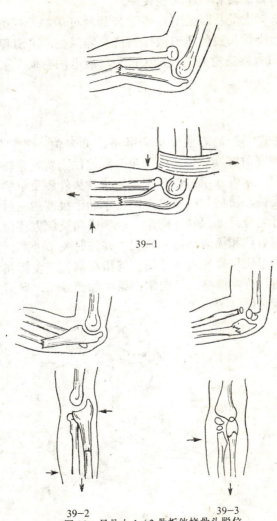

39—1

39—2   39—3
图39 尺骨上1／3骨折伴桡骨头脱位

3. 前臂上段有骨擦音及假活动。肘外侧可摸到突起的桡骨头。

4. 前臂旋转和屈肘功能丧失。

5. 前臂上段及肘关节正侧位 X 线片可了解骨折类型。

6. 如桡骨头脱位压迫或挫伤桡神经深支，可出现手腕不能伸直，虎口背侧感觉减退或消失征象，肌电图有助于了解桡神经损伤性质。

治疗

整复

1. 伸直型：局麻或臂丛麻醉下、仰卧位、患肢外展 80°左右，肘伸直前臂旋后位。两助手分别握住上臂及手腕部，作对抗拔伸牵引。术者双手拇指分别抵住桡骨头外侧及掌侧用力向尺侧、背侧推按，使桡骨头复位。同时下助手极度屈曲肘关节，尺骨骨折多可复位，如尺骨仍向掌，桡侧成角及侧方移位，在助手保持前臂旋后位和极度屈肘的情况下并使肘关节外翻。术者双手拇、食分别捏住尺骨骨折远近端、拇指在掌侧，食指在背侧，将尺骨远端向尺背侧推挤，并向掌侧徐徐加大成角，然后向背侧反折，使骨折对位（图 40）。

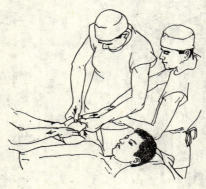

矫正尺骨桡侧移位

图 40 伸直型孟氏骨折复位法

2. 屈曲型: 麻醉及助手准备同上。患肘呈半屈位，前臂旋前位，对抗拔伸牵引，术者拇指向内前方按压桡骨头，助手将患肢伸直，并将前臂旋后位,桡骨头即可复位。如尺骨仍向桡骨侧移位，术者双手拇、食指作尺桡骨间隙夹挤分骨，并向尺侧推挤向桡侧移位的尺骨骨折远端，或用反折法整复尺骨骨折移位。

3. 内收型: 准备同上。患肘伸直位，对抗拔伸牵引。术者1手拇指向内侧按压桡骨头，其余4指扳提肘内侧，另1手握住前臂用力外展，以整复脱位的桡骨头和向桡侧成角的尺骨骨折（图41）。

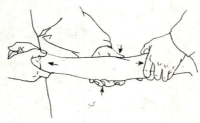

图41 内收型整复法

固定

1. 伸直型: 复位后，将长方形压垫放置在桡骨头前外侧，呈弧形压位桡骨头，分骨垫放在骨折处，外包以棉垫。将4块小夹板放置好，外侧夹板近端须压住桡骨头部的压垫，3根连筋带捆扎，使肘屈略小于90°，前臂旋后位悬吊于胸前（图42）。

2. 屈曲型: 复位后，肘伸直。前臂旋后位，将长方形压垫放置于桡骨头后外侧，外包以棉垫，用前臂超肘关节的小夹板或硬纸壳固定（图43）。2—3周后改肘半屈位固定。

3. 内收型: 复位后，除压垫放置在桡骨头外侧，余同屈曲型固定法。

4. 闭合骨圆针固定法: 在局麻或臂丛麻醉下，桡骨头复位后，消毒铺巾，骨圆针自鹰嘴端钻入尺骨近端，手法复位尺骨断端后，骨圆针穿入骨折远端，小夹板或石膏托固定，肘屈

90°，前臂旋后位悬吊胸前。

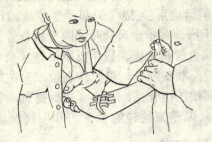

42-1　伸直型小压垫放置部位

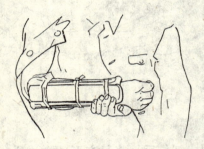

42-2　伸直型小夹板固定外形
图 42　伸直型孟他其氏骨折固定法

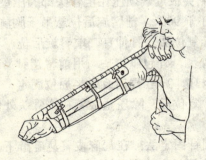

图 43　屈曲型小夹板固定法

药物

按 3 期用药原则。

练功

早期作手的握拳活动和腕关节、肩关节的各方面活动；中期作肘关节屈伸活动；后期作前臂旋转活动。

2.10　尺、桡骨干骨折

发病

尺、桡骨干骨折比较常见，多发生在儿童及青壮年。骨折多由间接暴力所致，一般桡骨骨折线在上，尺骨骨折线在下，以横形骨折和斜形骨折为多见。扭转暴力所伤者，尺骨骨折线多在上端，以螺旋形较多；直接暴力伤者，尺、桡骨骨折线多在同一平面上，以粉碎和横断形为多见。如桡骨骨折在中上$\frac{1}{3}$交界处，则骨折近端由于旋后肌的作用，而呈旋后、外展位，骨折远端因旋前肌的牵引而呈旋前位。

诊断要点

1. 有明显的外伤史。

2. 前臂肿胀，疼痛，瘀血斑，前臂有成角或短缩畸形，旋转功能丧失。

3. 局部压痛，冲击痛，有假活动和骨擦音。

4. 前臂正侧位 X 线片可明确骨折部位及移位情况。

治疗

整复

旋转移位是尺、桡骨骨折的主要矛盾，夹挤分骨手法，可以有效地纠正旋转移位，使尺、桡骨断端象单根骨折一样，相互稳定、便于对位。整复时，患者仰卧或坐位，两助手分别握住肘上部和手腕部。中下$\frac{1}{3}$骨折，前臂中立位；中上$\frac{1}{3}$骨折，前臂旋后位。对抗拔伸牵引，以纠正成角及重叠移位。术者双手拇指和其余4指分别捏住骨折部的掌背侧，夹挤分骨，使靠拢的骨折断端分开到最大限度，同时双手拇指由背侧推按成角的骨折断端，其余手指提拉向掌侧移位的另一端，缓慢地作折顶手法（图44），

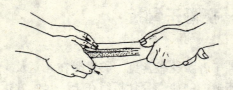

44—1 加大成角

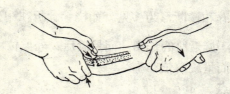

44—2 顶按折端,扳回成角

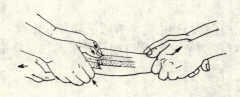

44—3 折端对位

图44 尺桡骨双折用折顶法纠正重迭移位

使骨折断端对顶复位。然后术者两手紧握骨折部位使前臂作掌背侧及尺桡侧的摇动，使骨折断端紧密接触。桡骨在上$\frac{1}{3}$骨折，近

端易向桡背侧旋转移位，远端则向尺掌侧旋转移位，术者在双手分骨的同时，1手捏住骨折远端向桡背侧推按，1手捏住骨折近端向尺掌侧推按，可纠正移位。

固定

两个分骨垫，置于两骨折端之掌背侧。两块方形压垫，分别置于骨折端的掌背侧。4块小夹板放在前臂掌背侧和尺桡侧，3根连筋带捆扎，前臂悬吊胸前。上 $\frac{1}{3}$ 骨折，前臂旋后位，中下 $\frac{1}{3}$ 骨折前臂中立位（图45）。

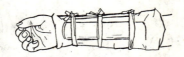

正位

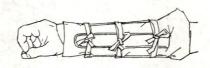

侧位

图45 尺桡骨骨折小夹板固定

药物

按3期用药原则。早期如前臂肿胀严重，可内服复元活血汤（1）加减。

练功

整复固定后，注意夹板松紧度，防止因夹板过紧造成前臂缺血性肌挛缩或坏死。早期作手指屈伸及握拳活动；中期作肘及肩关节的活动；后期作前臂的旋转活动锻炼。

2.11 桡骨远端骨折

发病

桡骨远端骨折常见。多发生在老年，如发生在青少年，则为骨骺分离，常为间接暴力所伤。由于跌倒姿势不同，骨折可表现为伸直型和屈曲型（图46）。巴通氏骨折（Batong）系桡骨远端掌侧骨折合并腕关节向上脱位，属屈曲型骨折脱位。直接暴力所伤多为粉碎性骨折。

诊断要点

1. 有外伤史，尤其是跌倒伤。

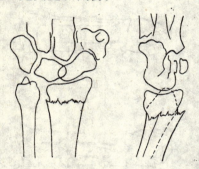

46-1 骨折断端向掌侧成角,骨折线未进入关节

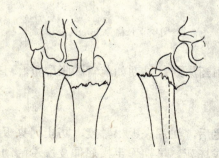

46-2 骨折远端向背侧移位,骨折线未进入关节

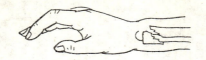

46-3　史密斯氏骨折移位

图 46　桡骨远端骨折

2.　腕部肿胀、疼痛、伸直型呈"餐叉"畸形。

3.　局部挤压痛，有骨擦音和假活动，腕部功能丧失。

4.　腕部正侧位 X 线片可明确骨折类型。

治疗

整复　以伸直型为例

1.　在局麻下，患者坐位或仰卧位，前臂中立位。助手双手握住前臂中部。术者双手握住手腕部，使双拇指按压于骨折远端背侧，余 4 指抵于骨折近端掌侧，行拔伸牵引，纠正旋转及重叠移位。在持续牵引下，双拇指向掌侧按压，余 4 指向背侧端提，同时，突然使腕部掌屈尺偏，纠正向桡、背侧移位。术者再以 1 手保持掌屈尺偏位，1 手拇指在桡骨背侧，由骨折近端向骨折远端按压，纠正残余移位（图 47）。

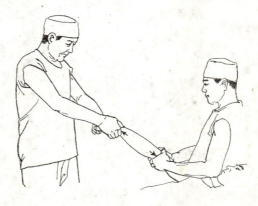

47-1　在牵引下矫正重迭及旋转移位

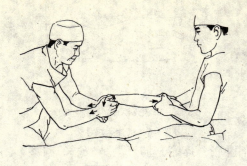

47-2　而后猛力牵抖,使骨折段对位,同时迅速尺偏掌屈

图 47

2.　准备同上。一助手握患肢手部，另一助手握住前臂，对抗牵引。因骨折远端容易旋前，故牵引时,手腕应稍旋后 10—15°。术者立于外侧，1 手握前臂下段向桡侧提托，另 1 手握腕部向尺侧推按，纠正桡侧移位。术者再以双手拇指向掌侧按压骨折远端背侧，余 4 指抵住骨折近端掌侧，向背侧端提，纠正向背侧移位。然后，术者双拇指在桡骨背侧，由近向远重复按压 1—2 次，使其完全复位（图 48）。

注意：开始牵引时，远端要顺势向桡背侧牵引数分钟，待嵌

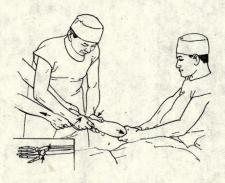

48-1　矫正桡侧移位

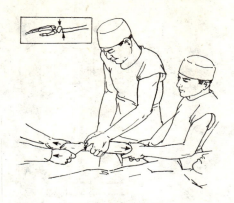

48-2 矫正掌、背侧移位

图 48 桡骨远端伸直型骨折复位情况

插松解后，再顺前臂纵轴牵引。术毕、术者要用双手掌分别置于前臂下端桡尺侧，作相对挤压，使下尺桡关节复位。

固定

棉垫包裹，以小夹板固定，桡，背侧板远端超过腕关节，尺、掌侧板平齐腕关节，可限制腕关节背伸桡偏活动，3根连筋带捆扎固定。前臂中立位，悬吊胸前（图49）。

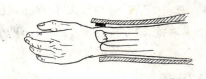

正位

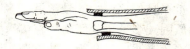

侧位

49-1 小压垫与小夹板放置部位

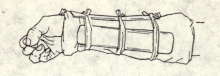

①正位

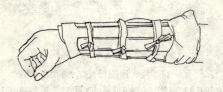

②侧位

49-2　①～②小夹板固定之外形

图49　克雷氏骨折的固定法

药物

按 3 期用药原则。

练功　以伸直型为例

固定后练习手指屈伸活动和腕关节的掌屈尺偏活动，肩肘关节活动不受限制；解除外固定后，行腕关节屈伸活动和前臂旋转活动。

2.12　腕舟状骨骨折

发病

腕舟状骨骨折在腕部损伤中比较常见，多发生于青壮年。间接暴力是常见的原因，多见于跌倒伤。直接暴力所引起的骨折较少见。根据骨折夹角大小，可分为 3 种类型：Ⅰ型 < 30°，Ⅱ型 30°—50°，Ⅲ型 > 50°。根据骨折部位分为：结节骨折、腰部骨折及近端骨折。

诊断要点

1. 有明显外伤史。

2. 腕部鼻烟壶肿胀、疼痛，第一，二掌骨冲击痛。

3. X 线片，除腕部正侧位外，尚需摄握掌斜位片。如体征疑为骨折而 X 线片阴性，可暂制动两周后，再拍片，如有骨折，此时骨折端骨质已吸收，骨折线清晰可见。

治疗

整复

舟状骨骨折往往移位很少，一般不需整复。如有移位骨折则需整复。整复时患者仰卧，一助手握住前臂，使肘屈 90°，另一助手 1 手握住拇指，1 手握住其余 4 指，沿前臂纵轴方向拔伸牵引。此时，患者前臂处于轻度旋前位，手腕处于平伸尺偏位。术者立于外侧面向远端，双拇指按压鼻烟壶部，余指握住手腕部尺侧和掌侧，助手使患者手腕部轻度背伸桡偏，术者双拇指向掌、尺侧按压，助手根据骨折夹角大小顺势使手腕作相应的掌屈尺偏位：Ⅰ°轻度尺偏，Ⅱ°：中度尺偏，Ⅲ°：重度尺偏。

固定

硬纸壳固定法：复位后，鼻烟壶部放置小压垫，上盖硬纸板，胶布贴住，外包棉垫，用特制硬纸壳裹住手腕部桡背掌侧（图 50），尺侧放置塑型的一根小夹板，绷带"8"字形包扎，使手腕部根据骨折夹角固定在一定的掌屈尺偏位上，以有利于骨折断端的稳定，前臂中立位悬吊胸前 1—3 个月。

药物

按 3 期用药原则。因骨折愈合较慢，故内服接骨丹（11）时间宜长。

练功

早期肩、肘活动不受限制；中期轻度地练习手指的屈伸活动；骨折愈合解除外固定后，方可练习握拳及腕部屈伸功能。

注意

1. 骨折夹角：即舟状骨骨折线与桡骨下端尺倾关节所成的角度。

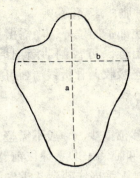

a. 中线：
上自前臂中段
下至拇指指间关节
b. 最宽处：
能包绕手掌背部
图 50　硬纸壳示意图

2. 掌屈度：即手掌的背侧与前臂背侧向掌侧屈曲的角度，一般在 30°。

3. 尺偏度：即第三掌骨与前臂纵轴尺偏的角度。轻度尺偏位，即尺偏度小于 10°；中度尺偏位，即尺偏度在 10°—15°；重度尺偏位，即尺偏度在 20°左右。

2.13　第一掌骨基底部骨折

发病

第一掌骨基底部骨折，多见于跌倒伤和撞击伤。可分单纯基底部骨折和掌骨基底部骨折合并腕掌关节脱位（Bennett 骨折）。前者以横断型多见，骨折远端受拇长屈肌、拇短屈肌与拇内收肌的牵拉、骨折近端受拇长展肌的牵拉，骨折向桡背侧成角畸形（图 51）；后者，内侧三角形小骨片与大多角骨的关系不变，外侧骨折端，因拇长展肌的牵拉和拇短屈肌的收缩由大多角骨关节向外侧背侧移位，并向掌侧屈曲。

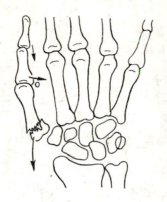

图 51　拇指掌骨基底骨折（箭头表示肌力牵引与骨折移位方向）

诊断要点

1. 有外伤史。
2. 局部肿胀，疼痛，向桡背侧成角畸形，拇指功能丧失。
3. 局部压痛，有假活动、骨擦音和冲击痛。
4. 正侧位 X 线片可了解骨折类型。

治疗

整复

患者坐位，术者一手握住腕部，拇指放在骨折部的背侧，按住突出部位，另手握拇指，在掌指关节屈曲的情况下，进行对抗牵引，并使掌骨头尽量外展，但指骨勿外展，骨折即可复位。

固定

外展夹板固定法：小夹板塑形成 30°外展形状，两个小压垫，1 个放在骨折突起部位，1 个放在掌骨头掌侧，棉垫衬里。将弧形夹板放置前臂桡侧及第一掌骨桡背侧，夹板弧形成角部正对腕关节，夹板近端用宽胶布固定，夹板远端用窄胶布与掌骨头压垫环绕固定，使第一掌骨呈外展位、拇指屈曲位（图 52）。如骨折并脱位者固定不稳定时，可加用拇指末节指骨骨牵引，以维持骨折复位（图53）。

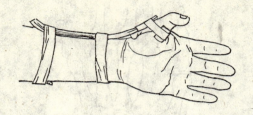

图 52　拇骨掌骨基底骨折夹板固定

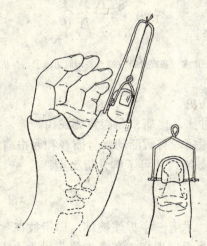

图 53　骨牵引固定法

药物

按 3 期用药原则。

练功

早期练习 2—5 指屈伸活动和肘肩关节活动；中期练习拇指屈曲活动；后期练习拇指伸屈展收及腕关节屈伸旋转活动。

2.14 掌骨骨折

发病

掌骨骨折临床较为多见，多发生在青壮年。多由传达暴力引起，如跌倒伤、拳击伤。亦可由直接暴力引起。掌骨骨折最易发生在掌骨颈部，以第4、5掌骨为好发部位，多为横断骨折。其次为掌骨干骨折，基底部骨折较少见。因屈指肌的牵拉，骨折多突向背侧成角畸形。

诊断要点

1. 有明显的外伤史。
2. 掌背部肿胀、疼痛，皮下瘀血，局部突起。
3. 掌骨有时短缩、手指功能丧失。
4. 局部压痛，有骨擦音，假活动和冲击痛。
5. 手部正斜位 X 线片可了解骨折类型。

治疗

整复

1. 掌骨颈骨折：患者坐位，术者一手握住手掌部，一手握住患指，在牵引下屈曲掌指关节成 90°位，此时近节指骨近端关节面移到掌骨头的掌侧面，这样，侧副韧带紧张，有利于稳定骨折的掌骨头。术者握患指之手，随之向手背侧推挤近节手指，同时另手按压骨折近端，骨折即可复位。(图 54)。

2. 掌骨干骨折：局麻下，患者坐位，术者 1 手握手腕部，1 手握持患指，行对抗牵引。然后双拇指按压手背突起处，纠正成角畸形。再以双拇、食指在掌背侧分别夹挤掌骨间隙，纠正侧方移位。如为多发性掌骨干骨折，整复时，先在手掌部握 1 绷带卷，使手成功能位，用胶布将绷带卷固定。然后用手法依次整复移位的骨折，即整复 1 处，使用胶布条贴在指背侧，远端牵引粘贴，逐一进行。各指的纵轴线须指向舟骨结节。

3. 掌骨基底部骨折：移位较轻者不需整复；如移位和成角

较重，整复手法同掌骨干骨折。

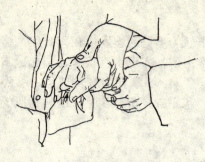

54-1　整复手法

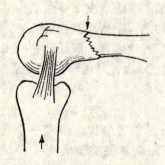

54-2　用力方向及作用示意

图54　掌骨颈骨折整复方法

固定

1．掌骨颈骨折：复位后，用竹板或铝板塑形成"匸"形，即在相当于掌指关节和近侧指间关节处各塑成直角形。棉垫衬里、放置在手背及手指的背面，使掌指关节保持直角位，用胶布粘贴固定（图55）。

2．掌骨干骨折：用木板固定法：复位后，在骨折部背侧两骨间隙放置分骨垫，并在掌背侧放置棉衬垫。再在手背侧及掌侧各放1块木板，用胶布固定，最后用绷带包扎（图56）。不稳定性单根骨折（斜形或螺旋形），复位后，在掌侧放置塑形竹板或

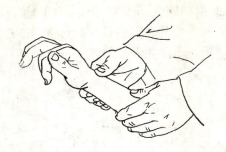

图 55　直角小夹板放置法

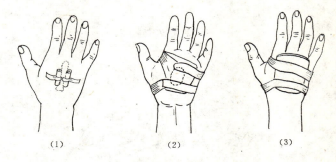

(1)　　　　　　　　(2)　　　　　　　　(3)

(1)分骨垫的放置与胶布固定

(2)掌侧夹板毡垫（点线），胶布固定

(3)背侧夹板与胶布固定

图 56　第三掌骨干斜形骨折

铝板，夹板之弧形使手指保持功能位，并紧贴手指掌侧和手掌部，先用胶布固定，后用绷带包扎，再在患指背侧粘贴胶布，将胶布远端绕过夹板远端贴住。在骨折部背侧两骨间隙粘贴分骨垫和棉衬垫、外盖硬纸壳、绷带包扎固定（图57）。

3.　掌骨基底部骨折，固定法同掌骨干小夹板固定法。

药物

按三期用药原则。

练功

早期避免患指和腕关节屈伸活动；3—4周解除外固定后，逐渐进行手指和腕关节的功能锻炼，只可主动活动，不可被动强行扳拉手指，以免加重手指关节僵硬。

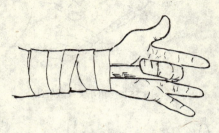

57-1　患指胶布粘贴牵引

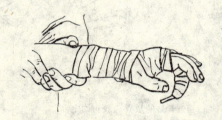

57-2　包扎固定外形（侧位观）

图57　掌骨干骨折钩形夹板加胶布牵引固定法

2.15　指骨骨折

发病

指骨骨折比较多见，直接暴力所造成的骨折，常为横形或粉碎性骨折。间接暴力为指端遭受撞击，暴力传导而致骨折，常引起斜形或螺旋形骨折。根据骨折部位，又可分为近节，中节和末节指骨骨折。

诊断要点

1．有明显外伤史。

2. 患指肿胀、疼痛。骨折移位者，有侧突畸形，同时伸屈活动受限。

3. 局部挤压痛、有假活动、骨擦音和冲击痛。

4. 手指正侧位 X 线片可明确骨折类型：近节指骨干骨折因骨间肌和蚓状肌牵拉而向掌侧成角，而指骨颈骨折，骨折远端向背侧旋转，可达 90°；中节指骨骨折如在屈指浅肌止点近侧，则向背侧成角，如在肌止点远侧，则向掌侧成角；末节指骨基底背侧撕脱性骨折，则表现锤状指畸形（图 58）。

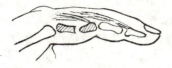 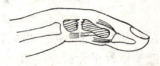

58-1 近节指骨骨折断端向掌侧成角　58-2 中节指骨近段骨折断端向背侧成角

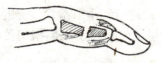 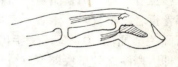

58-3 中节指骨中段骨折断端向掌侧成角　58-4 末节指骨底背侧撕脱骨折、"锤状指"

图 58　指骨不同部位骨折之移位

治疗

整复

因手指功能精细而灵巧，指骨骨折应准确整复，如遗留畸形，则影响手指的外型及功能。

1. 近节指骨骨折，指阻麻醉下，患者坐位，术者左手拇、食指捏住骨折近段，右手 3—5 指紧握骨折远段、对抗牵引，再以拇指分别捏住骨折的掌背侧，屈曲近侧指关节，同时拇指向背侧推顶骨折断端，纠正掌侧成角。伴有侧方移位者、右手拇食指再分别置于骨折两侧，进行挤压推按，纠正侧方移位。近节指骨颈骨折整复时，宜用折顶手法，将骨折远端向背侧牵引，双手拇、食指分别捏住骨折远近端的掌背侧，然后迅速屈曲手指，屈曲时应将近端的掌侧顶向背侧，骨折即可复位（图59）。

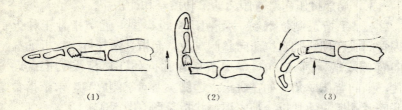

(1)移位情况　(2)整复方法　(3)整复后情况

图 59　指骨颈骨折

2. 中节指骨骨折：根据骨折部位和成角移位情况，整复手法同近节指骨干骨折。

3. 末节指骨骨折：移位不大者，可不予整复。有劈裂或侧方移位者，可用拇食指对挤掌背侧或内外侧，以纠正移位。基底部骨折者，整复时，术者一手握持患指近节和中节指骨，使近侧指间关节屈曲 90°位，一手拇食指捏住末节，使远侧指间关节过伸，撕脱之骨折块即可复位。

固定

1. 近节、中节指骨骨折。

(1) 不超关节固定法：根据骨折成角移位方向，在掌背侧或外内侧，放置小压垫，胶布贴住，棉垫包裹，两块瓦形纸壳或4块小夹板不超关节，胶布拉紧固定（图60）。

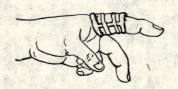

图 60　不超关节的局部硬纸壳固定法

(2) 功能位固定法：铝板或竹板按照患指功能位塑型，根据骨折移位和成角方向放置压垫、棉垫衬里，内外侧放置短夹板，铝（竹）板安放合适，用胶布固定、绷带包扎。不稳定性骨折除用局部外固定外，可加用指骨胶布条牵引（图61），以稳定骨折断端。

2. 末节指骨骨折：

（1）劈裂成侧方移位骨折，复位后，用两块小夹板或两块硬纸壳，胶布粘贴固定即可。

（2）基底部骨折：铝板或竹板塑形，使患指近侧指间关节屈曲 90°位，远侧指间关节过伸位，胶布粘贴固定（图62）。3 周后更换直夹板，近端不超过近侧指间关节，远端至手指末端，棉压垫呈梯形，放置指腹前半部分，夹板放置患指掌侧，胶布粘贴固

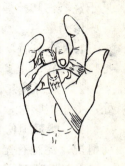

图 61　近节指骨骨折整复
后牵引固定方法

定，使末节手指处于背伸位。固定期间可以进行近侧指间关节的屈伸活动，3 周后去外固定。

药物

按 3 期用药原则。

练功

早期除患指外，其余 4 指不限制活动。手指伸直位固定者，除锤状指外，一般不超过 2—3 周，即应改为屈曲功能位固定；解除外固定后，积极进行患指的屈

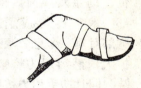

图 62　末节指骨背侧撕脱
骨折固定法

伸功能锻炼，但避免强行手法板拿，以免加重指间关节的粘连挛缩。

2.16　肋骨骨折

发病

肋骨骨折多发生于老年人，其次为壮年。造成骨折的原因分

为直接暴力、间接暴力、混合暴力和肌肉收缩力。骨折多为闭合性。可为1根或多根肋骨的1处骨折，亦可为1根或多根肋骨的多处骨折，后者因数根肋骨游离，形成浮动胸壁，发生矛盾呼吸，对呼吸和循环系统产生严重影响。开放性气胸时有所见，多见于锐器伤和枪弹伤，是比较严重的创伤，临床应予重视。

诊断要点

1. 外伤后，局部疼痛、肿胀、可有瘀斑、深呼吸、咳嗽、打喷嚏和转动上身均使疼痛加重。

2. 局部压痛，两手前后或左右挤压胸廓，或1手按压骨折处，令患者咳嗽，均引起剧痛，有时有骨擦音。

3. 严重损伤者，注意患者血压和心脏检查，以明确内脏损伤情况，注意有无皮下气肿和矛盾呼吸等现象。

4. 胸廓X线片可帮助观察骨折类型及胸内并发症情况。

治疗

整复

有移位的肋骨骨折，整复时患者坐位，助手双手前后挤压于上腹部和腰部。术者1手放置骨折部位，1手按于胸部对侧，令患者深吸气，尽量使胸围扩大，然后用力咳嗽，术者挤压骨折端，同时助手用力挤压上腹部，骨折即可复位。如为凹陷性骨折，术者双手应挤压骨折部位的两侧，以使骨折复位（图63）。

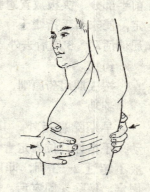

图63 肋骨凹陷骨折
对挤整复法

固定

1. 硬纸壳绷带固定法：硬纸壳1块，棉垫衬里放置骨折部位，胶布粘贴住，外用绷带围胸缠绕数圈，将骨折部位和上下邻近两条肋骨全部固定（图64）。

2. 胶布固定法：适用于第 5—9 肋骨骨折。备胶布宽 5 cm 左右，比病人胸廓半周长 10cm。患者坐位，双臂抬起，深呼气之末，尽量使胸围缩小。术者先在骨折部后侧，超过中线 5 cm（即健侧肩胛中线），贴紧胶布，由后绕过骨折部向前跨越正中线 5 cm（超过锁骨中线），然后迭瓦式（重叠 $\frac{1}{3}$—

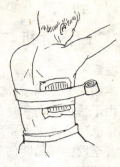

图 64　肋骨骨折纸壳、绷带固定法

$\frac{1}{2}$）向上和向下各增加 2—3 条，一直将骨折部位和上下邻近两条肋骨全部固定（图 65）。

药物

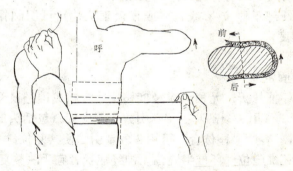

图 65　肋骨骨折胶布固定法

初期活血化瘀，行气宽胸止痛，内服复元活血汤（1）加减（可加桔梗、杏仁、贝母、瓜蒌、苏子），咳血者加三七、白芨、仙鹤草、藕节；中期宜服接骨凡（11）；后期待骨折愈合解除外固定后，外贴伸筋膏，内服伸筋片。

练功

单纯肋骨骨折者，固定后，可行走活动，限制两上肢过大幅度的活动，以免固定脱落。伤情重者，应卧床休息，待病情稳定后，可下地活动。

2.17　颈椎骨折与脱位

发病

本病主要是间接暴力所致，如重物打击头顶、坠落伤或撞击伤。由于暴力方向和受伤姿势不同，可分为屈曲型和伸直型。受伤部位以环枢椎多见。如骨折脱位严重，可产生脊髓、神经的压迫，甚至发生脊髓断伤致高位截瘫，治疗困难，预后较差。

诊断要点

1. 有典型的外伤史。

2. 颈部疼痛，病员往往双手托扶头部。

3. 颈项肌僵硬，头颈部屈伸及旋转功能受限。

4. 有的病人有脊髓神经刺激症状。

5. 颈部正侧位 X 线片（或张口正位片）可明确骨折脱位部位及程度。

治疗

整复固定

1. 环椎骨折：无移位或轻度移位，脊髓或神经根无明显压迫症状者，可用头颈部牵引架牵引或头颈支架（包括头部）固定3—4个月。有明显移位者，可用头颅牵引法使其复位。

2. 环椎脱位：环椎半脱位无神经症状者宜手法整复。

（1）环椎一侧半脱位：复位前先行颈部推拿按摩以松解颈项部肌肉痉挛僵硬。患者俯卧，上助手右手掌托住枕骨下方、左手掌放在颌下；下助手双手下拉两肩，顺势对抗牵引。术者立于患侧，双手拇指按压第二颈椎棘突与后弓上。上助手在牵引下，将倾向患侧的头颈逐渐旋正，并向背侧过伸。同时术者双手拇指用力向前按压，往往闻及复位声。上助手轻轻回旋头颈部，使下颌回居中线。术毕，用头颈牵引架或颌枕布带牵引（图 66）。

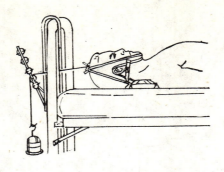

图 66 颌枕带滑动牵引法

（2）环椎双侧半脱位：准备同上。因双侧脱位头颈前倾畸形，故先沿患者躯干纵轴方向对抗牵引。术者立于右侧，双拇指按枢椎棘突及后弓。上助手在牵引下将头颈部左右活动，继将患者头颈逐渐背伸。术者双手拇指稳健地向前按压，即可闻及复位声（图67）。

（3）颈椎关节的半脱位或暂时性脱位：多因屈颈位遭受暴力，或急刹车时极度屈颈所致。整复准备同上。一侧颈椎关节半脱位棘突偏离中线，故术者1拇指应放在倾斜的棘突上按压，另手拇指按压在脱位的下1个颈椎的棘突上。在持续牵引下，上助手将倾向患侧的颈部朝对侧屈曲旋转并向背侧过伸；同时术者双拇指将上下两个棘突向中线挤压，使之复位。双侧性半脱位，上助手在持续牵引下将患者颈部背伸，同时术者双拇指按压脱位椎

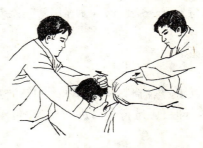

67-1 助手拔伸法

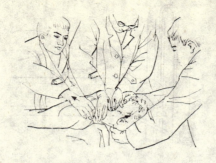

67-2 使颈后伸,同时按压向后突之棘突

图 67 环椎双侧半脱位整复法

体的下 1 个棘突，即可复位。

(4) 颈椎体的压缩性骨折：手法适用于无脊髓神经压迫症状者。患者仰卧，头颈部伸出床头。助手固定两肩，术者 1 手托住后枕部，1 手拉住下颌部，顺势对抗牵引，并逐渐使颈后伸，即可复位。术毕用头颈牵引架牵引固定。

(5) 颈椎关节屈曲性脱位：多见于颈 4、5 和颈 5、6 之间，可能为瞬间脱位，亦可能为小关节突交锁，但都伴有严重的脊髓或神经根损伤。前者可用中立位枕颌布托或头颈牵引架牵引，防止再脱位。后者应首先牵引，以整复交锁的小关节突与解除神经的压迫，切勿单纯采用过伸位复位，以免加重脊髓神经的损伤。应采用颅骨牵引，先顺势牵引，重量 10 公斤左右，复位后，改中立位牵引，维持量 2～3 公斤，4～6 周解除牵引。

药物

按 3 期用药原则。

练功

早期仰卧木板床，限制头颈部活动，四肢活动不受限制；解除牵引或固定后，即可下地行走，进行头颈部的屈伸旋转活动。

2.18 胸腰椎压缩性骨折

发病

胸腰椎压缩性骨折，在脊柱损伤中较为常见，多为高处坠落损伤或弯腰时重物砸伤所致。骨折多发生于青壮年，老年人因骨质疏松轻微外伤即可发生骨折，如跌倒伤。一般发生于胸椎11～12或腰椎1～2部位，骨折多为1个椎体，亦有2个椎体。因暴力大小、受伤姿势及年龄、体质原因，骨折可分屈曲型和伸展型，稳定型和非稳定型，无脊髓神经损伤型和脊髓神经损伤型。

诊断要点

1.　有外伤史。如坠落损伤或重物砸伤。

2.　腰背部疼痛，轻度肿胀。屈曲型局部后突畸形，棘突间隙增宽。

3.　局部有压痛和叩击痛。咳嗽、喷嚏时疼痛加重。不能坐立。

4.　如有脊髓神经损伤则有其节段以下的感觉、肌张力、肌肉运动、生理反射、病理反射以及大小便的改变。

5.　因腹膜后血肿刺激造成肠麻痹，出现肠胃气滞血瘀症状，如腹胀痛，呕恶，二便不利。

6.　X线片检查可明确骨折的类型和性质。

治疗

整复固定

1.　稳定型胸腰椎压缩性骨折:

(1) 功能锻炼法:患者仰卧木板床，骨折部位垫软枕。待疼痛缓解后，进行腰背肌锻炼。第一步，五点支撑法:患者先屈肘伸肩，后屈膝伸髋，用两肘、两足和头部五点支撑，将腰部和臀部腾起，使脊柱过伸。第二步，三点支撑法:两肘屈曲，两手交叉胸前，用两足和头部支撑，整个身躯离开床面。第三步，弓桥支撑法:患者用双手和双足作支撑，全身离开床面成弓形。第四步，飞燕点水法：患者改俯卧位，先作抬头挺胸，同时两臂后伸，使头颈及胸部抬起，离开床面；然后，膝关节伸直，双下肢同时抬起，离开床面。以上步骤，循序渐进，反复锻炼，一般4周下地作腰背肌后伸活动锻炼。此法安全简便，效果可靠（图68）。

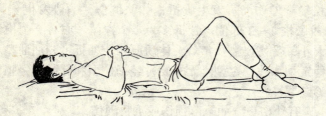

68-1 整复后之卧床

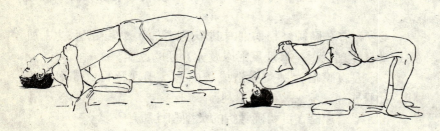

68-2 五点练功法   68-3 三点练功法

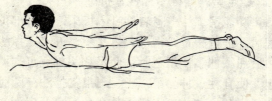

68-4

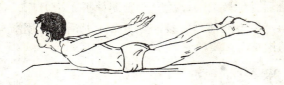

68—5

图 68 胸腰椎压缩骨折的功能锻炼方法

（2）**手法整复法**：适宜青壮年及体力劳动者。

①俯卧位整复法：应用镇痛剂。一助手立于患者头侧，用双手拉住患者两腋下。另助手立于患者足侧，双手握住患者双踝，对抗拔伸牵引。术者立于患者身旁，先用双手按摩腰部软组织，使肌肉松弛。再用双手掌重叠放于骨折后突部，令患者深呼吸，当患者吸气时，术者缓缓按压，反复数次，纠正骨折后突畸形。

②双踝悬吊牵引法：患者俯卧床上，双踝包以棉垫，将双踝缓缓悬空吊起，使胸腰部过伸，利用患者体重将压缩骨折拉开。同时，术者用双手撑按压骨折后突部，使之复位。术毕，用脊柱夹板外固定，或用"工"字形腰背支具固定。

2. **胸腰椎骨折脱位**：手法整复较困难。如果用单纯过伸动作解除关节交锁，比较困难，甚至反使椎体分离，引起脊髓神经损伤。整复时，患者俯卧位，先在水平位用力拔伸牵引，按压纠正后突畸形（勿用暴力），使腰部过伸，骨折脱位方可纠正。术毕，仰卧后伸位休息。

药物

早期，伴有肠胃气滞者，用顺气活血汤加减；伴有气滞血瘀，腑气不通者，用大成汤加减，或用番泻叶代茶饮；中期，服用接骨丹；后期，服用伸筋片。久病体弱者，服壮腰健肾汤（51），外用伸筋膏或热敷灵。

练功

早期宜卧床休息，翻身时，胸腰部保持过伸位；中期在床上作腰背肌后伸锻炼，1日数次；后期骨折1个月后，可离床作腰后伸活动，但不能前屈弯腰；骨折2个月后，可逐渐进行腰部的屈伸活动锻炼。

2.19 股骨颈骨折

发病

股骨颈骨折较为常见，多发生于老年人。由于老年人骨质疏松，轻度外伤即可引起骨折。青壮年股骨颈骨折少见，但引起之暴力较大。按损伤机制可分为内收型和外展型；按骨折部位可分为囊内型和囊外型；按骨折线可分为横形、斜形和螺旋形，或分为稳定性和不稳定性骨折。因股骨颈血运差，骨折不愈合率较高，尤其是囊内不稳定性骨折愈合率更低。

诊断要点

1. 有外伤史。老年人多见于跌伤，青壮年多见于坠落和车祸伤。

2. 患髋疼痛，但肿胀不著，多数不敢站立和行走，有时表现为膝关节前内侧疼痛。

3. 患肢多有轻度的屈膝屈髋及外旋畸形。有移位骨折者患肢缩短1—2 cm。

4. 腹股沟中点压痛，患髋活动受限。大粗隆部或足跟部冲击痛。

5. 骨传导音降低（听筒放置在耻骨联合，叩击内踝）。

6. 髋关节正侧位 X 线片可明确骨折类型。

治疗

整复

患者仰卧位。用 0.5%普鲁卡因 10 毫升注入髋关节囊内，第一助手双手拉住两腋部；第二助手双手掌按压两髂前上棘。术者立于患侧，1 手握踝部，另一肘窝挎住腘窝部，使患髋半屈曲位，膝关节屈曲 90°位，然后用力挎提腘窝，下压踝部，并稍加摇晃，再将患肢内旋伸直外展 30°位。测量双下肢，如等长表示已复位。第二助手由按压骨盆改为抵住对侧骨盆，术者用拳或足跟顺股骨颈方向用力叩击股骨大粗隆部，使断端嵌插（图 69）。

固定

1. 外展长木板固定法：

木板上平腋下 6—7 肋部位，下至足跟，木板塑形成外展 30°。棉垫衬里；长木板放置在髋部外侧，使木板突面正对大粗隆部，绷带包缠固定，使患肢保持内旋外展 30°位（图 70）。术毕，患者仰卧漏洞床，臀部垫气圈，便于大小便时不移动臀部。

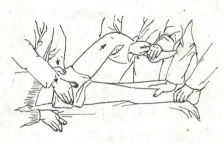

69-1 髋半屈位拔伸

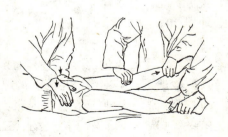

69-2 内旋、拉直、外展

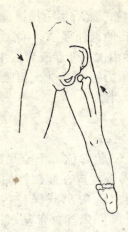

69-3　整复股骨颈骨折叩击手法、用力方向及作用示意

图 69　股骨颈内收型骨折闭合整复法

2. 多针固定法

整复后，大粗隆部消毒铺巾。局麻，在大粗隆下 2 cm 处朝股骨头中心点（股动脉和腹股沟韧带交叉中点外下 1 cm），方向钻入 1 枚粗骨圆针约 8 cm 深。在进针处向上向下各偏斜 10—20°左右交叉钻入两枚粗骨圆针。拍摄正侧位 X 线片，认为满意后，无菌纱布覆盖针尾。足部穿丁字鞋，保持患肢外展 30°中立位。

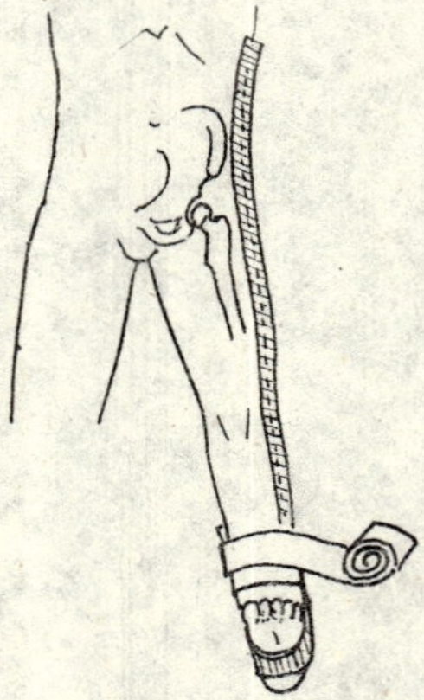

药物

图 70　超关节夹板固定法示意

本病多系老年人，而青壮年创伤亦较重，故全身反应较严重。早期辨证用药，调理全身是治疗本病的重要措施。肠胃气滞，大便干结者，内服大成汤（7）加减；肺气不宣，咳嗽气喘者，内服苏子降气汤（52）加减；患髋

疼痛肿胀较重者，内服复元活血汤（1）加减。中期内服接骨丹（11）；骨折愈合后，内服伸筋片（50），外用2号洗药熏洗（47）。

练功

复位后，限制患髋活动，不能随意翻身，可作足趾和踝关节的屈伸及股四头肌的舒缩活动。骨折愈合后，先行髋膝关节的不负重伸屈活动，但是患髋不得内收和外展。以后，逐渐下地，由扶双拐到扶单拐行走，最后弃拐负重活动。复查时，如有股骨头坏死征象，应延缓负重时间。

2.20 股骨干骨折

发病

股骨干骨折较为常见，多由较大暴力所造成，因此骨折断端移位明显、软组织损伤严重。主要是直接暴力所伤，表现为横形、斜形、粉碎形骨折；也有间接暴力所伤，多为斜形、螺旋形骨折。小儿可为青枝形骨折。中段骨折最多，上段或下段次之。上段骨折近端向前、向外旋转移位，远端向后、向内、向上移位；中段骨折远端多向内、向上移位，断端向前外侧成角畸形；下段骨折远端向后倾斜移位或向后成角，严重者可压迫或刺伤腘动脉、静脉和胫神经。

诊断要点

1. 有明显外伤史。

2. 患肢肿胀疼痛，多数伴有短缩、成角，或旋转畸形。

3. 局部挤压痛，跟部冲击痛，有骨擦音和假活动。

4. 因创伤重，内出血较多，成人一般出血在1000毫升，可引起休克。

5. 移位较大的骨折可能损伤坐骨神经和股动脉、静脉。应检查足背和胫后动脉及足趾活动情况。

6. 大腿正侧位X线片可明确骨折部位和类型。因可能伴有同侧髋关节脱位，临证时应注意髋关节的检查。

治疗

股骨干骨折的治疗应根据患者年龄及骨折类型而采用不同的方法。

整复固定

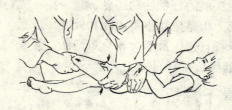

图71　小儿股骨干骨折整复法

1. 手法复位双下肢过头皮肤牵引法：适宜5岁以下儿童，有移位的不稳定性骨折。局麻下，患儿仰卧，助手双手按住髂前上棘固定骨盆。术者1手握住患肢膝部，对抗拔伸牵引，纠正重叠移位。另1手拇指和其余4指分别握住骨折断端，根据移位方向进行挤压，纠正侧方移位（图71）。术毕，小夹板固定加双下肢过头悬吊皮肤牵引（图72），或小夹板固定加长木板外固定3周（图73）。

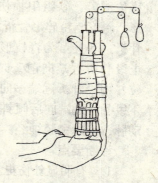

图72　患肢局部小夹板固定
加双下肢悬吊皮牵引

2. 手法复位皮肤牵引加局部小夹板外固定法：适宜6—15岁少年有移位的骨折。准备同上，增加1助手，1手握踝部，1手握膝下，使患髋半屈曲位对抗拔伸牵引，纠正重叠移位。术者双手根据骨折移位方向进行推按，纠正侧方移位（图74）。术毕，小夹板固定，水平位皮肤牵引（图

75)。或屈膝位皮肤牵引4—6周（图76）。

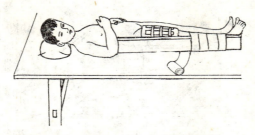

图73　小儿股骨干骨折单纯夹板固定法

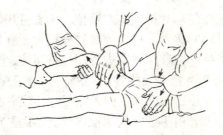

图74　儿童股骨干骨折整复方法

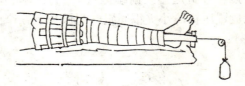

图75　患肢水平位皮牵引

3.　手法整复骨牵引加局部小夹板固定：适宜成人有移位的骨折。在局麻或全麻下，患者仰卧位，患髋屈曲30～60°，外展20—40°，屈肘70—80°。一助手用宽布带经会阴部前后侧绕过，布带两头达健侧肩上方，用手握住。另一助手双手按住髂前上棘以固定骨盆，第三助手双手握住患肢膝关节下部行对抗拔伸牵引，以纠正重叠移位、如不能纠正，术者可用折顶手法纠正

之。斜形或螺旋形骨折，骨折面背靠背，可用回旋手法使之复

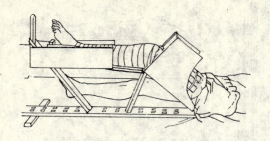

图 76　屈膝直脚架皮牵引

位。横断骨折或短斜形骨折的侧方移位，术者可用双手指或手掌进行整复。如肌肉发达者，可用双前臂分别置于骨折部位的内外侧或前后侧，根据骨折移位方向进行端提挤压使之复位。上段骨折，髋关节屈曲外展角度大些并略加外旋，助手握住近端向后、向内推按，术者握住远端向前、向外端提；中段骨折，髋关节稍屈曲外展外旋，术者用 1 手向内侧推挤骨折断端，然后用双手在断端前后或内外夹挤；下段骨折应尽量屈曲膝关节，术者双手握住腘部作支点将骨折远端向前端提（图 77）。术毕，根据骨折移位成角情况放置压垫，小夹板固定。患肢放在牵引架上，行骨牵引（图 78）。

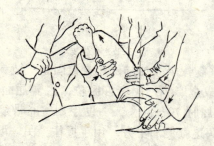

77—1　股骨上 1／3 骨折整复法

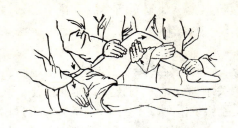

77-2　股骨下1/3骨折整复法

图77　成人股骨干骨折闭合整复法

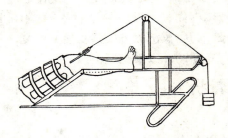

78-1　股骨中下段骨折股骨髁上牵引(勃朗氏架)

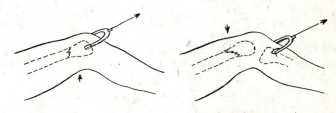

(1)屈曲型骨折在股骨髁上穿针　　(2)伸直型骨折在胫骨结节穿针

78-2　股骨下段不同类型骨折应在不同部位施行骨牵引

图78　股骨骨折骨牵引

药物

早期因内出血较多，大腿肿胀较重，应重用活血化瘀药物以利于消肿和预防感染，如复元活血汤（1）加减；中期和后期可按常规用药。

练功

由于下肢长时间固定和牵引，易产生肌肉萎缩（特别是股四头肌）和膝踝关节僵硬，影响肢体功能的恢复，故整复固定后，应积极进行功能锻炼。早期不影响上肢活动，可练习足趾踝关节的屈伸活动；约2—3周骨折稳定可取半坐位，双臂支撑抬起臀部，练习髋关节和膝关节的伸屈功能，使下半身连同患肢上下活动，带动牵引一起滑动；3—4周开始，双手拉吊环，健足作支撑，抬起臀部；4—5周，双手扶床架，健肢站起；后期骨折临床愈合后，去掉牵引或长木板，保留小夹板作不负重的患肢功能活动，并行按摩和药物熏洗促进关节功能的恢复；骨折骨性愈合后，下床弃拐行走活动，以锻炼肌肉。

2.21　髌骨骨折

发病

髌骨骨折为关节内骨折。多见于老年人。间接暴力和直接暴力皆可致骨折。以前者为多见，如跌倒伤，常为横断形骨折，骨折多发生在中$\frac{1}{3}$或下$\frac{1}{3}$，一般移位较大；后者以打击伤为多见，常为粉碎性骨折，一般移位较小（图79）。

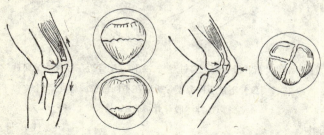

79—1　间接外力骨折　　　　79—2　直接外力骨折

图79　髌骨骨折的发生与移位

诊断要点

1. 有明显外伤史，如跌扑伤或打击伤。

2. 因膝关节内积血，膝前肿胀较重，伴有疼痛瘀血斑，膝关节伸屈功能丧失。

3. 膝前压痛，波动，移位之骨折可触及骨折间隙或游离的骨折块。

4. 膝关节正侧位 X 线片可明确骨折类型。

治疗

因属关节内骨折，故整复应解剖对位。

整复固定

1. 无移位骨折：不需整复，穿刺抽净关节内积血后，厚棉垫包裹，长木板放置膝外侧或后侧，使膝关节保持略屈曲位，绷带缠绕固定。

2. 有移位骨折：

(1) 手法整复抱膝圈固定法：适用于移位不大的骨折。先根据髌骨大小，用绷带或软藤做成圆圈，用绷带缠绕数层，另扎连筋带 4 根，木板 1 块，上自大腿中部，下至踝部，木板中部两侧各钉两枚铁钉。整复时，患者仰卧位，伸膝。局麻下，抽净关节内积血。术者立于患侧，1 手固定骨折远端，1 手拇、食、中指用力向下推挤骨折近端，使其与骨折远端靠拢。同时使两骨折块向内外侧互相错动，以使断裂的筋膜挤出骨折间隙，待有骨擦音感觉，表示骨折已复位 (图 80)。然后 1 手拇、食、中指捏按骨折块的上下端，1 手拇指触及髌骨前方，如感觉不平时，表示骨折端有前后移位，可用拇指按压向前突起的骨折断端。最后双手拇、食、中指用力挤紧骨折断端。棉垫衬里，放置盘形硬纸壳，将抱膝圈压住硬纸壳套在髌骨边上。木板放置在膝关节后侧，腘窝间衬以棉垫，使膝关节略屈位。4 根连筋带于内、外侧的上、下方分别捆扎在 4 根铁钉上，绷带缠绕固定。固定期间应经常注意检查抱膝圈的位置及固定的松紧度 (图 81)。

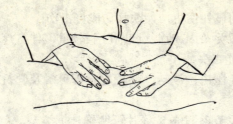

图 80 髌骨骨折整复方法

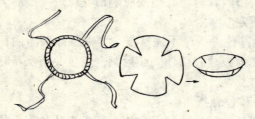

81--1 抱膝圈、盘形纸壳

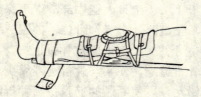

81-2 侧面观

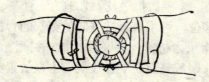

81-3 正面观

图 81 髌骨骨折固定方法

(2) 闭合穿针加压固定法: 适用骨折移位较大手法整复失败

者。常规消毒、局麻下，从上下端骨折块内侧分别向外侧贯穿 1 根克氏针，2 根针应与骨折面平行，纱布保护针孔，然后一助手双手拉拢克氏针内外侧两端，使骨折断端靠拢。术者拇、食指挤压髌骨前方，纠正髌骨前后移位。用制备好的两块带孔木块分别套入克氏针两端，并向中间用力推挤，使两骨折断端紧靠，胶布粘贴固定木板。术毕，长木板固定略屈膝位 2—3 周。

药物

因关节内积血较重；即使抽吸亦易再渗。故初期除用大量活血化瘀药外，需加渗湿利水药。如薏仁、防己、木通、车前子等。中期和后期按常规用药。

练功

早期卧床休息，但不影响上肢健肢及腰背部的活动。患肢抬高练习足趾和踝关节屈伸活动；2 周后开始行股四头肌舒缩活动和膝关节屈伸活动，活动范围不超过 15°；3 周后，肿胀消退，下地不持重扶双拐行走；4—5 周，解除外固定，逐渐加大膝关节的主动屈伸活动范围，并可下地扶单拐行走。在此期间配合中草药熏洗效果更好。

2.22 胫腓骨骨折

发病

胫腓骨骨折比较多见，尤其多见于儿童和青壮年。因胫腓中下 $\frac{1}{3}$ 交界处血运差，骨质脆弱，故容易发生骨折，且骨折后不易愈合。间接暴力可引起斜形或螺旋形骨折；直接暴力多为横形或粉碎性骨折，胫腓骨骨折多在同一水平位（图 82）。因胫骨前内侧皮下组织很薄，骨折断端易刺破皮肤，形成开放性骨折，因肌肉的牵拉和体位的关系，骨折远端易外旋移位，骨折近端向前内侧成角。挤压伤易出现小腿肿胀，严重者造成筋膜间室高压综合症。

诊断要点

1. 有明显的外伤史或疲劳史。

2. 小腿肿胀，疼痛、功能丧失、严重者可有短缩、成角及外旋畸形。

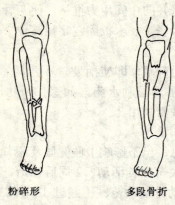

粉碎形　　　　　　　多段骨折

图 82　胫腓骨干骨折常见类型

3. 局部压痛和跟部叩击痛，严重者可有骨擦音和假活动。

4. 检查足背、胫后动脉搏动情况，判断有无腘动脉损伤；检查足趾屈伸情况，判断有无神经损伤。

5. 小腿正侧位 X 线片可明确骨折部位和类型。

治疗

胫腓骨干骨折的治疗原则，主要是恢复其长度和负重功能，因此凡骨折的成角、旋转和重叠畸形均应纠正，以预防创伤性踝关节炎的发生。

整复

患者仰卧位，在局麻下，上助手双手握住小腿上端，下助手双手握足踝部，对抗牵引，以纠正重叠及成角畸形。术者 1 手握住骨折近端，另 1 手握住骨折远端，使远端对合近端。同时施以挤按端提手法纠正侧方移位（图 83）。然后令下助手轻轻摇摆骨折远端，使骨折断端紧密接触。

固定

根据骨折部位和成角、移位方向放置压垫，胶布粘贴，棉垫衬里，小夹板 5 块放好，连筋带捆扎。长板根据骨折部位放置小腿外侧。上 $\frac{1}{3}$ 骨折，长板超膝部；下 $\frac{1}{3}$ 骨折，长板超踝部。用绷带包缠固定。

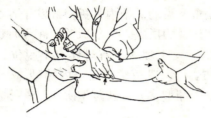

图 83　胫腓骨干骨折整复方法

固定时应注意几点：

1.　小夹板塑形应注意胫骨有突向前外侧的弯曲度。

2.　外侧夹板上端易压伤腓总神经。

3.　后侧夹板下端易压伤跟腱和跟后部。

4.　不稳定性骨折应加跟骨牵引。

5.　小夹板固定松紧度要随时调整，防止筋膜间室高压综合征的产生。

药物

胫骨中下 $\frac{1}{3}$ 骨折因血运差，愈合慢，故应着重补肝肾、壮筋骨。早期小腿肿胀较重伴有水泡者，除重用活血化瘀行气药外，宜加用清热解毒药，如桃仁承气汤（8）合五味消毒饮（5）加减；中期内服壮腰健肾丸（51）或接骨丹（11），后期内服伸筋片（50）。外用 2 号洗药熏洗。

练功

早期上身可坐起，并练习足趾屈伸活动和股四头肌舒缩活动；骨折稳定后去除木板和牵引，练习膝关节和踝关节屈伸活动；后期骨折愈合后去除小夹板，扶双拐下地活动，逐渐改单拐练习持重，以弃拐行走。

2.23 踝部骨折

发病

踝部骨折是最常见的关节内骨折，好发于青少年，多因奔跑行走时扭伤的间接暴力所致。由于踝关节跖屈时稳定性差，故易产生内外翻损伤，发生骨折，有时伴有半脱位。根据暴力的大小、方向和受伤姿势，骨折常分为：内翻型、外翻型、外旋型、压缩性骨折。以内翻型多见，外翻型次之。直接暴力所致骨折多是开放性。

诊断要点

1. 有明显外伤史，尤其扭伤史。
2. 踝部肿胀，疼痛，有瘀血斑，严重者有水泡。
3. 局部压痛，能触及骨擦音。
4. 踝关节内翻或外翻畸形。
5. 根据踝部的正侧位 X 线片和体征，可进一步判断骨折类型。X 线片应包括小腿下 $\frac{1}{3}$ 部位。

治疗

踝部骨折因属关节内骨折，故需解剖复位。骨折的同时，软组织损伤也较重，故须筋骨并重，以利其负重和活动。

整复

1. 患者仰卧位，神经阻滞麻醉。上助手双手握小腿，下助手 1 手握足背，1 手握足跟，顺着原来骨折移位方向对抗拔伸牵引。外翻型骨折，由外翻牵引逐渐变成内翻牵引（图 84）。内翻型骨折，由内翻牵引逐渐变成外翻牵引（图 85）。同时术者双手分别在踝部两侧相对挤按，使之复位。外翻型骨折，内侧手掌在踝关节上方，外侧手掌向内推挤外踝，反之亦然。合并胫腓下联合分离者，令下助手将足轻轻旋转，同时术者双手掌用力挤按双踝，使分离消失，距骨外脱位得以复位。然后上助手在牵引的同时向后按压小腿，下助手向前提拉足部，并逐渐背屈 90°，使向后脱位的距骨恢复原位，同时使向前张口的内踝复位。必要时，以拇指向前上方推挤内踝后下方，纠正内踝残余移位。

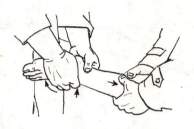

图 84 踝外翻骨折整复法

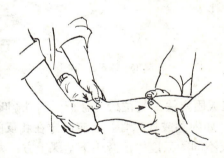

图 85 踝内翻骨折整复法

术毕，足中立位，术者 1 手握足前部，1 手握踝部，将足被动屈伸数次，借助距骨对踝穴的模造，恢复关节面的形状。

2. 三踝骨折的整复方法：后踝骨折块小于胫骨下关节面$\frac{1}{3}$时，可单纯手法整复。按上法先整复内外踝骨折，再整复后踝骨折。术毕，下助手用力挤压内外踝，术者 1 手握小腿下端向后推按，1手握足部向前提拉背屈。由于后关节囊的牵拉紧张，使后踝骨折复位，同时向后半脱位的距骨复位。后踝骨折块大于胫骨下关节面$\frac{1}{3}$时，踝关节不能背屈，因越背屈距骨越向后移位，后踝骨折块向上移位越大，故手法整复有困难。应使用长袜套悬吊牵引或跟骨牵引、通过悬吊牵引使后踝逐渐复位（图 86）。

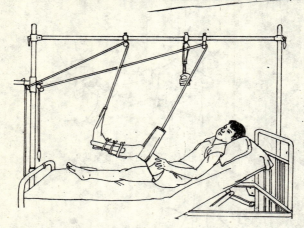

图 86　袜套悬吊牵引

固定

1.　小夹板固定法：复位后，骨折无内外翻畸形，应将足固定在中立位，如内翻或外翻骨折，应固定在相反的位置上。5块夹板用火烤成不同的弧度，前两块下至踝上方，内、外、后侧夹板下至足跟部。压垫放置在外踝下（外翻型骨折）或内踝下（内翻型骨折）、胶布粘贴、棉垫衬里，5块夹板放好，3根连筋带细扎固定。然后，从足跟底穿过下道连筋带两侧结扎固定内外侧夹板远端，使足保持90°背屈位。

2.　硬纸壳固定法：压垫及衬里放置法同上。将两块硬纸壳修剪成上宽下窄的形状，上自小腿下$\frac{1}{3}$段，下至踝下部。两块硬纸壳叩于踝部内外侧，两根连筋带捆扎，再在跟底部放置一块方形硬纸壳，棉垫衬里，1根连筋带从跟底经踝部两侧穿过下道结扎好的连筋带拉紧结扎，绷带包缠固定足背屈90°（图87）。

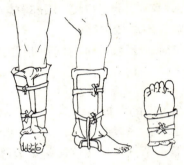

(1)正面观　　(2)侧面观　　(3)足底面观
图87　踝部瓦形纸壳固定法

药物

按3期用药原则。早期踝关节肿胀重者，内服复元活血汤(1)加减。

练功

早期，小腿抬高，上身坐起。积极练习足趾的屈伸活动，膝关节活动不受限制；中期逐渐练习踝关节的屈伸活动，但防止重复受伤机制的活动；4周后，除去外固定，积极进行踝关节的不负重屈伸活动，以防止踝关节粘连。同时有利于骨折的模造塑形，使关节面光滑。

2.24　跟骨骨折

发病

跟骨骨折比较常见，多见于成年人。坠落伤是其常见原因。骨折常发生在跟骨体和结节部。跟骨结节关节角一般为40°，因骨折多为压缩性骨折，故跟骨结节关节角变小，足弓塌陷，跟骨增宽。根据骨折的部位，可分不累及和累及跟距关节骨折两大类。后者属关节内骨折，常发生创伤性关节炎。

诊断要点

1. 有明显外伤史，尤其坠落伤。
2. 足跟部肿胀，疼痛，足弓变浅，跟部增宽，常有瘀血斑。
3. 跟部挤压痛，不敢持重站立。
4. 跟部侧位和轴位 X 线片可明确骨折类型。

治疗

整复固定

1. 不累及跟距关节的骨折。

（1）跟骨结节骨折：患者俯卧位，一助手握住小腿，另一助手握住足前部，使膝关节直角屈曲位，踝关节蹠屈位。术者用克氏针横向穿入跟骨结节内，套入牵引弓，先向后牵引，以松解骨折面的交锁，然后再向下牵拉，使骨折复位；对于跟骨结节横形骨折，准备同上，术者用拇、食指在跟腱部用力向远端推挤骨折片。术毕，用小夹板外固定：跟骨两侧放置梯形压垫。两块弧形夹板超踝关节固定两侧，前侧弓形夹板下至足端，后侧夹板置于跟上。足底放一木板，足心部垫高，棉垫衬里，连筋带捆紧固定，使足保持极度蹠屈位，膝关节略屈位（图 88）。

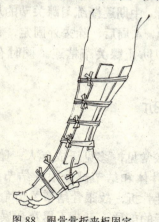

图 88 跟骨骨折夹板固定

(2) 接近跟距关节的跟骨体骨折：因跟骨体压缩性增宽，且跟骨体后半部向上移位，故整复时，患者仰卧位，膝部垫高成屈曲位。一助手握住小腿，术者用双手掌相对挤压，以纠正侧方移位。然后1手握住足前部，1手握住足跟结节部，行拔伸牵引，使足极度蹠屈，使骨片复位并恢复跟距角和足弓（图89）。术毕，用上法固定，或用木板鞋固定法（用1cm厚的木板做成鞋底状，足弓部高起以适应正常足弓），先用棉垫包裹足部，硬纸壳覆盖足背和跟骨结节部，木底鞋放置足底部，连筋带"∞"字形捆扎固定（图90）。术后踝部后侧用沙袋垫高，使关节略屈位。

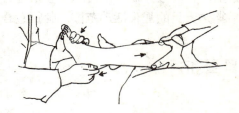

图89　跟骨骨折整复法

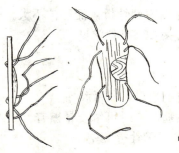
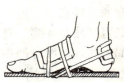

木制鞋底板（正、侧面）　　木制鞋底板纸壳固定法

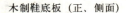

图90

2. 累及跟距关节骨折。此种骨折最常见。跟骨体部因压缩而粉碎塌陷，跟骨结节上升，跟骨体增宽外翻，跟距关节下陷，如复位不良，可致严重的创伤性关节炎。整复方法同上 (2)，以恢复跟骨结节关节角和跟骨体的宽度。

药物

按 3 期用药原则

练功

原则上应是活动宜早，负重宜晚。早期抬高患肢，使膝、踝关节保持屈曲位，可作足趾的屈伸活动和股四头肌的舒缩锻炼；中期骨折稳定后，在夹板控制下，可不负重下地行走，作足部的蹠屈活动；后期加大足的屈伸活动范围，骨折愈合牢固后，方可负重行走。

2.25　蹠骨骨折

发病

蹠骨骨折是足部最常见的骨折。多为直接暴力所伤。如重物砸伤和车辆轧伤；间接暴力伤次之，如扭伤。前者可为横断形和粉碎性，后者可为斜形。又可为分基底部、骨干部和颈部 3 种类型。骨折断端易向蹠侧成角，远断端易向蹠侧移位，也可向侧方移位。第 5 蹠骨基底部多发生撕脱性骨折，而移位不大。合并蹠跗关节脱位比较多见，以第 1 和第 5 蹠骨常见。

诊断要点

1. 有明显外伤史，或疲劳史。
2. 足背肿胀、疼痛，有瘀血斑，不敢持重。
3. 局部压痛，蹠骨冲击痛，有时可触及骨擦音。
4. 足部正斜位 X 线片可明确骨折类型。

治疗

第 1 蹠骨头与第 5 蹠骨头为足的 3 个着力点之 1，且 5 根蹠骨排列又构成前足的横弓，因此,蹠骨骨折后，应力求恢复原来的形状。

整复

1. 2人整复法：患者仰卧位，局麻下，助手握住小腿中下段，术者用纱布包缠患趾，1手向足背方向成20°—30°拔伸牵引，以纠正重叠移位，再转向跖侧方向成10°—15°牵引。同时，另一手拇指由骨折部位跖侧向背侧推挤骨折远端，以纠正跖侧成角畸形。然后术者用另1手拇、食指置于骨间隙，相对夹挤分骨，矫正侧方移位。若合并跖趾关节脱位时，应先整复脱位，再整复骨折（图91）。

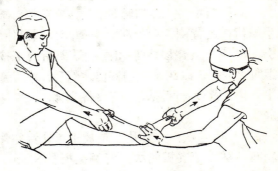

91-1　牵引

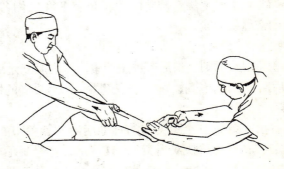

91-2　矫正　侧成角及重迭

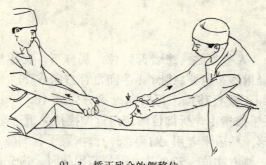

91-3 矫正残余的侧移位

图91 蹠骨骨折复位法

2. 1人整复法：患者仰卧位，局麻下，术者位于患足内侧，双手拇指在足背侧，食指在足蹠侧，分别捏住骨折远近端，用力牵引，以纠正重叠移位.再用捏近端拇指向下按压，用捏远端之食指向上提托，以纠正蹠侧移位。然后，术者双手拇、食指分别捏住蹠骨蹠背侧骨间隙，进行夹挤分骨，以矫正侧方移位。

固定

1. 小夹板固定法：分骨垫2个放于蹠骨背侧骨间隙，棉垫衬里，胶布粘贴。小夹板两块，背侧夹板长8 cm，蹠侧夹板长6 cm，绷带包扎固定，患足跟后部用沙带垫高。

2. 硬纸壳固定法：棉垫衬里，足背侧和蹠侧各置硬纸壳1块，用绷带缠绕固定。

药物

按3期用药原则。伤后若肿胀严重，可内服复元活血汤（1）加减；后期用活血止痛散（45）熏洗患足，以利功能的恢复。

练功

术后抬高患肢，作踝关节的背伸活动和膝关节的屈伸活动；骨折稳定后，不持重扶双拐步行；4周后，穿带足弓垫的木底鞋练习行走。如无木底鞋，可待骨折牢固愈合后再下地行走，以免骨折延迟愈合或畸形愈合。

3 脱位

3.1 概说

发病

多由直接暴力或间接暴力引起。

亦可因体质虚弱、发育不良、关节囊或关节周围的韧带松弛等引起。

若脱位未经完全治愈，关节周围的韧带及关节囊未完全修复，则易反复发作成为习惯性脱位。

关节本身有病变，如结核、化脓等，可引起病理性脱位。

脱位分类

按脱位的程度，可分为全脱位和半脱位。

按脱位的方向，可分为前脱位、后脱位、上脱位、下脱位和中心性脱位。

按脱位的原因，可分为外伤性、病理性、习惯性、先天性脱位。

按脱位后的时间，可分为新鲜性（2～3周之内）、陈旧性（已超过2～3周仍未复位）脱位。

按脱位的关节是否有伤口与外界相通，可分为开放性、闭合性脱位。

诊断要点

1. 一般症状。局部疼痛，肿胀，关节活动障碍。

2. 特殊体征

畸形：如肩关节前脱位有方肩畸形；肘关节后脱位有靴形畸形等。各种脱位各有特定畸形。

关节盂空虚：脱位后可造成原关节盂内关节头脱出而空虚。

如下颌关节脱位，在耳屏前方可触及一凹陷。

弹性固定：脱位后肢体被周围痉挛的肌肉、韧带等固定在特殊位置上，虽仍有轻微活动，但被动活动时可有弹性阻力。

并发症

常可见骨折、血管损伤、神经损伤、创伤性关节炎、骨化性肌炎等并发症。必要时，应拍 X 片或做其他检查，以明确诊断。

治疗

手法复位

1. 外伤性脱位：在适当麻醉下，应尽早进行复位。复位时，应先明确诊断，清楚脱位的机理与方向，尽量利用杠杆原理复位。

2. 陈旧性外伤性脱位：因时间已久，其关节内外血肿机化，周围软组织产生疤痕粘连，造成了整复的困难。近年来，采用新疗法，提高了疗效。治疗时，在麻醉下牵引时间要长些，牵引力量由轻到重，由小到大。在牵引下缓慢、稳健、有力地进行脱位关节屈伸、收展、回旋等各方向的活动，使其疤痕与粘连逐步得以松解，然后再进行复位，可提高成功率。

固定

复位成功后要适当固定，以利于软组织的修复，防止再脱位。一般固定 2～3 周。陈旧性脱位固定时间略长。

复位固定后，可进行适当功能活动与药物治疗，详见总论。

3.2 肩关节脱位

发病

肩关节是由较大的肱骨头与较小的肩胛骨关节盂构成。其活动范围大，关节囊又较松弛，在关节的前下方无肌肉遮盖，故受外伤时，肱骨头容易由此处发生脱位。最常见的是前脱位和下脱位（图 92）。

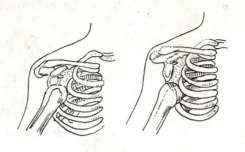

前脱位　　　　　　　　　下脱位

图 92　肩关节脱位

诊断要点

1. 有明显的外伤史，患肩疼痛，肿胀，活动受限。

2. 患肩呈方肩畸形（图 93），常在腋下、喙突下或锁骨下摸到脱出的肱骨头。

3. 检查时，将患侧手掌放在健侧肩部，肘关节不能贴紧胸部；或将肘关节贴紧胸部，则手掌不能放于健侧肩部，称为杜加氏征阳性。

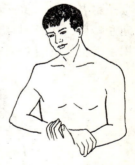

图 93　右肩"方肩"畸形

4. 肩关节脱位常伴有肱骨大结节撕脱骨折；或伴有腋神经损伤。必要时拍摄 X 片或作神经损伤的有关检查。

治疗

整复

一般不需麻醉。

1. 足蹬法：患者仰卧床上，术者对坐于患侧床沿，双手握住患者腕部，将患肢伸直外展 30°。用足底（左侧脱位用左足，右侧脱位用右足）蹬于患者腋下。足蹬手拉，徐徐用力，在此持续拔伸牵引的基础上，再使患肢外旋内收；同时，足跟轻轻用力向外侧支撑肱骨头。当听到咯噔的复位声和复位感，即为成功。此法适用于下脱位（图94）。

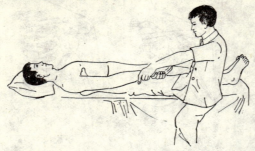

图94　肩关节脱位脚蹬整复法

2. 膝顶法：患者坐在长凳上。术者与患者同一方向立于患侧。以左侧脱位为例，术者左足立地，右足踏在患者坐凳上。将患肢外展 80～90°，并以拦腰状绕过术者身后，术者以左手握其腕，紧贴于左胯上。右手掌推住患者左肩峰，右膝屈曲，将膝顶于患者腋窝，同时右手推、左手拉、右膝顶。术者并徐徐用力向左转身。然后，右膝抵住肱骨头用力一顶，即可复位。此法适用于下脱位（图95）。

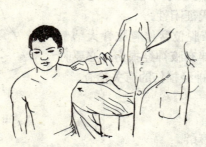

图95　肩关节脱位前面观,膝顶手拉法

3. 杠抬法：准备长 1 米、直径约 5 cm 的木杠一根，木杠中部用毛巾或棉花包绕。让患者坐凳上，一助手将此木杠中部放于患者腋下，另一助手握患侧腕部顺势向下牵引。术者抬木杠另一端，与第一助手同时用力上抬木杠。在上提下拉对抗牵引下，持续用力，当听到复位声，即为成功（图96）。

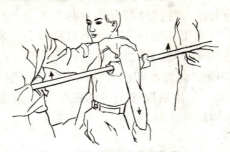

图96 肩关节脱位杠抬整复法

固定

复位成功后，将患肢上臂内收内旋，屈肘小于90°，贴于胸前，用绷带包扎固定（图97）。

陈旧性脱位的处理：

肩关节脱位3周后未能复位者，肩周围已产生粘连，时间愈久，复位愈困难。若时间尚短，肩关节僵硬程度尚不严重者，可试行闭合手法复位，若不成功再考虑手术治疗。

复位前数日，可先服用活血化瘀

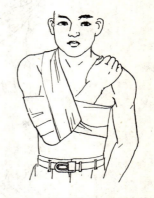

图97 肩关节脱位绷带固定法

与软坚的中药，促使粘连挛缩的软组织变得软一些。内服药物如下：

当归9克 赤芍12克 土元9克 红花6克 威灵仙12克 穿山甲6克 花粉12克 木香6克 青皮9克 血竭3克 桑枝15克 甘草6克 水煎服 每日1剂 连服3～5剂。

复位时先用2号洗药烫洗，或用酒糟，或用醋糟加热外熨1～2小时。

复位应给予有效麻醉。患者仰卧，术者两手环握其肩部，下助手握其腕部做各方向的被动活动，并做肩部环转等，活动范围可逐渐加大，使局部粘连尽量松解。然后采用牵拉端托复位法（图98）进行复位。复位时需有另一助手在患者健侧双手环抱患侧腋下（或用宽布带环绕）与下助手对抗牵引。术者环握肩部的双手，其拇指顶于肩峰，余指向外板拉肱骨头。在以上协同作用下，其体征与畸形消失，即已复位。有时听不到明显的复位声。可拍 X 片证实。复位后要按上述固定法加强固定。后期更要加强功能锻炼，以防再度粘连。

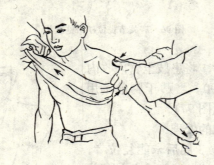

98-1　肩关节脱位患者坐位整复法

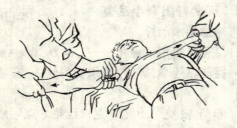

98-2　患者卧位臂外展 90°整复法肩关节脱位牵拉端托复位法

图98　陈旧性肩关节复位法

3.3　肘关节脱位

发病

肘关节由肱骨下端的滑车、肱骨小头与尺骨上端的半月切迹、桡骨小头构成。按尺、桡骨上端关节面脱位的方向，可分为前脱位、后脱位和侧脱位。后脱位最为常见,前脱位甚少，故此只介绍后脱位。

诊断要点

1. 有外伤史（多为臂外展背伸、肘关节伸直位受伤）。

2. 肘部肿胀、疼痛,活动受限。若伴有骨折时，肿痛重或局部有瘀斑。

3. 肘关节弹性固定于半屈位（约130°），尺骨鹰咀尖有明显后突畸形，肘前窝饱满，可触到圆滑的肱骨下端。肘后三角正常关节消失。

4. 若合并侧方移位时，可摸到尺骨鹰咀偏向一侧。X片可观察有无骨折。

治疗

手法复位

1. 牵拉推板法：患者坐位（或卧位），一助手握患肢上臂下段。术者立于患侧，1手握其腕上部，沿前臂纵轴向下牵引。另一助手握肘关节，用拇指推肱骨下端向上向后；其余4指在肘后拉尺骨鹰咀向前向下。同时将肘关节逐渐屈曲，听到复位声即为成功。（图99）。

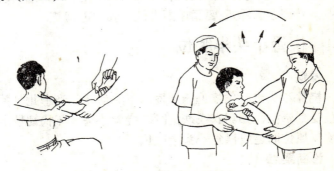

图99 肘关节后脱位牵拉推板法

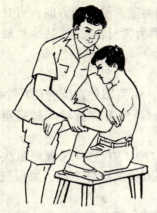 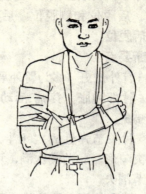

图 100　肘关节脱位膝顶拔伸法　　图 101　肘关节脱位,肘"∞"形绷带固定

2.　膝顶拔伸法：患者端坐，术者立于伤侧前面，1 手握其上臂，1 手握其腕部，同时以 1 足踏在患者所坐凳子上，并将膝部顶在患肢肘窝内，屈肘 90°，膝用力前顶。握腕之手顺患肢前臂纵轴用力牵拉，并逐渐屈肘，即可复位（图 100）。

固定

复位成功后，使患肘屈曲小于 90°，用肘"8"字绷带包扎，前臂用长方形纸壳垫托，并缠绕绷带悬吊于胸前（图 101）。固定 2～3 周。固定期间除限制肘的屈伸活动外，其他活动可不必限制。外固定去除后，要循序渐进地加强功能锻炼。

3.4　桡骨小头半脱位

发病

桡骨小头半脱位多见于 4 岁以下的幼儿。当患儿肘关节在伸直位受到牵拉，如穿衣或跌倒时，桡骨小头被环状韧带卡住，阻碍恢复原位即造成桡骨小头半脱位。

诊断要点

1.　患肢有被牵拉的病史。

2.　患儿肘部或前臂疼痛，不愿活动患肢，尤其不敢上举。

3. 肘外侧桡骨小头处压痛明显，前臂常呈旋前位，不敢旋后，被动屈肘时患儿疼痛哭闹。

4. 肘部无明显肿胀、畸形。X线无异常。

治疗

手法复位

家长抱患儿正坐，一助手（或家长）1手握住其上臂固定。以右侧伤肢为例，术者右手握患儿腕部，左手拇指按压桡骨小头外侧。术者右手慢慢向下牵拉，并将前臂旋后，同时左手按压桡骨小头，然后屈曲肘关节。当听到或感到轻微的复位声，便已复位。这时患儿肘部疼痛消失，亦能屈肘或上举取物。若一次未成功，可再重复上述操作一遍。复位后，一般不用外固定，可嘱家长在近期内避免牵拉患肢，以防发生再脱位（图102）。

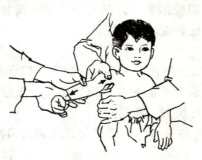

102-1 顺势拔伸,拇指按住桡骨头

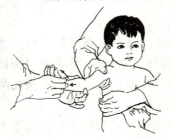

102-2 拔伸前臂旋后,拇指按压

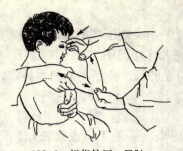

102-3　拇指按压，屈肘

图 102　桡骨头半脱位整复法

3.5　下颌关节脱位

发病

下颌关节脱位多因张口过大，如大笑，打呵欠，拔牙或咬硬物等所致。前脱位最常见，又可分为单侧前脱位、双侧前脱位。若反复发作往往形成习惯性脱位。

诊断要点

1.　双侧前脱位者，下颌向前突出，口半开，不能主动闭合或张开。上下齿列不能对合，语言不清，流涎不止，吞咽困难。在两耳屏前方可摸到一凹陷。

2.　单侧前脱位者，下颌向健侧倾斜，口角歪斜。在患侧耳屏前方可触及一凹陷。

治疗

手法复位

1.　口内复位法：令患者坐矮凳，头倚墙。术者立于患者前面，先将两拇指裹以纱布数层，并将两拇指伸入患者口腔内，分别置于两侧下臼齿的咬合面上。其余 4 指在两侧托住下颌体与下颌角。

复位时，先将两拇指同时向下按压，用力逐渐加大。其余各指配合拇指紧紧地握住下颌体向下向后推送。若听到弹响声时，两拇指迅速滑向臼齿两侧，以防被咬伤。当症状及畸形消失，即复位成功（图103）。

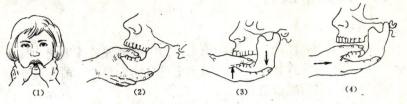

图 103　下颌关节脱位整复法（口内法）

若单侧脱位，亦可用此法，只是按在健侧的拇指不需用力即可。

2.　口外复位法：术者立于患者前方，双手拇指分别置于两侧下颌骨下颌支的后上方，其余4指把住下颌骨体部。然后双手拇指由轻而重向下按压下颌支，并慢慢向后方推送，即可复位。

固定

可用4头带固定。用1条宽纱布绷带，两端纵形剪开一段，即每端成为两个头。并将中间剪一长约3 cm的洞，兜在下颌处。把两端对应的两个头分别在头顶与后枕部打结（图104）。

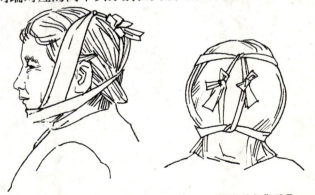

104-1　固定后之侧面观　　　104-2　固定后之背面观

图 104　下颌关节脱位四头带固定法

一般固定3~5天。固定期间不吃较硬食物，勿张口过大。若是习惯性脱位应固定2周左右，并可内服十全大补丸等药物。

3.6 髋关节脱位

发病

髋关节为人体最大关节，稳定有力，故其脱位多因强大暴力所致。病人多为青壮年男子。临床上可分为后脱位、前脱位和中心型脱位，以后脱位最多见。

诊断要点

1. 有明显的暴力损伤史。伤后患髋疼痛，功能丧失，肿胀不明显。不同的类型可有不同的畸形。

2. 后脱位、患侧臀部高突，患腿长度缩短。髋关节呈屈曲、内收、内旋畸形。有时可合并髋臼骨折或坐骨神经损伤（图105～1）。

3. 前脱位：患侧腹股沟或会阴部高突，可触到股骨头。患肢可变长。髋关节呈外展、外旋、半屈位（图105～2）。

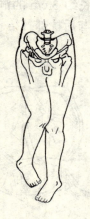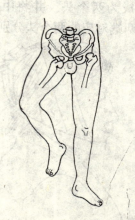

105-1 后脱位　　　　　105-2 前脱位

图105 髋关节脱位畸形

4. 中心型脱位：患肢缩短。多伴有髋臼骨折，X片可帮助确诊。

治疗

手法复位

可在硬膜外麻醉下进行。

1. 后脱位:

(1) 屈髋提拉法: 患者仰卧, 助手用两手按压患者两侧髂部以固定骨盆。术者面向患者, 骑跨在屈髋屈膝各 90°的肢体上。用前臂肘窝部或双手套握在伤肢腘窝部, 并逐渐提拉拔伸, 促使股骨头接近关节囊的破口处。在向上提拉的同时, 慢慢内旋髋关节, 以使股骨头滑入髋臼中, 可稍加摇晃。若听到咯噔复位声, 再将患肢慢慢伸直 (图 106)。

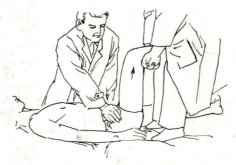

提拉整复法

图 106 髋关节后脱位提拉整复法

(2) 旋转法: 患者仰卧, 助手依上法固定骨盆。术者立于伤侧, 用 1 手握住伤肢踝部, 另 1 上肢以肘窝提托其患者腘窝部。在向上提拉的基础上, 将大腿内收, 髋关节极度屈曲, 使其股部紧贴腹壁。然后将患肢外展、外旋、伸直。在此连续过程中, 可出现咯噔复位声音 (图 107)。

2.前脱位:

(1) 牵拉推板法: 患者仰卧。一助手拉住患者两侧腋窝; 一助手握住患侧踝部。两人对抗拔伸牵引。术者立于健侧, 1 手板住髂骨部, 1 手推向前脱位的股骨头。在 3 人协同作用下, 可听到复位声（图 108）。

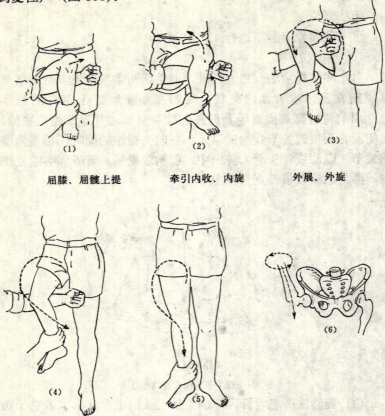

(1)　　　　　　　(2)　　　　　　　(3)

屈膝、屈髋上提　　牵引内收、内旋　　外展、外旋

(4)　　　　　　　(5)　　　　　　　(6)

伸髋、伸膝　　　继续伸直　　复位过程中,股骨干的径路

图 107　髋关节后脱位旋转复位法

(2) 反旋转法：复位准备与方法基本同后脱位的旋转复位法相似，只是旋转的方向相反（图 109）。

固定

复位后仰卧位，可用皮肤牵引或沙袋制动（即用 4～6 个沙袋紧贴患肢两侧放置）。后脱位者要维持髋部轻度外展、旋中伸直位。前脱位者则需保持患肢在轻度内收、内旋伸直位。皆应固定3~4周。

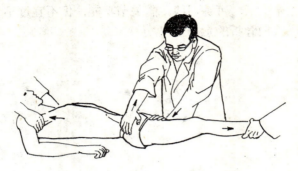

图108 髋关节前脱位牵拉推扳整复法

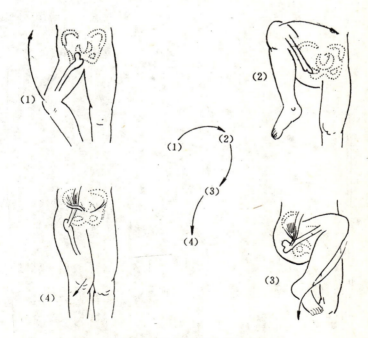

图109 髋关节前脱位反回旋复位法①~④

中心型脱位可用持续骨牵引或皮肤牵引，时间为 6～8 周，可有复位与固定两种作用。牵引初期酌情拍 X 片以了解复位情况。解除牵引后，可练习膝、髋关节功能，但不宜过早负重，要同时考虑髋臼骨折的愈合情况。

4 伤筋

4.1 理筋手法

手法的作用

理筋手法在临床上的应用范围很广，对骨折、脱位、伤筋皆可应用。其手法可以活血散瘀，消肿止痛，舒筋通络，祛风散寒，调和气血，活动关节,，解除肌筋挛急，促进损伤组织修复等作用。

常用的理筋基本手法及适应症

1. 按揉法

按，是用拇或食、中指的指腹，或用手掌根部，用力按压肢体特定部位、穴位上。其用力的大小，应根据病情的需要和病人耐受的程度而定。揉，是在按的基础上不离原位用手指或手掌进行左右或旋转的揉动，揉时要用腕力。临床上按、揉手法往往同时合并使用（图110）。

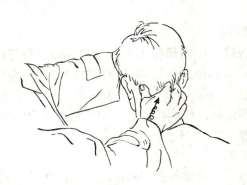

用指按揉两风池穴

图110 按揉手法示例

2. 推摩法

推，是用指腹（常用拇指）或手掌的根部，平稳的稍加按压，在肢体上缓慢地上下或左右推动。摩，是在推的基础上摩动、滑擦，较推法用力略小，速度稍快。两手法常常配合使用，上推时则下摩，下推时则上摩。部位小则用手指推摩，面积大则用手掌推摩。操作时要求有刚有柔，刚柔结合，达到体表感觉轻柔，内里力量刚劲，并非在表皮摩来擦去，徒伤皮毛（图111）。

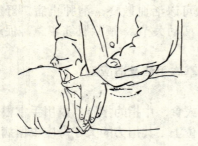

用手掌鱼际部推摩腰背筋

图 111　推摩手法示例

此法是治疗各种伤筋的常用手法，尤其对陈伤和劳损应用更多。

3. 拨络法

亦称拨筋。即用拇指加大用力与经络循行方向的横向揉动；或拇指不动，其他4指取与肌束垂直的方向，单向或往复揉拨，起到类似拨动琴弦的作用。手法的力量可轻可重，频率可快可慢。有解痉止痛，松解粘连等作用。适用于急、慢性伤筋而致挛缩和粘连者（图112）。

4. 捏拿法

即用拇指与其他各指相对钳形用力，将肌肉或韧带一紧一松的捏拿（图113）。捏时稍加用力，指劲要柔韧。拿时有上提之意，并非将肌肉提起。放松后手指不要离开体表。捏拿应顺肌肉的走行方向自上而下依次进行。此法能舒通气血，祛瘀止痛，缓解痉挛，松解粘连。常用于四肢及颈项部的陈伤和劳损。急性伤筋用此手法要轻揉。

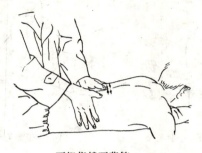

两拇指拨两背筋

图 112　拨筋手法

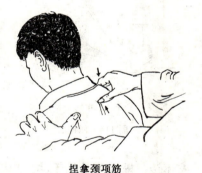

捏拿颈项筋

图 113　捏拿手法

5. 屈伸法

本法适用于关节有屈伸功能障碍者，是被动活动关节的一种手法。操作时 1 手握肢体远端，1 手握持关节部位，缓慢、均衡、持续而有力地做适当的屈伸活动。其活动度由小到大，逐渐增加，以病人能耐受为限度。使关节逐渐恢复至最大活动范围（图 114）。

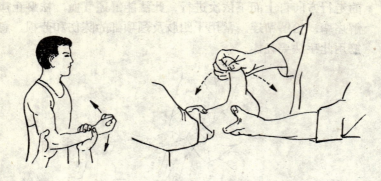

114—1　于肘关节　　　　114—2　于踝关节施用屈伸手法

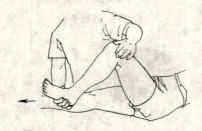

114—3　于膝关节

图114　屈伸法

6. 转摇法

即进行旋转或环转、摇摆晃动的手法。用手握肢体远端，被动地使其在某一方向或几个方向上摆动、旋转或环转（图115）。

操作时需轻揉、循序渐进，使活动范围逐步加大，以不引起剧痛为宜。本法可舒筋解痉，松解粘连，以恢复关节的正常活动范围。凡筋肉撕裂或断裂的新伤者禁用。

7. 叩击法

用手掌或拳捶击肢体。叩击时要有节奏，快慢适中，自左而右或自上而下反复叩击。用力轻巧而有反弹感（图116）。能疏通气血，祛风散寒，消除伤后瘀积或疲劳。治疗新伤或劳损，常与其他手法配合运用。

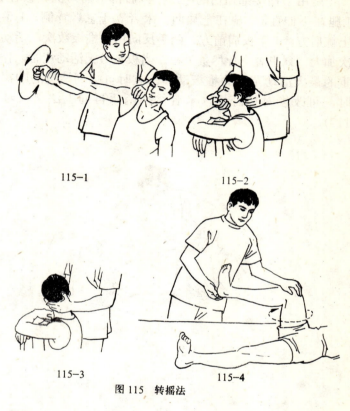

115-1

115-2

115-3

115-4

图 115　转摇法

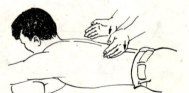

用双手小鱼际部叩击腰背筋

图 116　叩击法

8. 斜板法

是用于颈腰部损伤的手法。以腰部伤筋为例，患者右侧卧，1腿在下伸直，1腿在上屈曲。术者立于患者背侧，1手推髂前上棘后方，1手板肩前方。两手反向用力推板数次，活动范围逐次加大。嘱患者全身尽量放松。当板至最大活动度时，作一次稳重的最大活动范围的推板动作。有时可听到清脆的响声。必要时，可改换对侧卧位，术者倒换两手再同上法斜板对侧（图117）。

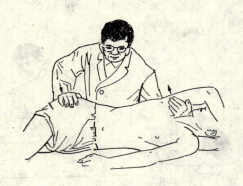

117—1

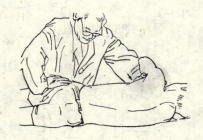

117—2

图 117 斜板法 腰部斜板手法

可用于颈部筋伤、落枕、腰部扭伤、腰部后关节错缝、滑膜嵌顿、腰部劳损等。可松解粘连和痉挛，使关节恢复正常功能。

9. 搓法

两手掌相对，分别置患部的对侧，两手来回搓动。可自上而下反复搓动多次，两手对挤的力量要平衡，动作轻柔、协调（图118）。

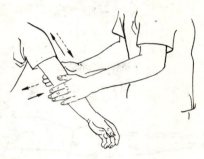

图118 搓法

本法常用作理筋结束时的手法，作为其他手法的调理。能使局部气血调和，筋脉舒松。可用于治疗四肢、肩、膝等的伤筋。

10. 滚法

常用的是掌滚，即手掌呈弧形、屈腕，将手的小指侧按于肢体上，进行反复滚动。沿肌肉走行方向、自上而下、自左而右地来回滚动（图119）。对陈伤和急、慢性劳损皆可使用，如肩背、腰、臀等面积大的部位更为适宜。可疏通经络，解痉止痛。

11. 牵抖法

患者仰卧或俯卧位，术者用手握住肢体远端（一侧或两侧肢体），沿肢体纵轴向下牵引，并有一助手拉住腋窝向上对抗牵拉。在牵拉的同时，术者做上下或左右的抖动，反复数次（图120）。

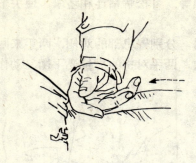

于腰背部施用滚法

图119 滚法

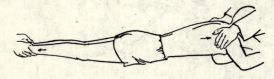

上下两端反向牵拉,牵力主要作用于腰部

120—1 牵法

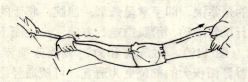

120—2 抖法

图120 腰部牵抖法

　　此法亦可作为理筋手法的终末手法。能舒筋解痉、松解粘连。可用于急、慢腰部伤筋、腰椎间盘脱出症、四肢屈伸不利等的治疗。

　　12. 腰部背伸法：有立位和卧位两种。

　　立位法即术者与患者背与背紧靠而立，两人之两手反扣，术者稍弯腰并用力将患者背起，使其双足离地，两足自然下垂。术者此时可作轻度上下跳跃的振动动作数次（图121）。

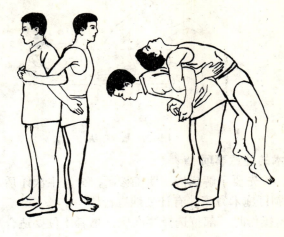

121-1   121-2

图121　腰部背伸法

　　卧位法又称板腿法，即术者1手板按于患者腰部，1手托起患腿，并迅速向后上抬拉，使其腰部过伸（图122）。

　　以上两法皆可用于急性腰扭伤或腰椎间盘突出症等。

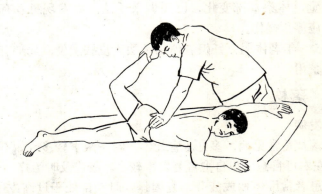

122-1

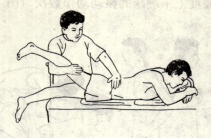

122-2

图 122　板腿手法

施术的注意事项

1. 首先要了解病情，明确诊断，分清主次矛盾，树立整体观念，制订施术方案，有计划地进行。

2. 操作时，部位选择要准确，患者体位要适合，助手配合要得当。

3.手法要熟练正确，做到柔和深透，持久有利，轻而不浮，重而不滞，轻巧灵活，连贯协调，软硬适宜，节奏规律。使患者感到酸、麻、木、热、胀或放射性得气感，则临床效果明显。

4.施术过程中嘱患者身体放松，并密切注意病人情况，询问其感觉，体察局部变化，以便调节手法。如发现患者有昏晕先兆，应停止操作。

5. 年老体弱、妊娠者慎用手法。皮肤感染，局部有挫裂伤等应禁用。

4.2　落枕

发病

落枕是常见病，多见于青壮年，春冬两季较多。如不经治疗1周左右可自愈，但自愈者复发率较高，故应及时治疗。

患者常因体弱或疲劳，复因睡眠时头部处于过高或过低位，使颈部肌肉牵拉而致病；颈项部受凉亦是常见致病因素。

诊断要点

睡眠后颈部出现疼痛，头常歪向患侧。转头时常与上身同时转动。颈项部可有条索状的肌肉痉挛与压痛。

治疗

1. 理筋手法

患者端坐。术者立于其背后，用拇、食、中指分别按压天柱、风池等穴约3～5分钟。再顺肌肉往下推摩数次，并以捏拿法捏拿肩部痉挛的肌肉2～3分钟。亦可将头部左右前后旋转与摇摆数次。

然后，1手托其头后部，1手托其下颏。用两手左右旋转其

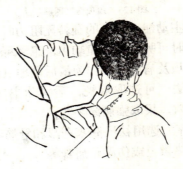

123-1 点穴按揉法

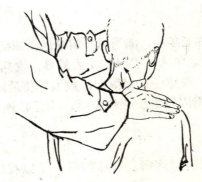

123-2 推摩颈项、肩胛筋肉

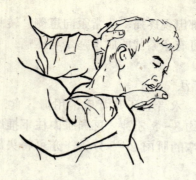

123-3　颈部斜板法

图 123　颈项伤筋理筋手法

头部，待患者能主动配合至头的旋转无阻力时，可突然向患侧做一稳妥斜板，有时可听到一清脆响声，患者可立感舒服。再以掌根部轻轻推摩颈项及肩胛部，作为最后调理（图 123）。

2. 针刺疗法：可选取落枕、后溪为主穴，绝骨（悬钟）、昆仑、风池为配穴，采取强刺激手法。

3. 药物治疗：选用祛风散寒利湿和舒筋活血等药物，参看总论篇章。外用热敷灵或伤湿止痛膏等。

4.3　肩关节周围炎

发病

肩周炎亦称老年肩、漏肩风、肩凝风、冻结肩等。此病多发于 50 岁左右的老年人，尤以妇女为最多。发病原因可为年老体弱，操劳过度；或感受风寒湿邪；或因外伤后固定时间过久等，皆可致肩关节周围软组织慢性炎症，广泛粘连，肩关节活动受限。

诊断要点

1. 早期患肩部疼痛，肿胀明显，尤以夜间痛重，活动受限。

2. 后期肿痛减轻，但活动障碍加重，甚至洗脸、梳头、穿衣等皆受影响。

3. 肩周围可有较广泛的压痛点，肩关节主动与被动活动，如内收、外展、后伸、内旋、上举等动作均受限制。

4. 病程可由数月至 1、2 年之久，有部分患者可自行痊愈，但因病程长而致肩部肌肉萎缩，甚至遗留肩关节强直。

治疗

1. 理筋手法

患者坐位，术者立于患侧，1 手握患肢腕部作牵拉、抖动、转摇等活动。用另手的拇与食、中指分别置于肩的前后。捏拿、按揉患肩，手力由轻到重，范围由小到大，两手配合同时进行。经充分活动后，再将患肢上举、外展、外旋、内收、后伸内旋等（图 124）。

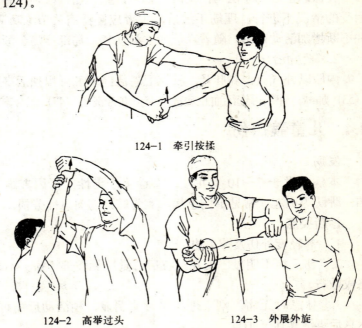

124-1　牵引按揉

124-2　高举过头　　　　124-3　外展外旋

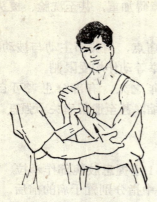
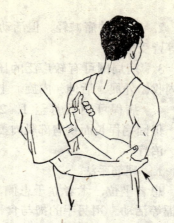

124—4　内收搭肩　　　　124—5　后伸内旋

图124　肩关节周围炎手法

　　在做以上各种手法与活动时，都可产生疼痛，故须在患者能耐受的情况下进行。理筋手法后，患者应坚持肩关节练功活动，并不断增加活动范围。随着功能的逐渐恢复，局部疼痛会渐减。

　　2.　药物治疗

　　内服以补气血、养肝肾、祛风湿、温经络，可用独活寄生汤（53）加减。外用可选活血止痛散（45）、2号洗药（47）配合熏洗。

4.4　儿童髋扭伤

发病

　　本病多发于7～10岁儿童，女性多于男性。可因奔跑、舞蹈、跳跃等引起。常见单侧患病，实为髋部筋肉急性劳损。

诊断要点

　　1.　有轻度外伤及劳累史。

　　2.　伤后症不明显，而在过夜后自觉一侧髋部疼痛。不敢走路或跛行。

　　3.　休息时无痛，刚下地走路时痛明显，稍活动后痛可减。休息后再活动痛又加重。

4. 患侧下肢可有变长，有的较健侧长 1.5～2 厘米。患髋肌紧张，可呈轻度外展外旋位。若被动内收内旋则产生疼痛，并有弹性固定样感。

5. 少数也有患肢变略短者，下肢略呈内收内旋位，而外展外旋受限。被动外展时疼痛。

6. 患肢屈伸一般不受限。无全身症状。X 片无异常发现。

治疗

1. 理筋手法

先令患儿俯卧，术者在患侧用手掌推摩 3～5 分钟，使患部肌肉松弛。再令其仰卧，助手两手按住患儿骨盆。术者 1 手扶握膝部，1 手握其踝部，使髋、膝屈曲。患肢变长者，此时在屈曲的基础上，将髋内收、内旋，然后伸直。如此反复操作 5～10 遍。其每次活动范围由小到大，力量由轻到重。以患儿能够耐受为限度，至两下肢等长为止。若下肢变短者，可将髋部屈曲、外展、外旋、伸直活动数遍，直至两下肢等长（图 125）。

手法后，嘱患儿休息 1～3 日，每天可在患髋部按揉或推摩 1 次。

2. 药物治疗

内服活血祛瘀片（54）、舒筋活血片（55）等。外用活血止痛散（45）煎水热敷。

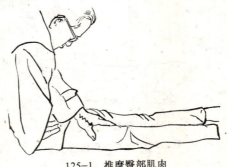

125-1 推摩臀部肌肉

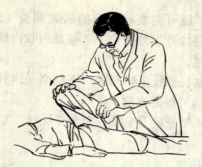

125-2　患肢屈曲内收、内旋

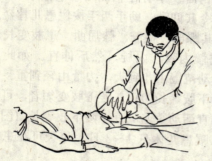

125-3　患肢屈曲外展外旋

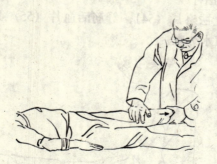

125-4　患肢内旋、拉直

图 125　小儿髋扭伤理筋手法

4.5 急性腰扭伤

发病

急性腰扭伤多因在劳动中用力不当，如搬抬重物时直腿弯腰容易扭伤，故为常见病。多发于青壮年。

诊断要点

1. 有急性腰扭伤史。

2. 局部痛重，咳嗽，打喷涕时可加剧。弯腰痛亦加重，伸腰痛常不增，休息痛减。往往腰不能挺直，多以两手撑腰。腰部活动受限，行走不便。

3. 在腰椎棘突间、棘突旁、骶棘肌等处有压痛点。

治疗

1. 理筋手法

患者俯卧，术者用两拇指自肩部起循脊柱两旁，自上而下进行按揉。当经过肾俞、志室、大肠俞、承扶、委中、承山等穴时可停留按揉三转，用本法自上而下重复操作 3 遍。然后 1 手按伤处，1 手扳拉患侧大腿下端，向后上方提拉 3 次，第 3 次稍用力重拉，有时可听到咯嗒声。最后，在脊柱两旁叩击数次。手法后，腰部制动，可卧硬板床休息 2 周（图 126）。

2. 针刺疗法

常用委中、昆仑、人中、肾俞等穴。行强刺激，局部压痛点可拔火罐。

3. 药物治疗

以活血化瘀，理气止痛为主，可内服复元活血汤（1）加减，或内服活血祛瘀汤（3）、跌打丸（56）等。外敷祛瘀消肿膏（57）。

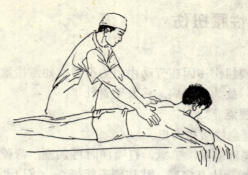

126-1　揉按

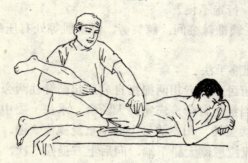

126-2　提腿

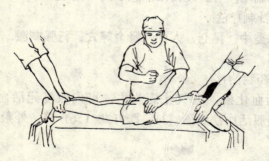

126-3　叩击

图126　腰部软组织损伤按摩手法

4.6 慢性腰肌劳损

发病

慢性腰肌劳损多因持续过久的弯腰、姿势不正、持续负重引起；也可是急性腰损伤未经充分适当的治疗迁延日久所致。皆能造成肾气虚弱，而易感风寒湿邪，邪阻经脉，局部筋肉挛缩、粘连水肿等。腰骶部先天异常者亦易发生本病。

诊断要点

1. 多有不同程度的外伤史或劳损病史。

2. 腰部常常隐痛，时轻时重，反复发作，劳累时加重，休息后减轻.部分患者有臀及大腿上部胀痛。

3. 因劳损的部位不同，可在腰椎棘突、横突、棘突旁、腰骶关节等处有压痛。

4. 部分患者的 X 片可显示椎体增生、骨质疏松、腰骶部先天异常等。

治疗

1. 理筋手法

可采用治疗急性腰扭伤的手法。先找出压痛点，自上而下逐个进行点穴按摩；亦可使用斜板法。但对老年患者或兼有风寒湿者，则不宜作提腿板动等较重的手法。以上手法可隔日作 1 次，10 次为 1 疗程。

2. 针刺疗法

以肾俞、命门、腰阳关、委中、昆仑为主要穴位，手法宜用补法。可加温针、艾灸、拔火罐等。

3. 药物治疗

以温经通络，补益肝肾为主。方用独活寄生汤（53）加减，也可服大活络丹（58），若有骨质增生者加服骨质增生丸（59），若兼风寒者可配用小活络丹（60），外贴镇江膏药（61）。

平时应避免过分劳累，预防寒湿，节欲房事，加强身体锻炼。

4.7 腰椎间盘突出症

发病

椎间盘由玻璃样软骨盘、纤维环和髓核 3 部分组成。纤维环为坚强有韧性的纤维软骨组织，和上下软骨盘及椎体连结在一起，有效地制止髓核向周围突出。髓核富有弹性，并被限制在软骨盘与纤维环之间，当髓核受到压力过大或其他原因时，可冲破纤维环而外突。经常向后突出，则引起神经根、马尾神经或脊髓的压迫症状。

本病好发于 20～40 岁青壮年，男多于女。多数因腰扭伤或劳累而发病。腰$_{4～5}$及腰$_5$～骶$_1$椎体间为好发部位。

诊断要点

1. 有或无明显外伤史。可突然发生腰痛，向下肢大腿后侧、小腿及足外侧等处放射。急性期痛剧，慢性者可时轻时重。

2. 腰部活动受限，其生理前曲消失，有侧弯，大多弯向患侧（图 127）。

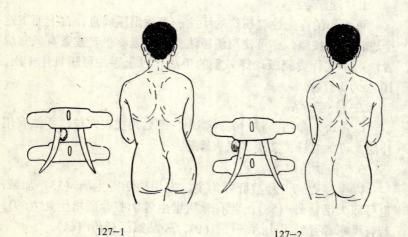

127—1   127—2

图 127 椎间盘脱出与神经的关系

3. 相应椎体棘突旁有压痛，可沿坐骨神经向下放射。

4. 患侧直腿抬高试验、足背屈试验可出现阳性。小腿肌紧张力、伸或屈趾肌力减弱，膝及跟腱反射减弱或消失。

5. X线检查：相应椎间隙变窄或前窄后宽。椎体边缘可有唇形增生等。碘油造影及CT检查皆可定位。

治疗

1. 急性期：应卧硬板床2周，轻度新鲜的脱出者有的髓核自行还纳，症状缓解。

2. 理筋手法：大多需经手法治疗。可采用推摩、斜板、牵抖法。术后卧床5～7天。如症状改变不明显，3日后再重复做1次。

3. 旋转复位法：症状较重或上述方法无效者可试用此法。以右侧腰腿痛、棘突向右偏斜者为例。患者端坐方凳上，1助手将其下肢与骨盆固定。术者立于患者右侧，右臂从患者右侧腋下穿过后右手扣住其颈后部，使其头部略前倾。术者左手拇指压向右偏斜的棘突上。然后，右手用力按压颈部使患者上身尽量前屈（约80°～90°），继而使其上身随着术者右手的板拉向右倾斜旋转，并连续向右后方旋转至最大限度。在此侧弯旋转的同时，左手拇指用力向左推按棘突。两动作互相协调下，可听到腰椎处有弹响声。最后使患者恢复正坐位，如未出现弹响声，可重复做1次。只要出现弹响，患者一般可立即感到痛减。术后卧硬板床休息5～7天（图128）。

4. 持续牵引法：可用骨盆带牵引，或用牵引床，每侧牵引重量10～20公斤，每次1～2小时，每天1次。同时配合局部按揉、针灸疗法、局部穴位封闭等。

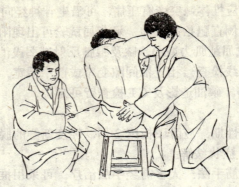

128-1

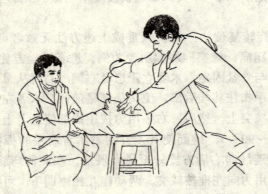

128-2

图 128　椎间盘突出旋转复位法

4.8　外伤性腰痛的中药治疗

外伤性腰痛的病因病机较复杂，可涉及腰部肌肉、韧带、骨骼、关节、椎间盘、神经等的病理改变。故临床多采用综合疗法。中药治疗是其中方法之一，但必须辨证施治，才能取得较好的效果。应根据急慢性损伤腰痛的症状与体征，弄清病机，辨证分型，确定治则，拟方选药。临证中常分以下几种类型辨证用药：

1. 偏气血瘀滞：

多有明显外伤史，腰痛如刺，痛有定处，痛处拒按，或有肿胀瘀斑。轻者俯仰不便，重者不能转侧。舌质紫暗，脉涩。可见于腰部肌肉、韧带等扭挫伤，急性腰肌劳损，急性腰椎间盘突出症，腰椎后关节紊乱等。

治宜活血化瘀、理气止痛。可用复元活血汤（1）或身痛逐瘀汤（62）加减。亦可内服活血祛瘀片（54）、跌打丸（56）、云南白药（63）等中成药。

2. 偏筋络不舒：

病程较久，腰部隐痛，有时连及背、臀、腿部，或有麻木重着感，时轻时重。适当活动后痛可稍减，活动过多疼痛加重。压痛点较广泛。此乃气郁血滞，久阻经络所致。可见于慢性劳损、腰背肌纤维炎，腰部结构先天畸形等。

治宜活血行气，舒筋活络。方用调荣活络饮（64）加减，可酌加川续断、穿山甲、乌药等。或内服舒筋活血片，外用狗皮膏（34）、镇江膏（61）。

3. 偏肝肾不足：

病程日久，腰痛以酸软为主，喜按喜揉，腰膝无力，遇劳更甚，卧则痛减。其中偏阳虚者，面色㿠白，手足不温，少气无力。舌质淡，脉沉细。偏阴虚者，则口燥咽干，心烦失眠，手足心热，舌红少苔，脉弦细数。可见于素体虚弱，筋骨不健，复受损伤或劳损者。

治宜补益肝肾，偏阳虚者，宜温补肾阳，方用右归丸（65）加减。偏阴虚者，宜滋补肾阴，方用左归丸（66）加减。若腰痛日久不愈，不易分清阴阳虚者，可服用青娥丸（67），加服舒筋活血片（55）、壮腰健肾丸（51）。

4. 偏风寒湿：

慢性腰痛，冷痛重着，静卧痛不减，阴雨天加重，得温则舒。舌苔白腻，脉沉而迟缓。可见于慢性劳损或陈伤患者，复感受风寒湿邪者。

治宜散寒祛湿，温经通络。方用麻桂温经汤（22）加减。亦可用小活络丹（60）、伸筋片（50）等。外用镇江膏（61）、坎离砂（48）。

5 骨关节感染

5.1 化脓性关节炎

化脓性关节炎临床多见于儿童，男多于女，以髋、膝关节多见，其次为肩、肘、踝关节，为单一关节发病。

发病

1. 暑湿：当夏秋之间，烈日暴晒，先为暑湿所伤，继而卧露贪凉，寒邪外束，则暑湿之邪客于营卫之间，因而发病。

2. 余毒：多因患过疮疡，疔毒，毒邪走散，注入经络关节而发病。

3. 瘀血：因积劳过度、外伤等，肢体受损，瘀血停滞，郁而化热，热毒注入关节而发病。

本病的致病菌多为金黄色葡萄球菌和溶血性链球菌，其次为肺炎双球菌、脑膜炎双球菌等。感染途径可为血行感染，也可因关节邻近骨髓炎并发或关节开放损伤感染。其病理表现：首先为滑膜充血，肿胀，白细胞浸润和渗出液增多。早期渗出液为浆液性，关节软骨尚未累及，如能及时治愈，关节功能可不受影响。若病变继续发展，滑膜肿胀，肥厚以致坏死，关节软骨遭到破坏，渗出液呈脓性，多遗留关节功能障碍。

诊断要点

1. 发病急，体温常可达到 38.5℃～40℃，畏寒，出汗、食欲减退等全身症状。

2. 受累关节肿胀、疼痛、皮温增高，患者被迫将关节处于松弛体位。如髋关节多处于屈曲、外展外旋位，膝关节半屈曲位，以减轻疼痛。

3. 由于关节囊内积液膨胀，而使囊腔扩大，加上肌肉痉挛，常发生病理性脱位或半脱位。

4. 化验检查：白细胞数和中性粒细胞数增高，血沉增快。

5. X线片表现：早期关节腔增宽，软组织肿胀。当关节面受到破坏时，则关节间隙变窄，附近骨质疏松，最后关节间隙消失，关节强直。

6. 关节穿刺和关节液检查对诊断有重要意义。穿刺液应进行细菌培养和药物敏感试验。

治疗

1. 早期

应根据关节液细菌培养和药物敏感试验的结果，选择大量而有效的抗生素。

对儿童和重症病人应注意降温、补液、纠正水及电解质代谢紊乱，增加营养，提高机体的抵抗力。

局部适当固定，防止关节受压而变形，缓解肌肉痉挛，减轻疼痛，防止畸形发生。

对小而表浅关节，每日或隔日作1次关节穿刺，吸尽关节积液，并用生理盐水冲洗，注入有效的抗生素。

对较大的关节，如膝关节，经穿刺后证实有积液和脓液后，选择两个穿刺点，用套管针进行穿刺，套管针进入关节腔后，拔出针芯，经套管插入直径 3 mm 的塑料管或硅管，再将套管退出，将塑料管固定于皮肤上。位置高的一根作为滴入管，低的一根作为吸出管，每日滴入抗生素和生理盐水 2000 ml 至 3000 ml，吸出管安置负压吸引器。如此可连续冲洗吸引，直至炎症完全控制为止。

必要时也可作关节切开引流，同时在刀口上、下各置冲洗吸引管1根，缝合切口，每日进行冲洗。

2. 后期

后期有关节脱位或半脱位者，可应用牵引进行复位，再以夹板或石膏固定。如果产生粘连、畸形等关节严重障碍、疼痛者，可考虑手术治疗。

3. 辨证用药：应以消、托、补三法治之。

急性期：应以清热解毒、活血通络为主，可用五味消毒饮
(5) 加减。

脓已成尚未破溃者，应以清热解毒、托里透脓为主，方药选
用透脓散加减 (68)。

后期已破，脓水清稀，肉芽淡白，疮口难愈，病程长，临床
表现气血两虚，应补气养血，可用八珍汤 (14)。

中药外治法：

早期外敷金黄膏 (20)、四黄膏 (28) 等。

收口期可用生肌玉红膏 (30)。

早期和溃后均可用解毒洗药 (69) 外洗患处，如溃破后熏洗
后常规换药。

5.2　化脓性骨髓炎

化脓性骨髓炎是由化脓性细菌引起骨骼感染。包括骨髓、骨
质、骨膜甚至累及骨周围的软组织。中医称为附骨疽。本病多见
于 10 岁以下的儿童，病人中 16 岁以下发病率为 90%，男多于
女。好发于四肢干骺端，以胫骨最多，其次为股骨、肱骨、桡
骨。常见的为金黄色葡萄球菌，约占 80%。

发病

急性血源性骨髓炎是由化脓细菌进入血流而引起。常见病灶
如疖痈、毛囊炎、扁桃体炎、中耳炎。也有查不到原发病灶的。
血源中的细菌是造成骨髓炎的先决条件，但必须具备诱发因素才
能造成骨感染。其因素：机体的抵抗力减弱，如久病体弱，过度
疲劳，着凉等；创伤造成局部骨内毛细血管的破裂，出血和瘀
血，使血流中断，细菌得以停留；细菌毒力有大小，细菌毒力大
者发病重，细菌毒力小者发病轻。

病理变化与转归：血源性骨髓炎，大都首先发生在长骨的干

骺端，此处属于松质骨，因儿童期长骨干骺端具有丰富的血管网，皆为终末小动脉，细而迂曲。血流缓慢，细菌感染后易在此处形成细菌栓子，停留繁殖，同时局部外伤造成骨组织内小的出血和细胞破坏，有利于细菌的繁殖，则形成感染病灶。开始为中性白细胞集聚和浆液性渗出，逐步变为脓性，病情如继续发展可出现以下结局：

1. 在机体抵抗力强或细菌毒力小的情况下，治疗得当，初发病灶可迅速被控制和吸收。

2. 致病菌毒力低或机体抵抗力强时，使病灶不发展，而转为局限慢性病灶，则成为局限性骨脓肿。

3. 炎症扩散，一般是在身体状况不佳或细菌毒力强的情况下，病灶蔓延。

病灶向外扩散，穿破干骺骨质，脓肿积于骨膜下，将骨膜剥离，形成骨膜下脓肿，有可能穿破骨膜形成皮下脓肿。

脓肿在髓腔内扩散，可形成广泛的骨髓炎。

脓肿侵入关节囊引起化脓性关节炎。

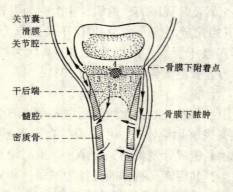

1.2.3 表示扩散方向；4.感染病灶

图 129 急性骨髓炎扩散途径

骨膜下脓肿形成时，被剥离的骨膜形成一层新骨，新骨逐渐增厚形成包壳，则骨干失却来自骨膜的血液供应，再加骨的营养血管栓塞，可产生广泛的骨坏死，形成与活骨完全分离的死骨（图129）。

诊断要点

1. 急性期

起病急，局部疼痛，全身不适、倦怠，继而寒战，持续高烧达（39℃～40℃），汗出而热不退。食欲不振，舌质红，苔黄腻，脉滑数。甚至有恶心呕吐，肝脾肿大等全身中毒症状。

随后患肢搏动性疼痛加剧，不能活动，呈环形肿胀，皮肤灼热，骨干骺端压痛明显，附近肌肉痉挛，关节屈曲，患儿拒绝检查。

化验血象增高，白细胞高达30 000以上，血沉增快，血培养为阳性。

X线片检查：早期无骨质改变，只显示软组织肿胀；两周后可见骨膜反应，干骺端处有骨质破坏；4周后死骨形成。

2. 慢性期

常有1个或多个窦道，反复排除脓液和死骨，瘘管周围皮肤增厚形成疤痕组织，色素沉着，如脓液排出不畅时，则局部肿胀，疼痛加剧，并有发烧和全身不适等症状。

合并病理骨折、脱位时，则出现畸形。

日久，患肢肌肉萎缩，全身消瘦，面色㿠白，神疲乏力，头晕盗汗。

X线片检查：可见死骨、空洞及包壳骨。有时看不到髓腔。

治疗

1. 急性骨髓炎，治疗的目的在于早期控制炎症发展，防止死骨形成。

早期，应选择大量有效的抗生素，有可能控制病变发展，使之愈合。

局部引流。诊断明确后，应用抗生素不能控制症状，并且在骨膜下或髓腔内穿刺吸出脓液，均应在局部钻孔，引流减压。在干骺端压痛最明显处，纵行切开，用骨钻在干骺端处钻多个孔眼。如果髓腔内脓液较多，可用小骨凿开窗，并将两根引流管置于髓腔内，作持续吸引冲洗用，选择有效的抗生素置于生理盐水内约 2 000ml 溶液中，进行引流冲洗，持续两周。

局部制动。患肢可用石膏托或皮牵引制动，以缓解肌肉痉挛，减轻疼痛。并可预防骨折和脱位。

补液维持水与电解质的平衡，可少量多次输血，应用大量维生素 C、高蛋白饮食。

中药治疗：

早期脓未成者，治宜清热解毒，化湿行瘀。可选用五味消毒饮（5）、黄连解毒汤（70）合方加减。

脓成未溃或排脓不畅者，应托里排脓，方用托里消毒饮（71）加减。

临床根据病情随症加减。如高烧、烦渴者可加生石膏、大青叶、败酱草等，疼痛明显者加乳香、没药；体虚者加人参、黄芪；阴虚火旺者加生地、玄参、丹皮、石斛等；神昏谵语者加安宫牛黄丸（72）。

中药外敷，可用金黄膏（27）等外敷。

2. 慢性骨髓炎

辨证用药：慢性骨髓炎多是病程日久，身体消瘦，气血两虚，脾肾不足，余毒未尽。治疗原则应益气养血，温肾健脾，托里消毒。方药可选用阳和汤加减。其中生黄芪 30 克，当归 15 克，赤芍 15 克，白芍 15 克，白术 9 克，熟地 30 克，白芥子 6 克，茯苓 9 克，补骨脂 9 克，黄柏 9 克，甘草 3 克。水煎服。鹿角胶 9 克（冲服）。

饮食不振者，可用香砂六君子汤（73）。气血两虚者应用八珍汤（14）。

外用药：可用大黄软膏（74），或生肌玉红膏（30）换药，同时也可撒上九一丹 (38)。以提脓祛腐，消肿生肌。

对经久不愈的慢性窦道以及死骨者，应行手术彻底切除窦道，清除死骨，以达到治愈的目的。

5.3 骨关节结核

骨关节结核中医称为"骨痨"或"流痰"。多见于 15 岁以下的儿童，男多于女。是常见的传染病之一。

发病

1. 直接病因：由结核杆菌侵入骨关节所引起，属继发病灶。其原发病灶多在呼吸系统和消化系统。

2. 间接病因：体质虚弱,先天不足，产后等。骨关节长期负重慢性劳损或外伤，致使局部骨质不健，抵抗力下降，易受结核杆菌的侵袭而发病。

肌纤维因素：肌肉附着丰富的骨骼则少发生。如髂骨、肩胛骨等。相反，没有或少有肌肉附着的椎体、跟骨、手足短骨则容易形成病灶。

终末血管因素：皮质骨结核少见，因皮质骨中血运丰富。而骨端及干骺端因血管口径小，又为终末枝，血流缓慢，故易发病。

年龄因素：儿童对结核菌的抵抗力较低，感染后易发病，而且易扩散。但因儿童代谢和修复能力强，治疗较容易。

根据骨关节结核病变和发展，可分为下列 3 种类型：

单纯骨结核：可发生于坚质骨和松质骨。坚质骨表现为骨质增生、骨膜增厚。松质骨结核表现为骨质破坏，产生结核肉芽组织，干酪样液化，死骨形成或空洞，无新生骨。

单纯滑膜结核：病灶局限于滑膜，多见于髋、膝关节。滑膜充血，水肿增厚，并产生大量结核渗出液。有时滑膜肉芽组织沿软骨边缘向内蔓延，造成软骨和骨面分离。

全关节结核：单纯骨、滑膜结核，未能及时治疗，病变发展可造成滑膜、软骨、骨都有结核感染，使软骨、骨相继出现不同程度的破坏，关节间隙变窄或消失。

诊断要点

1. 早期发病缓慢，症状不明显，继而少气乏力，全身倦怠，夜间疼痛明显，关节活动障碍，动则痛剧。

2. 中期受累关节逐渐肿痛，可有积液，不红不热，肌肉痉挛，潮热盗汗，失眠，胃纳差。

3. 晚期则病灶附近或远处出现寒性脓肿，脓肿很易溃破，流出稀水样或干酪样的坏死组织，疮口凹陷，形成慢性窦道长期不愈，患者日渐消瘦，精神萎靡，面色无华，导致气血两虚。

4. X 线片表现有诊断意义。在松质骨结核中有死骨型和溶骨型。死骨型多发现于松质骨中心，骨小梁模糊，密度增高或出现死骨。死骨吸收后出现空洞。如病灶在松质骨边缘，则表现为溶骨性改变，死骨较少；骨干结核表现为骨质增生如葱皮样；干骺端结核兼有松质骨与骨干结核的特点。

5. 化验：血沉增快，红细胞和血红蛋白降低。对早期诊断困难者，可作关节穿刺液细菌培养或病理检查。

治疗

1. 营养与制动：给充足营养可改善全身情况，增强抗病能力，有利于结核的恢复。制动能减少疼痛，防止病变扩散，有利于组织修复。

2. 使用足够的抗痨药物。

3. 辨证用药：

早期治宜温补和阳，散寒通滞化痰。可选用阳和汤加味治疗。原方加当归 15 克，白术 15 克。若形成脓肿者可加皂角刺 9 克，山甲珠 9 克，生黄芪 15 克。

晚期治宜补气养血为主，可用人参养荣汤（75）.如午后潮热,，口渴不欲饮，舌红少苔，脉细数，属阴虚火旺者，治宜养阴清热为主，可用抗结核汤（76），冲服大补阴丸（77）。如盗汗不止可加黄芪 15 克，浮小麦 9 克，煅龙骨 15 克。

验方：骨痨敌（78）对骨关节结核有较好的效果。四虫丸（79）、金蚣丸（80）也有一定的疗效。

外用药：脓肿未破可外用丁癣散（81）外敷。已破者可用凡士林油纱布，少许五五丹（82）或追毒丹（83）填入窦道。脓液少，伤口长期不愈合可用生肌玉红膏（30）换药。

THE ENGLISH—CHINESE ENCYCLOPEDIA OF PRACTICAL TCM

(Booklist)

英汉实用中医药大全

(书目)

VOLUME	TITLE	书名
1	ESSENTIALS OF TRADITIONAL CHINESE MEDICINE	中医学基础
2	THE CHINESE MATERIA MEDICA	中药学
3	PHARMACOLOGY OF TRADITIONAL CHINESE MEDICAL FORMULAE	方剂学
4	SIMPLE AND PROVEN PRESCRIPTION	单验方
5	COMMONLY USED CHINESE PATENTMEDICINES	常用中成药
6	THERAPY OF ACUPUNCTURE AND MOXIBUSTION	针灸疗法
7	*TUINA* THERAPY	推拿疗法
8	MEDICAL *QIGONG*	医学气功
9	MAINTAINING YOUR HEALTH	自我保健
10	INTERNAL MEDICINE	内科学

（京）112号

The English—Chinese
Encyclopedia of Practical TCM
Cheif Editor   Xu Xiangcai

14

ORTHOPEDICS AND TRAUMATOLOGY

English Cheif Editor   Lei Xilian

Chinese Chief Editor   Cao Yixun

英汉实用中医药大全

主编   徐象才

14

骨 伤 科 学

中文   英文

主编 曹贻训 雪希濂

*

高等教育出版社出版

高等教育出版社激光照排技术部照排

新华书店总店北京科技发行所发行

高等教育出版社印刷厂印装

*

开本 850×1168 1/32 印张 16.25 字数 420 000

1992 年 12 月第 1 版 1992 年 12 月第 1 次印刷

印数 0 001—4 273

ISBN7—04—003857—9/R · 16

定价 9.55 元